Manual of Otolaryngology

Diagnosis and Therapy

D1802889

Manual of Otolaryngology

Diagnosis and Therapy

Second Edition

Edited by

Marshall Strome, M.D.
Associate Professor of Otology and Laryngology,
Harvard Medical School; Chief, Division of Oto-
laryngology, Brigham and Women's and Beth
Israel Hospitals, Boston

James H. Kelly, M.D.
Associate Professor of Otolaryngology/Head and
Neck Surgery, Johns Hopkins University School
of Medicine; Chairman, Department of Oto-
laryngology/Head and Neck Surgery, Greater
Baltimore Medical Center, Baltimore

Marvin P. Fried, M.D.
Associate Professor of Otology and Laryngology,
Harvard Medical School; Surgeon, Brigham
and Women's Hospital; Surgeon in Otolaryngology and Associate Chief, Division of Otolaryngology, Beth Israel Hospital; Associate Surgeon
in Otolaryngology, Massachusetts Eye and Ear
Infirmary; and Associate in Otolaryngology,
The Children's Hospital, Boston

Little, Brown and Company
Boston/Toronto/London

Library of Congress Cataloging-in-Publication Data

Manual of otolaryngology : diagnosis and therapy / edited by Marshall
    Strome, James H. Kelly, Marvin P. Fried. —2nd ed.
        p.   cm.
    Includes bibliographical references and index.
    ISBN 0-316-81968-9
    1. Otolaryngology—Handbooks, manuals, etc.   I. Strome, Marshall,
1940–   . II. Kelly, James H. III. Fried, Marvin P.
    [DNLM: 1. Otorhinolaryngologic Diseases—diagnosis—handbooks.
2. Otorhinolaryngologic Diseases—therapy—handbooks.   WV 39 M2938]
RF56.M37   1992
617.5'1—dc20
DNLM/DLC
for Library of Congress   92-49902
                                                                                CIP

Printed in the United States of America

SEM

The authors extend their thanks to Beth Okurowski for her illustrations.

To our medical students and residents, whose intellectual curiosity and stimulation have earned them a place as special contributors to this text

M. S., J. H. K., M. P. F.

To Deena, Scott, and Randy—no man could have hoped for more

M. S.

To Alexander, Jamie, and Erin—with love

J. H. K.

To Rita, who has been with me all the way

M. P. F.

Contents

Contributing Authors

Marvin P. Fried, M.D.

Associate Professor of Otology and Laryngology, Harvard Medical School; Surgeon, Brigham and Women's Hospital; Surgeon in Otolaryngology and Associate Chief, Division of Otolaryngology, Beth Israel Hospital; Associate Surgeon in Otolaryngology, Massachusetts Eye and Ear Infirmary; and Associate in Otolaryngology, The Children's Hospital, Boston

Andrew C. Goldstone, M.D.

Instructor in Otolaryngology/Head and Neck Surgery, Johns Hopkins Hospital; Attending Otolaryngologist, Greater Baltimore Medical Center, Baltimore

Elizabeth Howell

Fourth-Year Medical Student, Harvard Medical School, Boston

James H. Kelly, M.D.

Associate Professor of Otolaryngology/Head and Neck Surgery, Johns Hopkins University School of Medicine; Chairman, Department of Otolaryngology/Head and Neck Surgery, Greater Baltimore Medical Center, Baltimore

Karen Drake Murray, M.A., C.C.C.

Speech-Language Pathologist, Speech and Hearing Department, Brigham and Women's Hospital, Boston

Jo Shapiro, M.D.

Instructor in Otology and Laryngology, Harvard Medical School; Associate Surgeon, Brigham and Women's and Beth Israel Hospitals, Boston

Marshall Strome, M.D.

Associate Professor of Otology and Laryngology, Harvard Medical School; Chief, Division of Otolaryngology, Brigham and Women's and Beth Israel Hospitals, Boston

David M. Vernick, M.D.

Assistant Professor of Otology and Rhinology, Harvard Medical School, Boston

Preface

Our goal in the preparation of the second edition of the *Manual of Oto-laryngology* was similar in many respects to that of the first edition: a concise, timely reference detailing the essentials of otolaryngology and head and neck surgery for students of the discipline. Pertinent new information, including artwork, has been incorporated and an entire new chapter on AIDS has been added. Unlike the contributors to the first edition, the primary contributors to this edition were, with one notable exception, either the editors or the full-time otolaryngology faculty of two Harvard institutions: the Brigham and Women's and Beth Israel Hospitals.

Throughout the revision process we had the support of many people, and though unnamed, they have our deepest appreciation. Our families deserve special recognition for their constant caring, counsel, and forbearance. We are more than fortunate that the Brigham Surgical Group Foundation continues to provide us with support not only for this effort but for research, postgraduate courses, and clinical activities.

Over the past 5 years we have had exposure to ever-increasing numbers of medical students, many of whom have chosen to pursue otolaryngology as a career. They have enriched, and continue to enrich, our academic lives. We hope this manual will meet their needs, as it is with them in mind that it is published.

M.S.
J.H.K.
M.P.F.

Manual of Otolaryngology

Diagnosis and Therapy

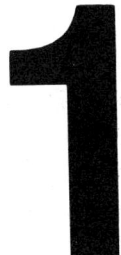

Emergencies

I. **Supraglottitis (epiglottitis)** is an acute infection involving the supraglottic larynx above the vocal cords to the tip of the epiglottis, including the aryepiglottic folds and the arytenoids. Swelling caused by infection in this critical part of the airway can lead to asphyxia and potentially death. Most cases in children are caused by *Haemophilus influenzae,* type B, whereas in adults a wider range of bacteria are causative (*Streptococcus pneumoniae,* beta-hemolytic streptococcus, and *Staphylococcus aureus*). In an adult, a viral etiology must also be considered. Early recognition and prompt intervention are critical to successful therapy.

A. **Signs and symptoms.** Supraglottitis in childhood is often characterized by abrupt onset and a relentless clinical course. The typical initial symptom is **fever** (temperature > 102°F), followed in a relatively short period of time by pain in the hypopharynx, often compromising the ability to swallow, and finally by **respiratory embarrassment**. The sequence of events from onset to a state of respiratory collapse may be as short as 4 hours. In other cases, the initial symptom complex may span 2–3 days. Differences in the clinical course are due to varied host resistance, airway size, and the virulence of the organism.

B. **Diagnosis**

   1. **The classic symptomatic triad of fever, dysphagia, and rapidly progressive respiratory embarrassment** strongly suggests the diagnosis of supraglottitis. In most cases, the symptoms are sufficiently classic to proceed directly to the emergency measure of securing the airway. Supraglottitis in the older child or adult, however, may be more difficult to diagnose and is not necessarily as rapidly progressive relative to airway obstruction as it is in the young child. In the absence of definite oropharyngeal pathology, the symptoms of neck pain, aggravated by swallowing or speaking, combined with low-grade fever and a muffled voice should alert the physician to the probability of supraglottitis.

   2. **Lateral x ray of the neck.** In cases in which the diagnosis is in doubt and the patient's condition stable, a lateral x ray should be obtained. X-ray findings of a swollen epiglottis and dilated hypopharynx establish the diagnosis.

3. **Indirect laryngoscopy.** The larger adult airway makes laryngeal occlusion unlikely during indirect laryngoscopy. This is not true, however, in the pediatric population. This examination should not be performed in the presence of hypoxia. The preferable current technique is use of the fiberoptic laryngoscope inserted transnasally. Placement of the tip of the laryngoscope well above the epiglottis (in the upper oropharynx) should not produce laryngospasm and allows excellent visualization of the supraglottis and possibly the level of the vocal cords. For those adults not requiring emergency measures, this technique allows for frequent evaluations of the airway.

4. **Points of caution in the diagnosis of pediatric patients**

   a. **A tongue blade examination or indirect laryngoscopy should not be performed** in hypoxic children with suspected supraglottitis. The intense pain and respiratory distress that are usually present make such an exercise difficult for the patient and may provoke acute respiratory arrest from laryngeal spasm, induced by tactile stimulus of the epiglottis.

   b. Children with supraglottitis may appear to have **meningitis.** They usually have high fever, a toxic appearance and, at times, nuchal rigidity. To position such a patient for lumbar puncture would further compromise the airway. One can make the differentiation clinically on two grounds: (1) patients with epiglottitis have respiratory signs and symptoms, which are not found in most patients with meningitis, and (2) patients with supraglottitis severe enough to cause nuchal rigidity also resist neck motion in virtually any direction—side-to-side, flexion, and extension.

C. **Management.** In most cases, the severity of respiratory distress requires stabilization of the airway by endotracheal intubation or tracheotomy. A decision as to the extent of airway compromise must be made, however. In some patients, especially adults, the compromise may be mild, requiring at most hospitalization for airway monitoring and administration of antibiotics, at times combined with steroids. In contrast to the pediatric population, intubation or tracheotomy is less often required in adults.

1. **Stabilization of the airway.** Once the diagnosis has been established, acute pediatric management usually proceeds to securing the airway. In major centers, nasotracheal intubation is the preferred method because it usually carries a lower complication rate than tracheotomy. With an endotracheal tube, however, unexpected extubation requires that an expert endoscopist be present for reintubation, if warranted. Ancillary services essential for managing small endotracheal tubes in children must also be available; close observation after intubation is as critical as the intubation process. From the time the diagnosis of supraglottitis is suspected until the airway is secured, a physician should be in attendance.

a. **Nasotracheal intubation.** Procedural techniques for intubation follow:

   (1) **General anesthesia by mask** (nitrous oxide and oxygen) induction is given and subsequently enhanced with halothane. Muscle relaxants are ill-advised in this setting.

   (2) **Invasive procedures,** even the institution of an intravenous line, should await intubation when possible.

   (3) **Oral intubation** is performed after a satisfactory level of anesthesia is obtained. The endotracheal tube size should be at least one size smaller than that normally used for a patient of similar size.

   (4) **The change to nasotracheal intubation** can be effected once the airway has been secured by oral intubation, cleared of all secretions, and the patient fully oxygenated. The nasotracheal tube usually remains in position 24–72 hours, depending on the clinical course. Patients seldom require reintubation if the tube is left in place for at least 24 hours.

   (5) **Extubation,** performed 24–72 hours after intubation, can be performed in the ICU. Endoscopy is no longer considered essential prior to extubation.

b. **Tracheotomy.** If expertise—medical, nursing, or both—is not available to maintain adequately a nasal endotracheal tube, a tracheotomy (see sec. **V.F.**) is preferable. Whenever possible, the procedure should be performed in the operating room with an endotracheal tube in place.

2. **Humidification.** During the period of mechanical ventilation, a humidified environment, with 30% inspired oxygen, is beneficial. In addition, humidification of the area around the tube helps prevent the development of thick local secretions, which could obstruct the small tubes in children. Suction and, when necessary, saline irrigation should be used both to remove secretions and check tubal patency.

3. **Antibiotic therapy.** Once the airway has been secured, antibiotic therapy should be initiated. Blood cultures should be obtained before beginning therapy to identify the bacterial organisms and their sensitivities. Such identification is of particular import in adults. Antigen studies on the serum will rapidly confirm the presence of *Haemophilus influenzae,* type B, in many patients.

a. **Choice of drug**

   (1) **Combination drug therapy** is the initial treatment of choice. In our experience, chloramphenicol and ampicillin can be administered simultaneously without adverse effect and usually with a prompt clinical response.

When the specific sensitivities become available, the antibiotic of choice is administered and other antibiotics discontinued.

(2) Chloramphenicol. In many parts of the country, *Haemophilus influenzae* is often resistant to ampicillin; consequently, the recommended antibiotic regimen is chloramphenicol, 100 mg/kg/day, in four divided doses administered intravenously. For very young patients (under the age of 18 months), the dose should be lowered to 50–75 mg/kg/day. When serum levels of chloramphenicol are known, they can be used to adjust the dosage.

(3) Ampicillin. If the pathogenic organism is sensitive to ampicillin, a dose of 200 mg/kg/day, in four divided doses administered intravenously, can be used.

(4) Second- and third-generation cephalosporins (e.g., cefuroxime, cefotaxime, ceftazidime) are excellent alternatives, particularly when ampicillin resistance is suspected or found.

b. Duration of antibiotic therapy. In most instances, 7 days of antibiotic therapy is sufficient and further therapy is not required. During the last 2–3 days of hospitalization, the patient is usually ambulatory and on a regular diet.

c. Use of steroids. Although steroids remain a controversial issue, they may be of value in certain patients in whom respiratory collapse is not imminent, i.e., in the adult patient and some children.

Dexamethasone is administered in the following dosage: 5 mg for the first 10 lb and 1 mg/10 lb thereafter up to a total of 20 mg as an initial dose. Half the initial dose is repeated in 6 hours and no more given.

D. Prognosis. If the steps of management previously outlined are observed, patients should recover without adverse sequelae. The prognosis for recovery to normal is excellent. If any question exists about the adequacy of the airway by the managing physician, early intubation must be performed. Failure to do so may result in respiratory arrest. Complications of intubation in this setting are infrequent.

II. Croup syndromes. Croup is an ill-defined cluster of diseases, characterized primarily by inspiratory stridor but sometimes by expiratory stridor as well. Anatomically, croup affects the subglottis, in contrast to supraglottitis, and displays a characteristic biannual epidemic character, usually peaking in the beginning of the winter season or late in the fall.

A. Viral laryngotracheitis. Viral croup, the most common of the croup syndromes, usually affects patients in the first 2 years of life. Bronchitis is specifically omitted from the name because distal inflammatory disease rarely occurs concomitantly. The disease typically occurs as a community-wide epidemic.

1. **Signs and symptoms.** Affected children appear to be ill but are not toxic, have a croupy cough, hoarse voice, and stridor that can be both inspiratory and expiratory. There is no significant dysphagia, throat pain, drooling, or preferred position. An elevated temperature is common but is not marked or spiking in character.

2. **Diagnosis.** The diagnosis of viral laryngotracheitis is most often clinical. The question of additional information from radiography has not been fully explored, although there appears to be no correlation between the x-ray findings and the degree of hypoxemia. Anteroposterior x rays of the neck, however, often help confirm the diagnosis when the characteristic subglottic tapered narrowing is visualized. Lateral soft tissue views assist only in eliminating other etiologic considerations (e.g., supraglottitis, foreign body). Endoscopy is considered only as part of the management protocol for advanced disease.

3. **Management**

   a. **Outpatient therapy** can be considered for most patients if the respiratory rate is less than 40 times/minute and if the patient is able to maintain oral hydration. Temporary relief may be obtained by using the bathroom shower to produce instant humidification. The use of a cool-mist vaporizer in the immediate environment is an important part of the therapy, particularly in the winter season with the associated dryness secondary to heating systems.

   b. **Inpatient therapy** is advised for children with respiratory rates greater than 40 and for those who are unable to drink adequate amounts of fluid.

      (1) **Intravenous fluids** and appropriate **humidification** of the inspired air permits a number of these patients to recover uneventfully. Despite these measures, however, some will still experience substantial respiratory distress.

      (2) **Medication**

         (a) Temporary resolution can be obtained by the use of **racemic epinephrine** nebulized with positive pressure, using a face mask. The dose for this agent is 0.25–0.50 ml mixed with 2 ml of saline. If administered by an experienced respiratory therapist, this agent typically produces striking improvement that lasts for varying periods of time.

         If racemic epinephrine is used, hospital admission is mandatory because of the risk of rebound airway obstruction in the hours following therapy. Racemic epinephrine can be administered as frequently as q30–60min, provided tachycardia does not contraindicate its use. The frequency of treatments required by the patient is a rough indication of how the clinical course is proceeding. A patient whose interval of therapy decreases from 4 hours to 1 hour is a candidate for more aggressive therapy.

(b) The use of steroids in this disease is an unresolved question. Although there is evidence that the use of steroids reduces edema in the supraglottic space when the edema is produced by trauma, the data for viral laryngotracheitis are more confusing. Several double-blind studies using low-dose steroids have not demonstrated efficacy, although two studies have demonstrated some efficacy if high-dose steroids are used.

If steroids are elected, they should be given early in the course of illness and in high doses: dexamethasone, 0.5–1.5 mg/kg, as a single-injection IM or IV, up to a total of 20 mg in one administration.

(c) Antibiotic therapy in viral laryngotracheitis is not indicated initially. If the course becomes protracted, however, consideration must be given to the probability of a secondary bacterial infection, and on that basis appropriate antibiotic therapy should be started. In this instance, ampicillin, 100 mg/kg, parenterally administered, is the initial drug of choice.

(3) Intubation and tracheotomy. Should intravenous fluids, humidification, and antibiotics fail to reverse the clinical status of the patient, the only alternatives remaining are intubation or tracheotomy to mechanically establish an airway. With careful, advanced planning, patients requiring airway assistance can be managed systematically and without confusion. Endoscopy should be performed in the operating room, initially defining the magnitude of inflammation, detecting the presence of any associated anomalies (e.g., subglottic stenosis), and removing inspissated secretions.

(a) Intubation. The area of narrowing in the airway occurs within a rigid space, the cricoid ring; therefore, it is imperative to use the smallest possible endotracheal tube consistent with good ventilation. In children, this typically means an endotracheal tube that is 0.5–1.0 mm **smaller** in outside diameter than would normally be used for that age or size child (Table 1-1). If a smaller than normal tube is not used, the risk of tracheal stenosis in the weeks following recovery is substantially increased. If intubation is the initial procedure chosen to establish the airway mechanically, a reevaluation is mandatory at 48 hours. If extubation is not feasible, tracheotomy becomes an important consideration.

(b) Tracheotomy. The initial choice between an endotracheal tube and a tracheotomy in croup is based on many of the same issues as for supraglottitis (see sec. **I.C.**). In croup, however, tracheotomy does offer the

Table 1-1. Size of bronchoscopes and tracheotomy tubes in children

Age	Bronchoscopes (mm × cm)	Tracheostomy tubes	
		Routine	Respirator
Premature	3 × 20	00	0
Newborn–3 mo	3.0–3.5 × 20–25	00 or 0	0 or 1
3–6 mo	3.5 × 25	0 or 1	1
6–12 mo	3.5–4.0 × 30	0 or 1	1 or 2
1–2 yr	3.5–4.0 × 30	1 or 2	1 or 2
3 yr	4 × 30	1 or 2	2 or 3
4 yr	4–5 × 30–35	2	2 or 3
5–7 yr	5 × 35	2 or 3	3 or 4
8–12 yr	5–7 × 35–40	3 or 4	4 or 5

Source: P. H. Holinger, J. A. Schild, and L. Weprin, Pediatric laryngology. *Otolaryngol. Clin. North Am.* 3:625, 1970.

distinct advantage of not placing a foreign body through the relatively immobile inflamed subglottis and should be considered early for slow resolution.

B. **Bacterial laryngotracheitis** is less common than viral, typically being caused by *Staphylococcus aureus, Streptococcus pyogenes, Streptococcus pneumoniae,* or *Haemophilus influenzae.* Clinically, the illness may be indistinguishable from viral croup but should be suspected when there is a persistent fever, elevation of white blood count, or lack of resolution with normal therapeutic measures. Tracheoscopy and cultures from the area identify the offending organism in most instances and guide appropriate antibiotic therapy. Occasionally, obstructing subglottic mucous casts or thick secretions necessitate their removal.

C. **Spasmodic croup** is a poorly defined entity consisting of croup symptoms, rapid in onset, usually occurring at night with a very short clinical course. An environmental change often effects resolution; steam and cool night air seem to be equally beneficial. Continuous symptoms for more than 24 hours would ordinarily rule out this diagnosis.

D. **Recurrent croup** suggests the possibility of a congenital anatomic abnormality, most often subglottic stenosis.

III. **Foreign bodies.** Cough and recurrent pneumonia, stridor, asthma, and respiratory arrest have all been seen as the result of aspirated foreign material. The symptoms relate primarily to the site of impaction. The hypopharynx is the area most frequently involved. Denture wearers or intoxicated patients are prone to aspiration of foreign bodies. Chicken and fish bones are the foreign bodies most often identified.

A. **Symptoms**

1. **Hypopharynx.** Most frequent among the presenting symptoms are pain on swallowing and persistent localized throat

discomfort. The patient can readily demarcate the involved area. Hoarseness is not a frequent occurrence, yet the voice may have a "hot potato" quality, sounding more muffled with larger foreign bodies.

2. **Larynx.** Impacted foreign bodies in the larynx often produce significant partial or total airway obstruction. The Heimlich sign, bringing the hand to the throat, is almost universally given. If complete obstruction occurs, the patient is unable to phonate, rapidly becomes pale, then cyanotic, showing increasing anxiety with subsequent agitation and then coma. Partial obstruction initially causes a cough, followed by hoarseness and stridor. Stridor may take several days to develop with smaller foreign bodies.

3. **Trachea.** Tracheal foreign bodies cause symptoms similar to those noted in the larynx. A brief but noteworthy coughing prodrome, followed by a quiet interlude, should suggest aspiration of a foreign body. Those that partially obstruct and change position may produce intermittent stridor, an audible thud or, if obstructing, ultimately cyanosis.

4. **Bronchus.** Objects usually lodge in the more distal air passages in children. The initial episode may go unnoticed. In 80% of cases, coughing, choking, or wheezing occurs alone or in combination. Not infrequently, however, the foreign body initially goes undetected. Therefore, unexplained recurrent pneumonia or localized asthma in childhood should always raise the suspicion of a foreign body.

B. **Diagnostic techniques**

1. **Indirect laryngoscopy** is especially beneficial in the evaluation of hypopharyngeal foreign bodies, which are most often located in the tongue base or piriform sinus. This technique is similarly beneficial in detecting laryngeal foreign bodies. It is the procedure of choice if there is a suspicion of a radiolucent aspirate (e.g., apple cores). In uncooperative patients, fiberoptic laryngoscopy via the transnasal route should be routine, not only for the hypopharynx and larynx, but also for the upper trachea.

2. **Radiography** can prove beneficial in the evaluation of radiopaque objects in the hypopharynx, larynx, trachea, and bronchi. Anteroposterior (AP) and lateral views of the neck, in addition to a lateral chest film with the arms held posteriorly, are necessary to assess the tracheobronchial tree. Fluoroscopy is mandatory, because 34% of radiolucent foreign bodies are not detected on routine x-ray studies within the first 24 hours. If the foreign body is not radiopaque, a region of obstructive atelectasis or emphysema can be noted fluoroscopically and augmented by changes in respiration.

C. **Points of caution**

1. **Total obstruction** with sudden aphonia while eating is an emergency situation, best handled by a sudden scapular blow. If this blow does not dislodge the foreign body, it should be followed immediately by the Heimlich maneuver. If both are unsuccessful, an emergency cricothyrotomy is indicated.

2. **Injudicious manipulation of a foreign body** in the trachea may cause subglottic impaction with acute obstruction. In the presence of an adequate airway, the patient should not be disturbed, and an endoscopy should be performed in a controlled manner.

D. Management

1. **Hypopharynx.** Removal of hypopharyngeal foreign bodies can be effected by having a cooperative patient hold the tongue, freeing the examiner's hand for a mirror-and-instrument extraction. If this fails, removal may require general anesthesia.

2. **Larynx.** Controlled laryngoscopy under general anesthesia is the most efficacious method of removal.

3. **Tracheobronchial tree.** Tracheobronchial foreign bodies should be removed endoscopically in the controlled operating room environment. Usually, the airway is secure in that only a portion of the respiratory tract is obstructed. Ill-conceived attempts at removal often cause further impaction of the object. A "safety zone" of time usually exists, allowing appropriate personnel, facility, and instruments to be prepared. A duplicate of the foreign object should be obtained, whenever possible, enabling the endoscopist to select the most appropriate instrumentation for removal. Topical vasoconstrictors, Fogarty catheters, preoperative steroids, and magnification are helpful adjuncts in selected instances.

IV. Neck infections compromising the airway

A. **Submandibular space.** (See Chap. 4, **V.A.4.**) Ludwig's angina is infectious involvement of the entire submandibular and sublingual space. Dental or periodontal infections are the most common sources of submandibular abscesses. It is not uncommon, however, for a submandibular gland infection to initiate a submandibular abscess. Initially, cellulitis may be limited to the sublingual space, and the abscess may be drained through the floor of the mouth.

1. **Anatomy.** The submandibular region is composed of two anatomic spaces: (1) the sublingual space, occupying the region above the mylohyoid muscle, and (2) the submaxillary space, lying external to the mylohyoid. These two spaces are in direct continuity posteriorly.

2. **Signs and symptoms.** If the tongue is elevated, but the neck is only minimally involved, respiratory compromise is not present. If infection penetrates through the mylohyoid, the disease process progresses rapidly. The submaxillary space becomes hard, and swallowing elicits pain. The temperature is elevated and, as the posterior tongue swells, respiration becomes labored.

3. **Diagnosis.** Dental and mandibular films are warranted to rule out a foreign body. A lateral x ray is most beneficial in assessing the degree of swelling in the tongue base.

4. Management. Therapy is directed primarily toward maintaining an airway and controlling infection. Appropriate antibiotics are given, especially for staphylococci and streptococci. Anaerobes must be considered. Antibiotics alone are the regimen of choice when respiratory obstruction is not present. High-dose penicillin intravenously or clindamycin intravenously (or both) is preferred. If respiratory obstruction occurs because of the posterior spread of infection to the tongue base or supraglottic larynx, a tracheotomy (see sec. **V.F.**) must be performed. Surgical management necessitates opening the tense space from the submental region into and including the tongue base.

B. Retropharyngeal space. (See Chap. 4, **V.A.2.**) Infections in the retropharyngeal space are most common in infants and children and arise from infection involving the nasopharynx, adenoids, and posterior nasal chambers, as well as the sinuses. Foreign bodies that penetrate the posterior pharyngeal wall can similarly be etiologic. Tuberculosis has produced these abscesses in adults.

1. Anatomy. The retropharyngeal space lies behind the hypopharynx and esophagus, extending from the base of the skull to the first thoracic vertebrae. Infections in this space can spread posteriorly to the prevertebral space that extends the entire length of the vertebrae or laterally into the mediastinum.

2. Signs and symptoms. The difficulty in diagnosing high abscesses in a child arise when lymphoid tissue, normally present in the nasopharynx, is enlarged. If an abscess is present, the patient's neck is usually held rigid and tilted away from the side of involvement. Pain is present, especially on swallowing. The child is febrile, the voice is muffled, and respiratory difficulty occurs relatively early in the course of the disease. Cellulitis secondary to adenitis occurs more frequently than a true abscess, and the symptomatology is less fulminant.

3. Diagnosis. Palpation can help delineate the true nature of a retropharyngeal swelling. When an abscess is suspected, palpation should be performed with the patient's head in a dependent position in the event of rupture. An abscess can be suggested by a lateral soft tissue film of the neck, with edema and secondary widening of the retropharynx being detailed and confirmed by fluoroscopy or computed tomography (CT) scan.

4. Management. Therapy includes antibiotics alone for cellulitis or in combination with surgical drainage for abscess formation. The surgical approach, either transoral or external, depends on the extent of the infection. An abscess extending below the level of the hyoid bone should have external drainage. Smaller superior collections respond to the transoral approach.

C. Pharyngomaxillary (parapharyngeal) space. (See Chap. 4, **V.A.3.**) Infections in the pharyngomaxillary area are common and arise from disease in the tonsils, adenoids, teeth and adnexa, parotid glands, and lymph nodes that drain the nose and pharynx. The posterior compartment may become contaminated via infection in the middle ear and mastoid (Bezold's abscess). Although not directly obstructing the airway, this most common of deep facial space infections can spread to contiguous areas, impinging on the airway in the pharynx or neck.

1. **Anatomy.** The pharyngomaxillary space is shaped like an inverted pyramid; the base is the base of the skull, and the apex is the hyoid bone. This space is divided by the styloid process into anterior and posterior compartments.

2. **Signs and symptoms**

   a. **Anterior** compartment involvement causes trismus (internal pterygoid muscle irritation) and swelling of the lateral pharyngeal wall.

   b. **Posterior** compartment infections cause less trismus than do anterior; however, infection here juxtaposes the great vessels of the neck with the potential for thrombosis or hemorrhage.

   c. **Common to both anterior and posterior** compartments are symptoms of fever, nuchal rigidity, odynophagia, parotid swelling, and pharyngalgia.

3. **Diagnosis.** A CT scan should define the extent of involvement. Lateral x rays of the neck may show concomitant posterior pharyngeal swelling. If vascular obstruction is suspected, orbital plethysmography can prove beneficial. Angiography may become essential if surgery is a consideration.

4. **Management.** Antibiotics, primarily cefoxitin in combination with gentamycin, must be administered intravenously in high doses. Surgical drainage when necessary is through an external incision in the submandibular region, going deep to the submaxillary gland and cephalad along the carotid sheath. Once recognized, surgery should be an early consideration.

V. **Trauma** causing respiratory embarrassment is seen with injury occurring in the area extending from the anterior oropharynx to the cervical trachea. Trauma can range from displaced dentures occluding the airway to tracheal separation. With severe trauma, there may be more than one region contributing to airway obstruction.

A. **Points of caution**

   1. Maintenance of the airway must be the primary management consideration.

   2. Motion of the neck must be restricted until injury of the cervical spine is excluded.

B. **Midface and mandible**

   1. **Initial considerations.** Obstruction of the airway can occur with mid- or lower-facial injury secondary to hemorrhage, edema, and posterior displacement of fracture segments. Foreign materials (e.g., denture fragments) are frequent causes of obstruction. No specific diagnostic respiratory obstructive patterns are manifested by these injuries and, therefore, the physician must

remain alerted to the frequently associated airway compromise. Proper management must first include the airway and then the fracture. The diagnosis should be established using clinical information, and appropriate measures should be taken to secure the airway. Time should not be wasted in first obtaining x rays or ancillary studies (e.g., blood gases).

2. Management

a. The oral cavity and pharynx must be cleared of debris, clot, and foreign body, either manually or by suction.

b. After cleaning, if the airway is still obstructed, simple repositioning of retrodisplaced segments should be performed. An oral or nasopharyngeal airway can maintain air flow until definitive fixation of the fractured segments is performed.

c. An emergency tracheotomy is rarely necessary for these injuries, but should be considered when swelling of the tongue base obstructs the airway.

C. Larynx. Injury to the larynx can occur from either blunt or penetrating trauma. A penetrating injury, associated with an open wound and air emanating from the site of impact, demands consideration of a laryngeal injury. Blunt trauma is more difficult to evaluate because the symptoms and signs may be slow to evolve.

1. Signs and symptoms. Subcutaneous emphysema, progressive airway obstruction, dysphonia, focal neck pain, loss of the thyroid cartilage prominence, and overt intralaryngeal mucosal lacerations can all be associated with significant laryngeal trauma. Dislocation of the cricoarytenoid joint must be considered, but in the acute stage, edema may mask this relatively subtle finding.

2. Diagnosis

a. Indirect laryngoscopy should be attempted initially, but may be difficult to perform in patients with multiple injuries.

b. Direct laryngoscopy. Flexible fiberoptic laryngoscopy can frequently clarify the nature and magnitude of the injury. When doubt exists, direct rigid laryngoscopy should be performed in the operating room with the airway secure. Disruption of normal anatomy and the presence of mucosal lacerations, foreign material, and cartilage injury should be documented. Cord mobility must be assessed and the arytenoids palpated. In massive trauma, injury to the trachea or esophagus often coexists; thus, endoscopic examination of these structures is indicated.

c. Radiographs. Plain films are of little value in assessing acute injuries, except for delineating the presence of subcutaneous emphysema. CT scans can aid in assessing the extent of laryngotracheal injury. Chest films assist in the evaluation of a pneumomediastinum or pneumothorax.

3. Management

a. Tracheotomy (see **F.**) is mandatory in the presence of an unstable airway secondary to laryngeal injury. Cricothyrotomy should be avoided if at all possible. Laryngeal fragments can easily be disrupted and infection spread if a cricothyrotomy is performed.

b. Acute laryngeal injuries with tissue disruption should be surgically explored and repaired at the earliest possible time. Mucosal lacerations must be meticulously repaired and cartilaginous fragments realigned and stabilized when necessary with nonreactive suture material or miniplates. Endolaryngeal stenting may be required to give intraluminal support.

Specific attention must be directed to the cricoid cartilage, since undiagnosed injuries at this site, once scarred, are very difficult to reconstruct. Unless there has been an obvious transection of the recurrent laryngeal nerve, considerations regarding function should wait. Vocal cord weakness often subsides spontaneously if the nerve has been contused, but should call attention to potential injury in the tracheoesophageal groove (i.e., great cervical vessels). Antibiotics (penicillin) should be used in open wounds.

D. Trachea. Although disruption of the airway with a laryngotracheal separation usually involves an open wound, rapid flexion-extension in sudden deceleration can produce the same injury.

1. Signs and symptoms

a. Upper tracheal injury has diagnostic characteristics similar to those of the larynx.

b. Subcutaneous emphysema should suggest a tracheal or esophageal disruption, although not signifying the magnitude.

2. Management

a. The esophagus must be examined for laceration, and the mediastinum should be evaluated for associated injury.

b. The mandatory tracheotomy should be placed as far from the site of injury as possible.

c. Tracheal separations must be repaired as soon as possible.

d. Debridement of obviously necrotic tracheal tissue may require a supraglottic laryngeal release to allow primary tracheal approximation.

E. Soft tissue of the neck

1. Points of caution

a. With blunt neck trauma, the primary consideration must be maintenance of an adequate airway.

b. The cervical spine deserves serious thought in the initial evaluation.

2. Signs and symptoms. Open or penetrating wounds of the neck are frequently associated with significant vascular involvement.

    a. An expanding mass within the neck raises the possibility of vascular injury.

    b. A patent airway can be jeopardized by progressive soft tissue swelling.

    c. Bleeding by mouth can indicate significant midneck vascular (carotid) disruption.

3. Diagnosis. When time allows, vascular radiographic studies are invaluable in the specific delineation of the site of injury. Cervical spine injuries must also be assessed by x ray.

4. Management

    a. Pressure tamponade should be performed initially. Indiscriminate clamping or ligation may cause associated nerve injury.

    b. Transoral bleeding can be controlled by pharyngeal packing; however, a tracheotomy (see **F.**) is mandatory prior to placement of the pack. Vaginal packing with a long instrument (e.g., a Kelly clamp) can be used.

    c. Lower neck trauma can be associated with injury to the intrathoracic vasculature, and these injuries require an emergency thoracotomy.

    d. Not all open neck wounds require exploration. If significant structural injury is suspected (Table 1-2), exploration is performed.

F. Tracheotomy: potential considerations

1. Indications

The need to establish an airway with a tracheotomy is due to airway obstruction or to ventilatory failure. Either can be acute or slowly progressive. The adage that when a tracheotomy is considered, it should be performed remains valid. It is far better to place a tracheotomy in a controlled operating room environment under local or general anesthesia than under duress with an anxious, obstructed patient and flustered personnel. The following outlines the indications for a tracheotomy.

    a. Obstruction

        (1) Trauma

            (a) Partial or complete obstruction of airway

            (b) Blunt injury with edema of the endolaryngeal or tracheal structures

Table 1-2. Indications for surgical exploration of neck wounds

I. Vascular injury
   A. Immediate indications
      1. Hemorrhage from neck wound
      2. Active transoral bleeding without visible source
      3. Chyle leak
      4. Expanding cervical hematoma
      5. Airway obstruction
      6. Widened superior mediastinum
      7. Absence of pulses
      8. Progressive CNS deficit from hypoperfusion
      9. Positive angiogram
      10. Bruit
   B. Delayed indications
      1. Major vessel thrombosis
      2. Occult hemorrhage
      3. Arteriovenous fistula
      4. Aneurysm or pseudoaneurysm
      5. Vertebral artery injury
      6. Thoracic inlet injury
II. Neurologic injury
   A. Jugular foramen syndrome (deficit of cervical sympathetic, fourth, fifth, sixth, and seventh nerves)
   B. Submandibular space injury with deficit to seventh and lingual nerves
   C. Horner's syndrome
   D. Brachial plexus deficit
   E. Hemiplegia
   F. Diminished visual acuity or contraction of visual fields
III. Respiratory and digestive tract injury
   A. Immediate indications
      1. Crepitus
      2. Stridor
      3. Aphonia or dysphonia
      4. Dysphagia
      5. Hyoid, thyroid, and cricoid cartilages painful to palpation
      6. Loss of thyroid prominence
      7. Positive endoscopy
      8. Positive contrast study
   B. Late indications
      1. Neck infection
      2. Mediastinitis

Source: Modified from M. May, et al., Penetrating wounds of the neck in civilians. *Otolaryngol. Clin. North Am.* 9:361, 1976.

   (c) Blood or foreign material in airway

   (d) Maxillofacial injury with aspiration and local edema

   (e) Collapse of airway and soft tissue support

(2) Foreign body

(3) Inflammation

   (a) Secondary to infection (e.g., supraglottitis)

   (b) Angioedema

(c) Allergic response

(d) Deep neck space abscess

(e) Secondary to caustic or thermal injury

(4) Congenital lesions

(a) At birth (e.g., subglottic stenosis)

(b) Aggravated by superimposed infection

(c) Progression of abnormality (e.g., laryngeal cyst, Pierre Robin syndrome)

(5) Neoplasia

(a) Hemangioma, lymphangioma

(b) Squamous cell carcinoma

(6) Paralysis or paresis of the vocal cord

(a) Bilateral

(b) Associated neuromuscular dysfunction

b. Ventilatory failure

(1) Retained secretions

(a) Depression of cough, postsurgical, pneumonitis, cystic fibrosis

(b) Aspiration of gastric contents

(2) Inefficient respirations due to depressed ventilatory stimulus of coma, central nervous system (CNS) disease, chest wall fracture or paralysis, chronic lung disease, head trauma

2. Method highlights. In most situations, placement of an endotracheal tube should be the primary mode of airway management when simpler measures fail. Circumstances arise when intubation is not feasible (e.g., massive injury to the lower midface, laryngeal fracture, or an acutely obstructing foreign body). If an open path to the airway is present, it should be cannulated with an endotracheal tube as a temporary measure. Especially in children, morbidity and mortality increase when a tracheotomy is performed in a struggling patient without initial airway control via an endotracheal tube or bronchoscope.

Cricothyrotomy (Fig. 1-1) should be used only as a temporary measure, until a controlled tracheotomy can be performed. A vertical incision is usually used for ease and rapidity in an emergency tracheotomy (Fig. 1-2). Sedation is contraindicated in acute obstruction, because respiratory collapse or total obstruction may ensue. Silk stay sutures placed through the tracheal wall and brought out through the wound may be invaluable should the tracheotomy tube become dislodged. Tracheotomy tape should be tied with the patient's head in flexion;

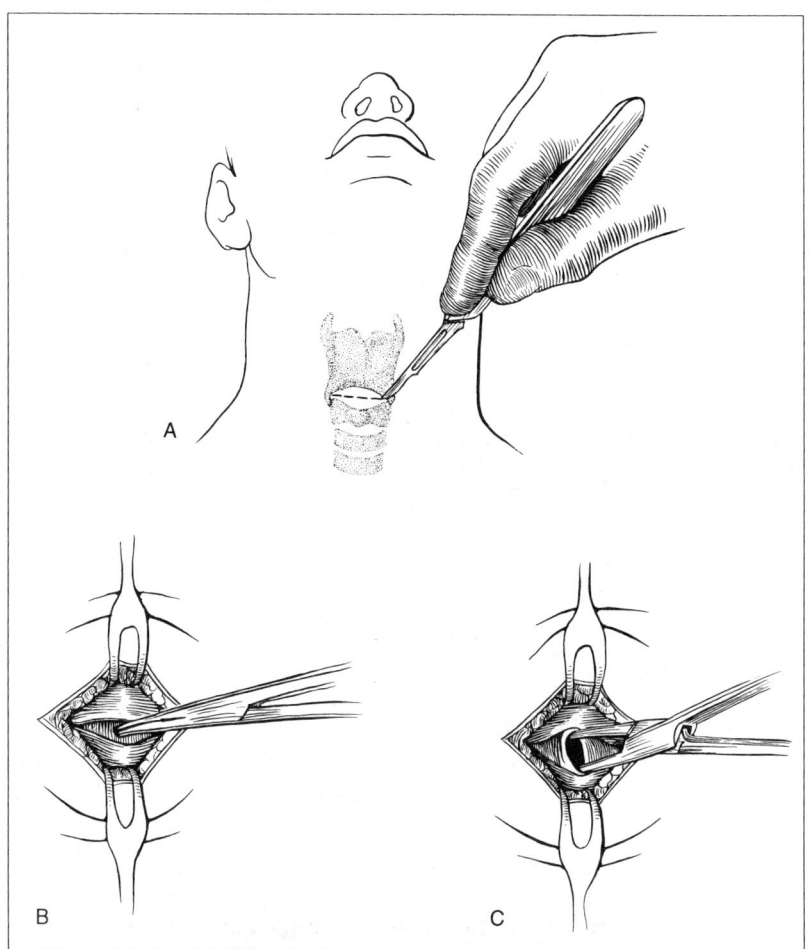

Fig. 1-1. Cricothyroidotomy. A. Incision directly over cricothyroid membrane. B. Subcutaneous tissue separated vertically. C. Cricothyroid membrane fenestrated vertically distracting cricoid and first tracheal ring.

otherwise, the tape will be too loose. After a tracheotomy, a chest x ray should be obtained to assess tube placement and to rule out a pneumothorax (see Figs. 1-1 and 1-2).

3. **Complications.** An emergency tracheotomy is hazardous under the best conditions. Prior control of the airway greatly diminishes the incidence of complications. The following complications are divided into immediate and delayed: those occurring within 24 to 48 hours after the operation, and those occurring after 48 hours.

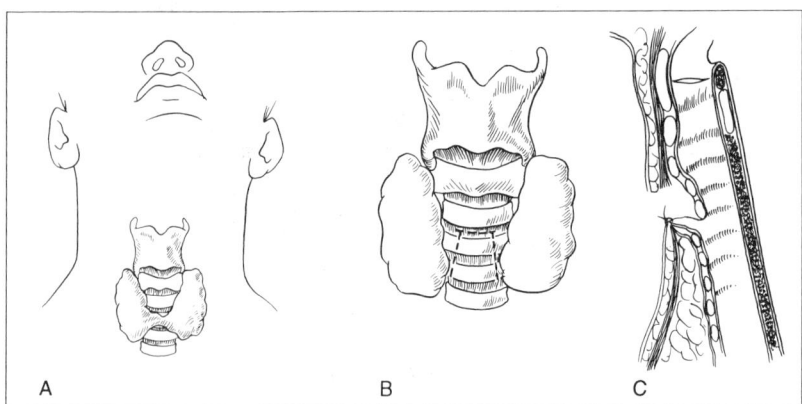

Fig. 1-2. Tracheotomy. A. Normal anatomy—depicting thyroid isthmus, trachea, larynx. B. Isthmus separated; anterior tracheal flap outlined. Flap is inferiorly based, involves two rings, and (C) is sutured to inferior skin flap. The tracheocutaneous suture is removed in 48 hours.

a. Immediate complications

(1) **Hemorrhage** may occur during the procedure from a prominent anterior jugular vein, an anomalous artery, or the thyroid gland.

(2) **Pneumothorax and pneumomediastinum** occur in more than one-third of emergency procedures, usually in patients with acute respiratory failure, as well as in those tracheotomies performed without an indwelling endolaryngeal tube. Avoidance is effected by minimum dissection of the pretracheal fascia and by controlled positive pressure. Often a pneumomediastinum needs no further therapy.

(3) **Immediate apnea** occurs in patients with hypercarbic respiratory stimulation in whom the hypoxic drive has been eliminated. On insertion of an airway, blood PCO_2 is diminished, and the respiratory stimulus is decreased or abolished. Controlled respiration may be needed in this situation.

(4) **Subcutaneous emphysema** sometimes results from tight incisional closure, aggravated by mechanical ventilation.

(5) **Atelectasis,** usually of the left lobe, occurs when a long tube is in the right mainstem bronchus. This condition is relieved by appropriate repositioning of the tracheotomy tube.

(6) **A poorly positioned or dislodged tube** occurs when the trachea is not cannulated under direct vision or the tube is not a proper length. Suturing the flanges to the neck

helps avoid accidental removal. This is a frequent cause of death in the initial postoperative period.

(7) Aerophagia may occur in children under the age of 3 and leads to gastric dilatation and cardiac arrhythmias. A nasogastric tube provides relief.

(8) Tracheoesophageal fistula rarely occurs as an immediate problem unless the tube is forced posteriorly and transects the trachea and esophageal wall.

(9) Recurrent laryngeal nerve paralysis occurs when the surgical dissection is off the midline, into the tracheoesophageal groove.

b. Delayed complications

(1) Hemorrhage may occur secondary to local granulation at the stoma. It can result from tracheal trauma from too vigorous suctioning, as well as dryness with associated crusting. More seriously, it may be due to erosion of a prominent vessel (e.g., the innominate artery) by the tracheotomy tube. The incidence of such can be decreased by placement of the tube at the second tracheal ring.

(2) Laryngeal stenosis is secondary to a tube placed into the larynx or the cricothyroid membrane and not lowered to the trachea.

(3) Tracheal stenosis occurs at the level of either the stoma or the cuff and is usually due to erosion (by motion, infection, and pressure).

(4) Tracheitis sicca most often occurs during the winter, when drying of the tracheal mucosa results in crusting. Adequate humidification is a must.

(5) Displaced tracheotomy tube is discussed in **a(6)**.

(6) Tracheoesophageal fistula, occurring as a delayed complication, is secondary to erosion by the tube or cuff, usually in the presence of a firm nasogastric tube. It can be a fatal complication in debilitated patients.

(7) Dysphagia and aspiration are usually secondary to loss of laryngeal competence and to irritation of the esophagus by the tracheotomy tube.

(8) Delayed decannulation is most often noted in children who rely on the open airway and who may require a gradual decannulation procedure (i.e., progressively smaller tubes). If airway obstruction is present with a plugged, fenestrated tracheotomy tube in place, the plug must be removed and the cervical airway reassessed.

VI. Acute angioneurotic edema (see Chap. 4, **V.B.2.**).

A. Allergic angioneurotic edema of any region of the larynx may occur as a response to a wide range of provocators, the most common of which are foods, inhalants, and drugs. A family history of asthma, hay fever, eczema, or angioneurotic edema may be used to differentiate hereditary and nonhereditary types. Aspirin is a common precursor; however, sensitivities to chicle, bee stings, house dust, cosmetics, and beef have also been reported. Iodine ingestion, as well as tetanus antitoxin and vaccines, induce the same responses.

1. **Signs and symptoms.** Laryngeal edema may occur after administration of penicillin, either orally or parenterally, and can be delayed 1–4 hours after exposure. Acute swelling is an anaphylactic reaction that can involve the epiglottis, arytenoids, ventricular bands, true vocal cords, or subglottis.

2. **Diagnosis** may be difficult. A family allergy history is invaluable. On indirect laryngoscopy, pale boggy edema of the entire larynx or a portion thereof is noted.

3. **Treatment.** In the early stages, subcutaneous epinephrine (0.3 ml) can rapidly reverse the swelling. Supplemental use of an antihistamine (diphenhydramine, 25–50 mg IV) or corticosteroid (e.g., dexamethasone, 5–10 mg IV) may be of value. If response to medical therapy does not occur, an airway must be established. The airway is best accomplished by endotracheal intubation. Cases of failure of intubation alone to control the airway have been reported, so the patient's airway must be carefully monitored, even after the endotracheal tube has been placed.

B. **Hereditary angioneurotic edema (HAE)** is a genetic disease of autosomal dominant inheritance in which there is a deficiency of the inhibitor of the first component of complement. The attacks begin in childhood, occur frequently, and diminish in the middle-age years. Mortality has been reported to vary from 5–50%.

1. **Signs and symptoms.** HAE differs from other forms of angioneurotic edema because of the presence of associated gastrointestinal symptoms (intermittent abdominal pain, nausea, vomiting, diarrhea), peripheral edema, poor response to standard epinephrine, steroid and antibiotic therapy, and more pronounced laryngeal involvement. Attacks are frequently brought on by trauma, stress, or anxiety, and have been aggravated by pregnancy and menstruation.

2. **Diagnosis** is aided by the laboratory measurement of C1 esterase, which is abnormally low. Also, C4 and C2 levels (other complement system components) may be depressed. Testing reveals no specific allergic substance. The same pale, swollen larynx found in allergic angioneurotic edema is seen on indirect laryngoscopy in complement-initiated angioneurotic edema. Once an attack begins, laryngeal edema may be slow to progress and may not reach maximum proportions for 24–48 hours, in contrast to the more rapidly progressing allergic variety.

3. **Management**

   a. **Acute** therapy, if the airway is endangered, often requires a tracheotomy. The trauma of intubation may aggravate the local laryngeal edema. As noted in **A.3.**, steroids, antihistamines, and epinephrine may not prove beneficial. In those patients with known HAE, close observation of the airway is mandatory. Purified C1 esterase inhibitor is available and effective in the acute situation.

    b. Maintenance measures are currently directed toward inhibiting plasma so that less C1 esterase is produced. Epsilon aminocaproic acid (EACA) is such an antiplasma substance, as is the analog of EACA, tranexamic acid. These two agents have been used in both short- and long-term therapy of patients with hereditary angioneurotic edema. Androgens, such as danazol or Stanazol, have also been successful therapeutically when used as a preventive measure.

VII. Acute airway problems of the newborn and infant. Respiratory distress in the newborn can occur from mechanical airway obstruction or from depression of physiologic respiration. Often the differentiation is difficult; however, slow, shallow respiratory efforts in a cyanotic child should suggest central, metabolic, or cardiovascular disturbance. What follows is a brief outline of some significant head and neck lesions causing mechanical airway obstruction.

A. Choanal atresia (see Chap. 4, **V.D.3.**). At birth and for the first 2–3 weeks of life, the child is an obligate nasal breather. Nasal airway obstruction, irrespective of etiology, can occlude the only functional air passage. This is a true emergency and must be dealt with rapidly. Choanal atresia can be either bilateral or unilateral. Bilateral obstruction causes symptoms from birth, while unilateral atresia may go unnoticed until the first upper respiratory tract infection, at which time the child becomes acutely symptomatic. The atresia is most often bony (90%), and the remainder are membranous, presumably secondary to a persistent buccopharyngeal membrane.

    1. Signs and symptoms. The neonate shows signs of nasal obstruction relieved with crying. A mucoid cast of the nasal chambers may be present. Persistent unilateral mucoid rhinorrhea should raise the suspicion of either atresia or a foreign body.

    2. The **diagnosis** of choanal atresia is confirmed by CT scan. Other associated skull base malformations are delineated as well. The standard advocated approach—passing a nasal catheter—can be misleading and is not recommended. The CT scan has replaced older contrast studies.

    3. Therapy

        a. Acute. A McGovern nipple (a baby bottle nipple with an open tip) or a conventional oral airway can be placed to maintain a patent airway until the nasal conduit can be established or until mouth breathing is acquired.

        b. Delayed management. Repair should be performed, in most instances, when the physical condition affords the administration of general anesthesia. Associated anomalies must be excluded. With the CHARGE syndrome (Coloboma, Heart disease, Atresia choanae, Retarded growth, Genital hypoplasia, and Ear anomalies) initial tracheotomy is the management. If corrected early, choanal atresia associated with CHARGE almost uniformly restenoses. Even in the child who rapidly acquires mouth breathing skills, an unrepaired bilateral atresia can alter the growth and development of the face. Surgery can be performed using microtechniques transnasally, and in selected cases the carbon dioxide laser may prove beneficial. Thick bony plates can require a transpalatal approach, and it remains the authors' procedure of choice. Stenting with plastic sheeting or tubing may be necessary for a period of 4–6 weeks to ensure mucosalization.

   c. Differential diagnosis. Other abnormalities causing nasal airway obstruction include encephalocele, meningocele, and adenoidal hypertrophy.

B. Congenital lesions of the mouth and pharynx rarely produce an acute airway emergency, but may precipitate respiratory distress by a combination of a lack of pharyngeal support and ineffective bolus transport with a predilection to aspiration. Such lesions include:

Cleft lip or palate (or both)
Pierre Robin syndrome (micrognathia, cleft palate, microglossia, and glossoptosis) (see Chap. 4, **V.D.1.**)
Oral hemangioma or lymphangioma
Treacher Collins syndrome (mandibulofacial dysostosis)

C. Laryngeal abnormalities. Although congenital lesions of the larynx represent the most common anomalies causing respiratory distress in the newborn, acute obstruction is rarely the cause.

   1. Laryngomalacia (or exaggerated infantile larynx) is the most common of these lesions. There is a lack of rigidity of the soft collapsible epiglottis, supraglottic structures, or both that easily occludes the airway during deep inspiration. Fortunately, this condition usually resolves by 18–24 months of age.

      a. Signs and symptoms. The stridor produced is usually high pitched, but the cry is clear and strong. Stridor is aggravated in the supine position.

      b. Diagnosis is made by direct laryngeal examination. The epiglottis appears narrow, curled, and elongated.

      c. Therapy. Bronchoscopy should be considered in severe cases because of the possibility of associated anomalies in the tracheobronchial tree. In spite of the potential for total airway obstruction, tracheotomy is rarely indicated. Micro-laser techniques can have a major therapeutic impact in this disorder.

   2. Atresia and web

      a. Atresia. Although rare, complete congenital obstruction of the larynx can occur, causing immediate airway distress in the newborn. The infant violently makes attempts at respiration, but to no avail. Direct laryngoscopy with possible intubation should be attempted. Often the atresia plate is cartilaginous, not allowing the endotracheal tube to pass. Tracheotomy must then be performed.

b. Webs. Laryngeal web formation occurs because of arrest of laryngeal development at the tenth fetal week. Total arrest causes atresia; webs of the larynx represent "partial" atresia. Most webs (75%) occur at the level of the vocal cords, with the remaining being equally divided between supraglottic and subglottic. Webs in the subglottis are frequently associated with cricoid abnormalities.

(1) Diagnosis. Infants with laryngeal webs have alterations in cry and in respiration. The magnitude of the symptoms varies with the extent of the web.

(2) Therapy. Often a thin membrane involves the anterior half of the glottis and can be incised endoscopically. Thicker webs may require repeated excision (e.g., with the carbon dioxide laser), dilatation, and stenting. Insertion of a metal or plastic laryngeal keel at the anterior commissure may be necessary to prevent reformation after thyrotomy has been performed.

3. Congenital subglottic stenosis may occur as an isolated abnormality and, after laryngomalacia, is the second most common laryngeal anomaly. The potential for significant airway obstruction is definitely aggravated with the first upper respiratory tract infection. Subglottic stenosis can be due to failure of development of the endolarynx, the cricoid cartilage, or both.

a. Signs and symptoms. Stridor may occur from birth, but can often be mild or absent until an infection intervenes. It is at this time that acute obstruction occurs.

b. Diagnosis should be suspect in all children with congenital stridor and in those infants with recurrent episodes of "croup." The diagnosis is made by direct inspection prior to intubation so that iatrogenic subglottic stenosis is not a consideration.

c. Therapy. Significant obstruction requires a tracheotomy. Resolution can be augmented by repeated dilatation, endolaryngeal excision via the laser, or open cricothyrotomy and insertion of autogenous cartilage or bone, depending on the degree of stenosis.

4. Laryngeal paralysis. Paralysis of the vocal cords in infants can be unilateral or bilateral, the latter being more common. Both types may be due to birth trauma with cervical injury, causing a transient state that usually clears in 4–6 weeks. Bilateral paralysis is frequently associated with a central nervous system disorder. It may be due to injury of the nucleus ambiguus (by hemorrhage or anoxia) or associated with meningomyelocele, Arnold-Chiari malformation, or cerebral agenesis.

Cases of hereditary bilateral abductor vocal cord paralysis have been reported in both normal and mentally retarded patients. Hypoxia, because of laryngeal obstruction, has been suggested as a possible cause of the associated retardation. Unilateral leftsided cord paralysis is more common than right because of coincident cardiovascular anomalies. It is compounded by the longer course of the recurrent laryngeal nerve on the left. Esophageal or paraesophageal abnormalities can impinge on the nerve, causing subsequent cord weakness.

a. Signs and symptoms. Unilateral lesions may be associated with very few symptoms, which include a weak cry and hoarseness. Stridor or respiratory compromise rarely occurs. Patients with bilateral cord paralysis may have a normal cry because of the symmetry and apposition of the vocal cords. Respiratory obstruction is not uncommon, especially in association with upper respiratory tract infection.

b. Diagnosis is made by direct laryngoscopy without anesthesia using the pediatric fiberoptic laryngoscope. Preoperative ultrasound can further define the condition.

c. Management. When obstruction is not a problem, the patient should be followed expectantly. With obstruction, tracheotomy may be necessary to establish an airway.

5. Neoplasms. The most common neoplasms in infants and children are papillomas and subglottic hemangiomas.

a. Papillomas are the most frequent laryngeal tumors of childhood and can be present at birth. They tend to recur and involve any region of the respiratory tract. The etiology is viral. Seeding to the distal respiratory tract has been noted primarily after surgical manipulation or tracheotomy. Spontaneous remission has been noted and can occur at any time. The lesions are benign, but malignant transformation has been associated with radiation therapy.

(1) Signs and symptoms include persistent hoarseness, a croupy cough and, occasionally, progressive airway obstruction.

(2) Diagnosis is best made by direct examination and biopsy.

(3) Management. Current therapy is directed toward maintenance of an adequate airway by periodic tumor removal and avoidance of a tracheotomy. The carbon dioxide laser is now the established treatment. In selected cases, microexcision and cryosurgery still have their proponents. Once a tracheotomy is placed, papilloma formation may occur at or near the stoma. Approximately 6% of children with severe respiratory difficulty require a tracheotomy.

b. Hemangiomas. Subglottic hemangioma may occur in isolation or in association with cutaneous lesions. There is a female preponderance by a ratio of 2:1.

(1) **Signs and symptoms.** These are often congenital lesions and may appear as recurrent episodes of "croup." Growth of the tumor usually ceases by 6 months of age, often followed by spontaneous regression. The symptoms are aggravated by crying, which causes engorgement of the tumor.

(2) **Diagnosis** can be made by radiography and confirmed by direct laryngoscopy. Biopsy remains controversial, but probably should be performed to rule out another tumor. Experience has shown subsequent hemorrhage to be rare.

(3) **Therapy.** If the lesion is small, the child should be followed expectantly, and often further intervention is not warranted. With progressive obstructive symptoms, CO_2 laser surgery must be considered as the initial treatment. With severe respiratory obstruction, tracheotomy below the level of the tumor may be necessary.

c. **Other laryngeal neoplasms** include lymphangioma (cystic hygroma) and congenital cysts (either supraglottic or subglottic).

Epistaxis

The warming and humidifying functions of the nose require that it have a good blood supply. The nose is supplied by both the internal and external carotid systems. The anterior and posterior ethmoid arteries arise from the internal carotid by way of the ophthalmic artery and supply the superior part of the nose. The greater palatine and sphenopalatine arteries derive from the external carotid by way of the internal maxillary artery. The superior labial is a branch of the facial artery, also from the external carotia. Numerous anastomoses communicate these two systems. A large concentration of vessels known as Kiesselbach's plexus, is found in Little's area on the anterior septum (Fig. 1-3). Over 90% of the patients who seek attention for epistaxis have bleeding from this region. Bleeding tends to be anterior in the young and posterior in the old. It is important that an attempt be made to identify the bleeding point, even if packing is necessary, so rational decisions can be made about the location of packing and specific artery ligation, if this becomes necessary.

I. **Differential diagnosis**

A. **Nasal trauma** is a common cause of epistaxis. Nasal fractures usually involve tears of the mucosa and bleeding. If an ethmoid artery is torn, there may be very brisk intermittent bleeding arising high in the nasal vault.

B. **Drying of the nasal mucosa** in cold, dry weather or increased stress (e.g., sneezing, nose blowing, or exercise) may be responsible for discrete bleeding from a single vessel.

C. **Hypertension** results in thickening of the arterial wall and decreased vasoconstriction, but is not per se a cause of epistaxis.

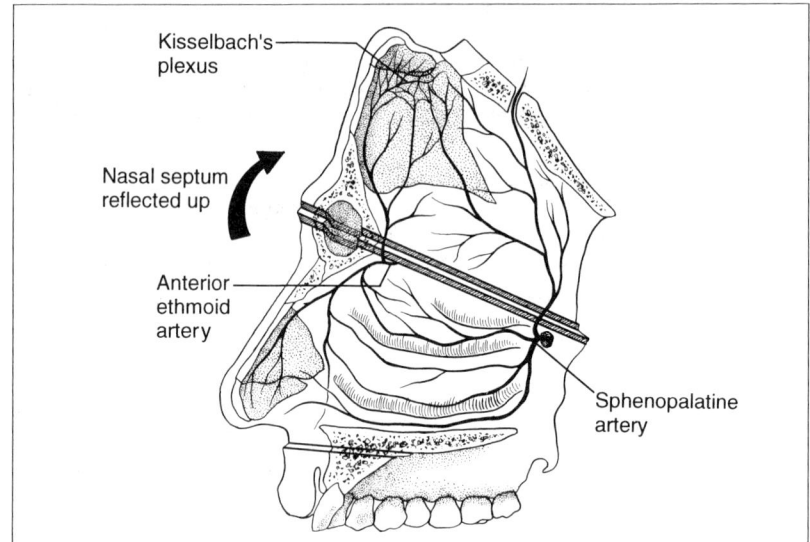

Fig. 1-3. Arterial supply to the nose. Drawing depicts septum rotated superiorly exposing the lateral nasal wall.

   D. A septal perforation often crusts and bleeds at its edges. Most perforations result from overvigorous cautery, but Wegener's granulomatosis and midline granuloma must be considered, as must cocaine use.

   E. Foreign bodies in the nose are frequently the cause of epistaxis in children. Nasal obstruction and purulent discharge often accompany the bleeding.

   F. Other causes. A generalized ooze or persistent or recurrent bleeding requires that one consider less common causes, such as:

   1. Hematologic disorders

      Anticoagulant use
      Antiplatelet drugs
      Clotting deficiencies
      Leukemia
      Thrombocytopenia
      Thromboasthenia
      Renal failure
      Hepatic failure

   2. Nasal tumor

   3. Sinus tumor

   4. Nasopharyngeal tumor

   5. Hereditary hemorrhagic telangiectasia

 II. Physical examination. The first person to examine the patient with epistaxis has the best chance of clearly identifying the bleeding point. The approach must be careful and systematic.

A. Equipment. Head mirror and light source (or head light), nasal speculum, bayonet forceps, suction with Fraser tip, 4–5% cocaine solution, and cotton or gauze pledgets.

B. Preparation. The doctor and patient should be gowned. The patient should blow his or her nose to clean it of clots and then sit upright.

C. Method of examination

   1. Patients presenting with bleeding

   a. Observe whether the bleeding is anterior or posterior and which is the predominant nasal chamber. The bleeding may appear to be bilateral if it is very posterior in origin or if there is a septal perforation.

   b. If the site of the bleeding is obscure, the nasal mucosa should be constricted, anesthetized, and cleared of blood by packing the nose with cottonoid strips that have been impregnated with 4–5% cocaine solution. An alternative to cocaine is a mixture of 4% lidocaine (Xylocaine) and 1:100,000 epinephrine. The strips should be left in place for at least 5 minutes. In the pediatric patient, a parent can assist, if necessary, by placing several drops of either solution in each nostril.

   c. When the packing is removed, the nose should be inspected again. The bleeding should have slowed or stopped, and it is usually possible to identify the bleeding point. Attention should be directed to the septum, the turbinate, and the meati between the turbinates as possible bleeding sites. An extreme septal deflection may make visualization impossible.

   d. Rigid fiberoptic nasal endoscopes, although not universally available, do allow for exact localization of a bleeding site and help direct specific local treatment or packing. This new technique clearly can minimize the amount of manipulation required.

   2. Patients in whom bleeding has subsided. If the bleeding subsides and the site of bleeding cannot be determined, the patient should be observed for several hours for recurrence.

III. Management. The bleeding should be controlled with the least possible manipulation and trauma. This is especially important when a clotting disorder is present, because manipulation has the potential to cause more bleeding. Even a successful pack causes additional trauma on removal.

   A. Packing

   1. Pediatric patients. The bleeding usually subsides when pressure is applied to the caudal end of the nose for several minutes with the head upright. If pressure is ineffective, silver nitrate application is preferred to electric cautery initially, because it is less likely to cause necrosis. Any cautery, however, should be judicious. Cautery can usually be performed quickly after topical anesthesia has been applied (see **B.1**.). Both sides of the septum should not be aggressively cauterized simultaneously, recognizing that this could result in a septal perforation. If packing is necessary, general anesthesia may be required.

2. Adult patients

   a. Light to moderately heavy bleeding

      (1) Manual pressure. As with the child, bleeding in the adult can usually be controlled with alar pressure for several minutes.

      (2) Cautery. If manual pressure is not effective, cautery is indicated. Before cautery, the interior of the nose should be anesthetized by cocaine (or lidocaine and epinephrine) packing. If the bleeding remains too brisk to cauterize effectively, a cotton-tipped applicator that has been dipped in 1:1000 epinephrine solution should be held against the bleeding site. A ring of surrounding mucosa can then be lightly cauterized, the applicator removed, and the bleeding site cauterized. A small piece of Surgicel or Oxycel should then be placed over the cauterized area.

      Postcautery instructions to the patient should include:

      No manipulation
      No nose blowing
      Open the mouth if you sneeze
      No straining, lifting, or strenuous activity for 1 week
      Elevation of the head of the bed for 1 week
      No hot food or drink for 1 week
      No smoking or alcohol for 1 week
      No aspirin for 1 week
      A cold-mist humidifier at the bedside
      Lubricating drops for the nose 3 times a day for 1 week
        (petrolatum or normal saline)

   b. Bleeding too brisk for effective cautery can also be controlled temporarily by injecting lidocaine with 1:100,000 epinephrine around the bleeding site. Similarly, lidocaine with 1:100,000 epinephrine can be injected into the pterygopalatine fossa.

   c. Bleeding from beneath the inferior turbinate is best managed by wedging a small piece of Gelfoam, Oxycel, or Surgicel beneath the turbinate. If this is ineffective, it is also possible to compress the bleeding site by fracturing the turbinate toward the lateral nasal wall. Alternatively, the turbinate can be fractured medially to expose the bleeding site for cautery. **Fracturing of the turbinate, however, should not be performed unless other measures fail,** because the nasal mucosa may be lacerated, adding an additional bleeding site.

   d. General oozing from the septum can usually be stopped by placing oxidized cellulose soaked in epinephrine over the bleeding site. Topical thrombin or Avitene applied to the bleeding site may also be beneficial.

e. Persistent bleeding from septal perforations can be controlled by placing a piece of Silastic on either side of the septum and sewing them together through the perforation. Avitene can be pushed into the perforated area between the two Silastic sheets.

B. Anterior packing. If cautery is unsuccessful, tamponade by packing may be necessary.

1. Anesthesia. Topical anesthesia with cocaine or lidocaine and epinephrine reduces the discomfort. Local infiltration, as for reduction of a nasal fracture, is also helpful (see Nasal Fractures, sec. **III.C.**). Nevertheless, packing is frequently unpleasant for both the patient and physician.

2. Method. Ideally, after the anesthesia has taken effect, usually 10–15 minutes, ½-in. iodoform gauze, well lubricated with bacitracin ointment, or petrolatum-impregnated gauze is carefully layered in the nose with bayonet forceps. The gauze should be packed firmly down toward the floor of the nose as it is layered. It should be manipulated under the inferior turbinate and layered on both sides of the middle turbinate. The packing should be firm, but not deforming, and should not extrude into the nasopharynx. A drip pad of 2-in. square gauze can be taped over the nostril. Care should be taken so the nasal vestibule does not swell, thereby causing alar necrosis. The packing should be left in place for 3–5 days. After that interval, it should be cautiously removed. General oozing may follow pack removal and last several minutes, but usually stops without further manipulation.

3. Alternate methods

a. Finger cot packs can be used to pack the nasal chamber. These are made by cutting the fingers from a surgeon's glove, filling each with gauze, and tying them closed with heavy sutures. They can be lubricated with bacitracin ointment and introduced with a bayonet. To prevent aspiration of a finger cot pack, all the sutures should be tied over a dental roll placed at the anterior nares.

b. Epistaxis balloons are also useful. Some are filled with air, others with normal saline.

c. Expandable sponge (Merocel) can be placed intranasally and affords compression to the bleeding site with minimal concern for pressure necrosis. These packs are also easily removable. Some are designed with hollow central tubes to maintain a patent nasal airway.

4. General instructions for the patient. In addition to the instructions after cautery listed in **2.a(2)**, the patient should:

Have an antibiotic (ampicillin or erythromycin), because the sinuses are obstructed

Have some medicine to dull the pain

Expect a headache

Expect epiphora and sometimes blood from the lacrimal punctum

Expect nasal drainage and obstruction for 1–2 weeks after the pack is removed

Have careful follow-up after pack removal for lysing of synechiae as they form

5. **Hospitalization.** An anterior pack can cause increased respiratory effort. In the elderly or critically ill, there is a risk of respiratory decompensation. Complete nasal obstruction, as with bilateral anterior packs or with most anteroposterior packs, is dangerous even in the young. Hospitalization of patients with anterior or posterior packs and careful observation are mandatory. Serial blood gas determination and oxygen may be necessary. The patient with a pack should not be sedated.

C. **Anteroposterior packing.** When the bleeding is posterior, an anterior pack may not provide sufficient tamponade. An anteroposterior pack is the conventional treatment in this circumstance (Fig. 1-4).

1. **Anesthesia** should include intranasal topical anesthesia, infiltrative anesthesia, and limited intravenous sedation only in the most uncooperative patients.

2. **Method**

   a. First, the posterior pack is prepared. A vaginal tampon, a piece of lamb's wool, or three 4-in.-square pieces of gauze may be used. The posterior pack is meant to fill the nasopharynx. Three long umbilical tapes or three heavy silk sutures are tied around the middle of the posterior packing material.

   b. A soft rubber catheter is introduced into the front of the nose, preferably in the side that is bleeding, until the end is visualized in the pharynx. A hemostat grasps the pharyngeal end of the catheter, bringing it out through the mouth. Two of the tapes or sutures are tied to the pharyngeal end protruding from the mouth. Pulling the nasal end then draws the posterior pack into the nasopharynx. Usually, it must be guided into the nasopharynx with a finger. Then the two tapes or sutures at the anterior nares are detached from the catheter and held with a clamp. The third tape or suture is left trailing from the mouth.

   c. The posterior pack provides a buttress for the placement of a firm anterior pack in the posterior third of the involved nasal chamber. The anterior pack is layered as described (see sec. **B.2.**).

   d. When the anterior pack is properly positioned, the two umbilical tapes or sutures attached to the posterior pack are tied over a dental roll or a piece of foam rubber placed at the anterior nares, preventing alar necrosis. The tape or suture

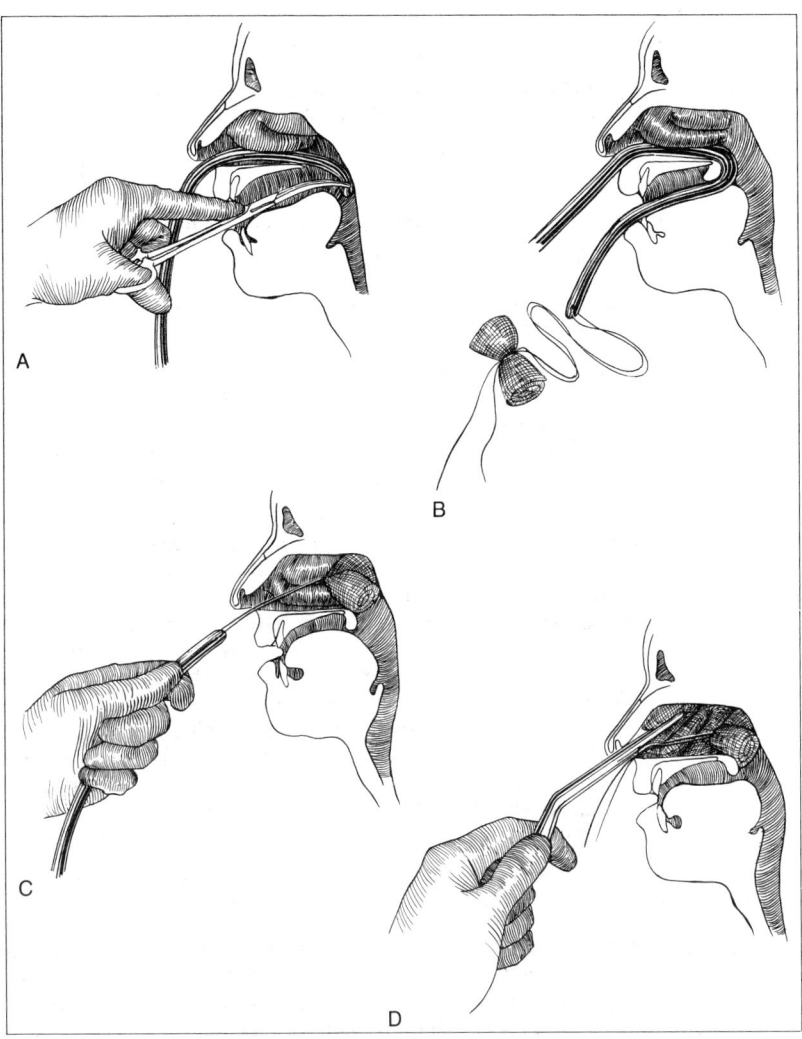

Fig. 1-4. Anterior–posterior pack for epistaxis. A. A red rubber catheter is passed through the nasal chamber into the oropharynx. B. Catheter is pulled through the oral cavity, and a sponge or dental roll is affixed to the catheter. C. Pack advanced with glove finger control into the nasopharynx. D. With an assistant holding the posterior pack taut, an anterior pack is placed. The ligature securing the posterior pack is then tied over a bolster.

trailing from the mouth is either taped to the cheek or cut sufficiently short so that it just protrudes into the oropharynx.

3. **Alternate method.** Control of posterior bleeding can also be effected by introducing a Foley catheter through the nose,

inflating the balloon when it is in the nasopharynx, and then drawing it up into the posterior choanae.

4. **Hospitalization.** The patient with an anteroposterior pack requires hospitalization and close observation.

   a. Daily monitoring of hematocrit and arterial blood gases is essential.

   b. Oxygen by mask is administered as needed.

   c. An antibiotic is required (ampicillin).

   d. Pain medication must be titrated carefully to avoid undue respiratory depression.

   e. Anteroposterior packing is always uncomfortable. Especially in the elderly, sedation reduces discomfort and cardiac stress must be balanced by a concern for hypotension from blood loss and respiratory depression from nasal obstruction and associated pharyngeal and palatal edema.

   f. The packing is usually removed in 5 days. The patient is prepared beforehand for repacking in the operating room, in case bleeding recurs. The tapes or sutures tied over the dental roll are cut and secured with a clamp. The anterior pack is carefully removed. Next, the tape or suture in the mouth is secured, the two tapes or sutures at the anterior nares released, and the tape or suture in the mouth pulled to deliver the posterior pack. There is usually a small general ooze after removal. If there is brisk bleeding, repacking should be performed in the operating room. However, bleeding following removal of an initially successful anteroposterior pack usually indicates the need for appropriate vessel ligation.

5. **Follow-up after discharge.** Careful follow-up after discharge is indicated to lyse synechiae as they appear.

D. **Arterial ligation.** If bleeding is not controlled with an anteroposterior pack, if there is rebleeding after the removal of packing, or if the patient is unable to tolerate the morbidity of the packing, the arteries supplying the nose can be ligated. This procedure is especially indicated in elderly individuals and those patients with chronic obstructive lung disease who cannot tolerate hypoxia induced by nasal obstruction. Ligation may involve one or more of the following arteries.

1. **The internal maxillary artery** and its branches are ligated in the pterygomaxillary fossa via a transantral approach. Ligation first requires a Caldwell-Luc procedure and then access to the pterygomaxillary fossa via the posterior antral wall.

2. In poor-risk patients, ligation of the **external carotid** using local anesthesia is often the surgical procedure of choice.

3. The **anterior and posterior ethmoid arteries** are ligated as they pass from the orbit to the ethmoid labyrinth.

E. Embolization. Use of angiography and embolization of the arteries is also a means of controlling troublesome recurrent epistaxis. This procedure should be considered in those patients who would be poor surgical candidates after routine measures have been tried. The very real possibility of inadvertent intracranial embolization and the cerebrovascular sequelae must be weighed against the benefits of this procedure and should be performed only by those skilled in this technique.

F. For hereditary hemorrhagic telangiectasia, a **septal dermoplasty** may be required. The mucosa of the septum and floor of the nose is removed surgically, and a skin graft is placed. Progesterone has also been shown to be effective.

Nasal Fractures

Nasal fractures are frequent. The prominent position of the nose makes it susceptible to isolated injury from birth onward (Fig. 1-5).

I. Anatomy. The upper third of the nose has bony support; the lower two-thirds, cartilaginous support. Superiorly, the nasal bones sit laterally on the nasal process of the maxilla and are joined above by the

Fig. 1-5. Nasal trauma. Direction of force depicted with anticipated fracture.

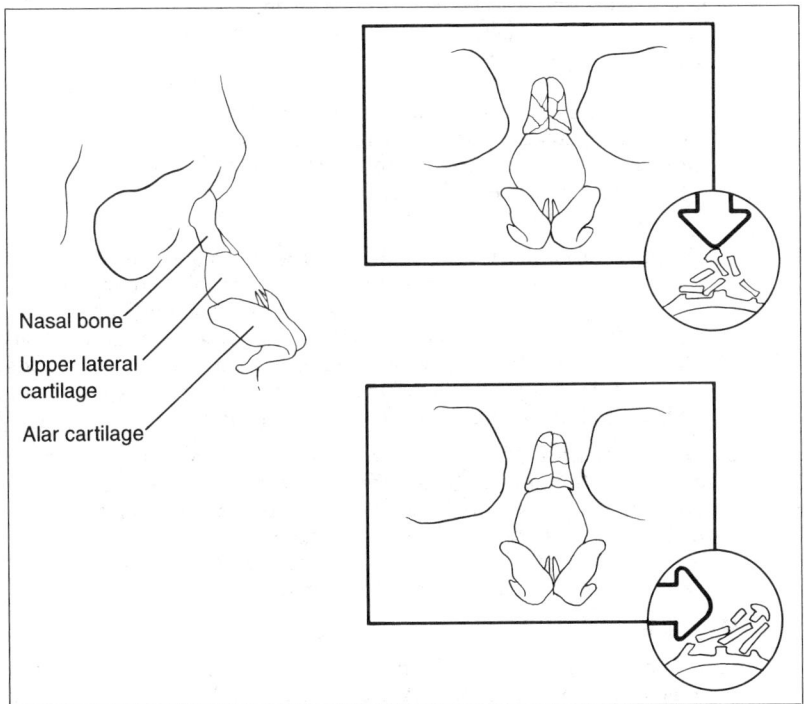

Nasal bone

Upper lateral cartilage

Alar cartilage

nasal process of the frontal bone. The paired upper and lower lateral cartilages provide support for the lower part of the nose. The nasal septum is cartilaginous (quadrilateral cartilage) anteriorly and bony (perpendicular plate of the ethmoid and vomer) superiorly and posteriorly.

II. Diagnosis

A. A detailed history is necessary. Included should be information about the date and time of the trauma, type of injury, epistaxis, prior nasal injuries or surgery, possible CSF rhinorrhea, and nasal obstruction. One must consider more extensive facial injuries (e.g., ethmoid, orbital, maxillary, and nasolacrimal apparatus). The patient should be asked about loss of consciousness as a consequence of intracranial injury.

B. Examination and palpation of the external nose can disclose deviation or depression, movement, degree of edema, ecchymoses, localized tenderness, crepitation, and subcutaneous emphysema. Examination of the inside of the nose may reveal blood or mucosal lacerations. The lining of the nose is closely adherent to the bony or cartilaginous framework; there will seldom be a fracture without blood, ecchymoses, or a mucosal laceration. This examination is easier if the mucosa is shrunk by packing the nose with 4–5% cocaine solution (or 4% lidocaine and 1:100,000 epinephrine) on cottonoid strips.

It is important to examine the septum. If there is a nasal fracture, the septum can also be fractured or dislocated. The septum alone can be injured. A septal hematoma will sometimes form. There is usually an associated increasing obstruction over the first 24 hours. Examination discloses a bulging area of the septum. The hematoma may later become an abscess. An untreated septal hematoma or abscess can result in collapse of the septum and in a saddle deformity due to dissolution of the cartilage. The diagnosis should be considered when there is fluctuance demonstrated on palpation of the suspected hematoma or abscess.

C. X rays are frequently obtained when there is a question of a nasal fracture. They are seldom helpful because nasal bony injuries often heal by fibrosis, leaving persistent radiologic evidence of an earlier fracture. Moreover, cartilaginous injuries cannot be visualized by x ray. The history and examination are the best methods of ascertaining the extent of the injury, although x rays may be helpful in delineating associated bony injuries.

D. Reexamination. If there is uncertainty, the patient should be asked to return in 2 or 3 days for reexamination, as the associated swelling subsides. This is especially important in children, recognizing that they can be difficult to examine, and an undiscovered fracture may result in distortion of the nose with growth. It may be necessary to examine the child under general anesthesia.

III. Management

A. Decision to reduce the fracture depends on an evaluation of both appearance and function. A boxer or football player is likely to have little concern about a slight deviation. An aesthetically perfect initial reduction may not be permanent due to contracture during healing. Most people cannot tolerate nasal obstruction or the loss of smell. For them a reduction is indicated.

B. Timing of reduction. Injuries seen shortly after trauma (1–3 hours) and without associated swelling may be reduced immediately. If the nose is very swollen, reduction should be performed 5–7 days after the injury. In children, an earlier reduction (2–3 days) may be necessary since healing is rapid. If there is a delay of more than 2 weeks in the adult, the injury should be given 6 months to heal and then correction should be performed using standard rhinoplasty techniques.

C. Anesthesia. In some cases, sedation before beginning the anesthetic infiltration is helpful. In the anxious adult, 5 mg of diazepam given slowly intravenously is usually sufficient. In children, general anesthesia may be necessary. The techniques for internal and external local anesthesia follow.

   1. Internal. The nose should always be packed for topical anesthesia; 4–5% cocaine solution on cottonoid strips (well wrung out) is introduced into each nostril and left in place for 5–10 minutes. It is sometimes helpful to repeat this procedure, since the anesthesia from the first packing can allow more complete packing the second time. The smallest possible amount of cocaine should be used for adequate anesthesia in order to prevent its adverse effects. Although 4 ml of 5% solution (200 mg) is often considered the maximum amount tolerated, dosage varies greatly among patients. The initial symptoms of cocaine toxicity involve the central nervous system. These symptoms include excitation and anxiousness, followed by an increasing respiratory rate and later respiratory collapse. The treatment of cocaine toxicity is by the intravenous administration of diazepam, 5–15 mg, or a short-acting barbiturate. A mixture of 4% lidocaine and 1:100,000 epinephrine can be substituted for the cocaine.

   2. External (Fig. 1-6)

   a. Two percent lidocaine with 1:100,000 epinephrine should be injected at the **infraorbital foramen** on each side. The foramen is palpable slightly medial to the midline of the lower orbital rim. Then, via an external and intranasal approach, the anesthetic should be infiltrated along each side of the nose from just above the medial canthus to the upper lip. Finally, one should infiltrate across the dorsum of the nose at the level of the medial canthi and across the upper lip. The anesthetic should be given 5–10 minutes to take effect. An initial wheal of local anesthetic should be injected to test the patient's sensitivity to epinephrine. Occasionally, an initial tachycardia will occur and subside.

   b. If there is great nasal discomfort, one can additionally inject anesthetic through the **greater palatine foramen** and **pterygopalatine fossa**. The greater palatine foramen is on the

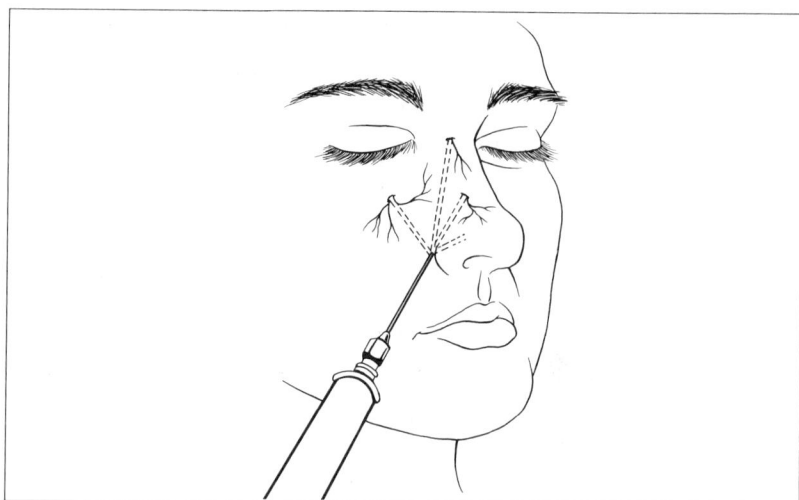

Fig. 1-6. External sites of injection for reducing nasal fractures. The nasal chambers are anesthetized with topical cocaine (4%) on pledgets.

lateral hard palate, just anterior to the junction with the soft palate. It is just medial to the anterior aspect of the third molar and can be palpated as a slight depression anterior to the hamulus. The distal 2.0 cm of the needle should be bent and advanced into the canal. If the needle is advanced too far, it can enter the orbit. An injection into the pterygopalatine fossa often slows or temporarily controls epistaxis.

D. Method

1. **External reduction.** The patient should bring recent photographs for comparison. The reduction is guided primarily by palpation externally and by intranasal inspection. If the nasal pyramid has shifted, firm pressure and intranasal elevation on that side will restore a more normal configuration. Depressed fragments should be elevated. A scalpel handle or nasal elevator is useful. If the entire nasal pyramid is displaced, an Asch forceps should be used to distract the fracture sites by placing one arm of the forceps in each nasal passage, pulling the nose away from the face, and then shifting it into an anatomic position. A large Kelly forceps with rubber tubing around each jaw can be used in place of an Asch forceps.

2. **Septal reduction.** After nasal reduction the septum often returns to the midline, but its position must be assessed. A light nasal pack should be placed to assist in support and to prevent hematoma formation.

3. **Suturing of open wounds.** A nasal fracture is often an open fracture since the mucosa is frequently torn. If the external skin is torn as well, it should be carefully sutured without sac-

rificing tissue. The excellent blood supply in the nose usually facilitates the healing of even severely traumatized tissue, but if there is an open injury, a broad-spectrum antibiotic should be considered.

4. **Splinting and packing.** The nasal pyramid is usually stable after reduction. There is little normal motion or distraction by muscles. An external splint is often applied, however, to protect the nose and to remind the patient to be cautious. It can be formed of soft metal or plastic. Tape is placed underneath the splint for padding and support. If the fragments collapse, internal support from packing the nasal chambers usually maintains their positions (see Epistaxis, sec. **III.B.**).

5. **Postreduction instructions to the patient**

   a. After the injury and again after the reduction, the patient should be instructed to:

   Sleep with the head elevated
   Apply ice for the first 12 hours
   Use a humidifier at night
   Sneeze through the mouth
   Refrain from blowing the nose
   Use lubricating drops (normal saline every 2–4 hours as needed)
   Refrain from vigorous exercise

   b. The patient should always be cautioned that it will take several weeks for the obstruction to decrease and that they can expect some infraorbital discoloration. Even an ideal reduction can be altered by scar contracture and may require a subsequent cosmetic procedure.

6. **Antibiotic prophylaxis.** If the nasal mucosa is opened, an antibiotic (e.g., ampicillin) should be given to diminish the possibility of secondary infection.

7. **Patient follow-up.** There should be careful follow-up to prevent the formation of synechiae, which are lysed as they appear. Initial follow-up examination should be 1–2 weeks after the injury, with repeat visits in 1–2 months.

Oropharyngeal Conduit

I. **Peritonsillar abscess,** also called **quinsy,** is a loculation of pus in the potential space surrounding the tonsil. It develops as an infection in a peripheral tonsillar crypt that penetrates the capsule, entering the connective tissue space between the capsule and the superior constrictor muscle. Another pathological mechanism can be an inflammation of the minor salivary glands (Weber's glands) located primarily at the superior tonsillar pole. The abscess occurs due to lack of drainage and location of pus. In this case, the tonsil may not be the primary cause of the infection. This may account for cases of peritonsillar abcesses in patients who have had their tonsils removed.

The infectious process generally remains localized to the peritonsillar area, but may break through the superior constrictor, gaining access to the deep spaces of the neck.

Peritonsillar abscess may follow an untreated or inadequately treated episode of acute follicular tonsillitis, occurring most often in adolescents or patients in their early twenties and affecting both sexes equally. The abscesses may be bilateral (7% of patients). Approximately 5% have had a prior episode. In many instances, a history of recurrent tonsillitis is not obtained. Approximately 70% of the abscesses are located in the superior pole of the tonsil, 19% are in the midtonsillar area, and 10% are either in combined areas or in the lower pole.

A. **Signs and symptoms.** A 3- to 7-day history of an extremely severe sore throat with associated dysphagia, odynophagia, trismus, and decreased oral intake is frequent. Speech is best characterized as being muffled or "hot potato" in quality. Usually, the patient's temperature at presentation is between 99 and 100°F. Except in the very young, airway obstruction is infrequent.

B. **Examination** reveals moderate to severe trismus, sometimes compromising an adequate intraoral examination. Copious mucus may cover intraoral structures. The oropharynx is inflamed, and the infected tonsil is swollen and usually displaced inferomedially, with similar displacement of the soft palate. Palpation of the area sometimes reveals fluctuance.

C. **Diagnostic studies** should include a complete blood count (CBC) with differential, Monospot testing, Gram staining, and aerobic and anaerobic cultures of aspirated material. Patients previously treated with antibiotics commonly have sterile cultures. If careful anaerobic cultures are performed, a significant percentage of these negative cultures will show anaerobic organisms. In untreated cases, group A beta-hemolytic streptococci have been isolated in approximately 25–50% of patients. Gram-negative organisms have also been isolated from peritonsillar abscesses and may play a major role in a chronic abscess.

D. **Differential diagnosis**

1. **Acute follicular tonsillitis with peritonsillar cellulitis** clinically may appear exactly as a peritonsillar abscess. The failure to aspirate pus differentiates the two. The therapy is similar.

2. **Infectious mononucleosis** appears as diffuse tonsillitis, usually without peritonsillar swelling. Increased adenopathy, a positive Monospot test, and atypical lymphocytes in a peripheral smear are often present. Petechiae are frequently seen on the soft palate.

3. **Traumatic aneurysms of the internal carotid artery** have no associated signs of infection. A pulsatile unilateral swelling, however, may appear in the region of the peritonsillar space.

4. **Parapharyngeal space infections** appear as an acute infectious process but often have significant associated upper cervical

swelling and tenderness. The lateral pharyngeal wall is more edematous than the area around the tonsil. This process is also unilateral.

5. **Parapharyngeal or tonsillar tumors** present with local pain and unilateral swelling, with either an intact or a necrotic mucosa. There are, however, no signs of acute infection (fever or elevated white blood cell count).

6. **Diphtheria** presents with diffuse pharyngitis after first involving the posterior pharyngeal wall. The tonsils are often covered with a dirty gray pseudomembrane (see Chap. 4, **III.B.**), which bleeds easily on manipulation.

E. **Management**

1. **Aspiration.** Cooperative adults who are not severely ill and are not developing complications can be managed with aspiration of the peritonsillar abscess and antibiotic therapy. Aspiration may be performed with an 18-gauge spinal needle inserted above the tonsil at the level of the junction of the uvula and the soft palate (Fig. 1-7). Topical anesthesia (e.g., benzocaine or lidocaine) can be used. Infiltrative anesthesia is usually ineffective due to the alkaline pH caused by the abscess. After aspiration the patient is placed on Augmentin 500 mg q8h because of the likelihood of a mixed bacterial flora and followed closely until the episode resolves. Should there be reaccumulation of pus or evidence of progression, such as increased trismus, further difficulty in handling secretions, or inadequate oral intake; the patient should be hospitalized, incision and drainage performed, and intravenous antibiotics administered. A negative aspirate may signify either disease of limited extent (e.g., peritonsillar cellulitis) or a failure to enter the abscess cavity.

Fig. 1-7. Peritonsillar abscess aspiration. A #16 or #18 spinal needle is introduced at denoted site—surgical drainage is rarely required.

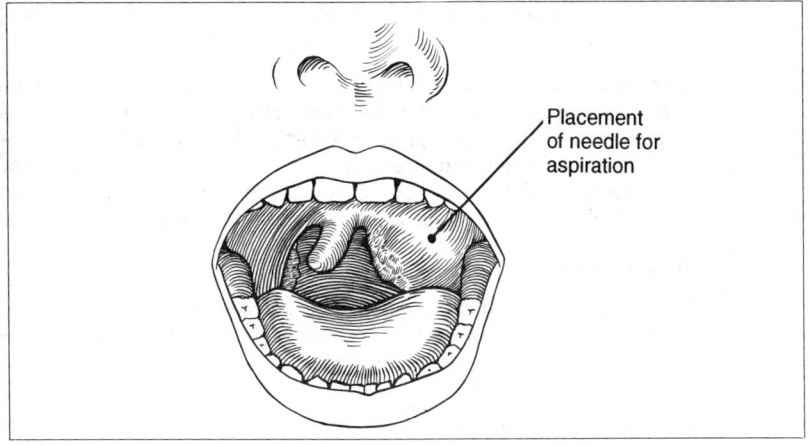

Placement of needle for aspiration

2. **Incision and drainage.** When an abscess is present, incision and drainage in a hospital setting are indicated in patients not responding to aspiration, in children in whom aspiration under local anesthesia would prove difficult, or in patients reaccumulating pus after adequate aspiration and antibiotic therapy. In an adult, after adequate topical anesthesia, a small incision is made through the mucosa at the level above the tonsil, near the junction of the uvula and soft palate. The coagulation status of the patient must be known because of potential bleeding. Using a blunt hemostat, the incision is spread until pus is encountered and is sufficiently opened to provide adequate drainage. This procedure should be performed with the patient in a sitting position. A similar procedure can be performed under general anesthesia if the patient is not a candidate for local drainage. In this situation, the patient is intubated and placed in the Trendelenburg position to prevent aspiration of pus. Acute tonsillectomy is usually performed if drainage requires general anesthesia.

3. **Acute tonsillectomy.** Tonsillectomy should be considered when the adequacy of incision and drainage is questioned on the basis of the clinical response. Inferior pole abscesses tend to reaccumulate following aspiration and are additionally difficult to evacuate with incision and drainage. The procedure is performed with general anesthesia, the patient having been intubated to prevent aspiration. There is controversy as to whether the uninvolved tonsil should be removed at the time of abscess tonsillectomy.

4. **Antibiotic therapy.** Unless the results of Gram staining indicate otherwise, the patient should be treated from the outset with penicillin (1,000,000 units IV q4–6h) or a first-generation cephalosporin. If the patient is allergic to penicillin, cephalosporin should be avoided, and clindamycin (600 mg IV q8h) should be used. Patients undergoing quinsy tonsillectomy should receive intravenous antibiotics 12–24 hours prior to the procedure, ensuring adequate blood levels and preventing bacteremia. Antibiotics should be continued for 10–14 days after surgical therapy.

5. **Instruction.** If the patient undergoes an acute tonsillectomy, he or she should receive routine instruction as to soft foods (approximately 1 week), pain medication (acetaminophen or codeine, 30–60 mg q4h), rest for 5–7 days, and observation for bleeding, which can occur 3 to 10 days postoperatively (see Chap. 4, **V.A.**). Bleeding must be reported immediately.

F. **Complications**

1. **Sepsis** can result from regional and distant seeding from the abscess. Septicemia occurs from progressive pharyngeal cellulitis or spread to the pterygomaxillary space (see Chap. 4 **IV.A.3.**).

2. **Laryngeal obstruction**

3. Dissection to deep fascial spaces

4. Pneumonia

5. Posttonsillectomy hemorrhage. The exact incidence of hemorrhage following tonsillectomy is unknown, but is thought to be between 1 and 5%. It may reflect a secondary infection in the tonsillar bed and, as such, the recommendation for postoperative antibiotics. The most common times for posttonsillectomy hemorrhage are during the first 24 hours and 7–10 days following the procedure, when the eschar separates from the bed. It must be emphasized, however, that *hemorrhage can occur at any time after tonsillectomy* until the tonsillar bed is well healed.

  a. Management. Any patient with posttonsillectomy hemorrhage should be thoroughly examined without delay. Unless the bleeding is immediately life-threatening, however, the examination should be deferred until an otolaryngologist is present, especially in a marginally tolerant patient and certainly in a child. This is essential if exacerbation of the bleeding and airway compromise are to be avoided.

  (1) Routine examination and management of light to moderate bleeding

  (a) Equipment needed. Proper lighting, suction equipment with a tonsil suction tip, and instruments to handle a potential crisis are key. These instruments include tongue blades, long forceps and hemostats, suture material (e.g., 2-0 or 3-0 chromic catgut on a taper needle), and tonsillar gauze sponges. Intubation equipment should always be available.

  (b) Anesthesia. Topical anesthesia, such as 4% lidocaine, can be used to facilitate the examination.

  (c) Technique. In the cooperative patient, the bleeding site can usually be identified after careful removal of the clot by forceps or suction. Most often the bleeding is slow and a large clot covers the tonsillar bed. Patients bleeding slowly or intermittently frequently swallow most of the blood and may not have outward signs of significant hemorrhage. Occasionally, no active bleeding is observed at the time of initial examination, but a clot is almost always present, denoting the specific site of the hemorrhage. The bleeding can usually be controlled by cauterization using silver nitrate. If silver nitrate is not effective, a solution of epinephrine and tannic acid, placed on a tonsil sponge and held for 2 minutes with pressure, will control most hemorrhages. More active arterial hemorrhages, however, may require either electrocautery or suture ligation of the involved bleeding vessel; both procedures are best done in the operating room.

(2) Management of severe hemorrhage. The most important consideration in managing severe posttonsillectomy hemorrhage is ensuring that the airway is secure. The vast majority of patients dying from posttonsillectomy bleeding do so not from blood loss but from aspiration and secondary obstruction. With a severe hemorrhage, control of the airway must take precedence over any manipulation of the tonsillar fossa. Intubation or tracheotomy is performed to secure the airway, and a firm pack is placed at the site to control blood loss until an operating room is readied. Most children with significant hemorrhaging need immediate operative management. When time permits, a hematocrit, blood typing, and cross-matching should be performed.

II. Traumatic hemorrhage.
Posttraumatic oropharyngeal bleeding occurs most often in young children who fall on objects they have put in their mouths.

A. Management of light to moderate bleeding. Bleeding from small vessels usually subsides spontaneously, but if it does not, the bleeding can be controlled by simple ligatures. Before ligation, the area should always be carefully inspected for the presence of a residual foreign body.

B. Management of severe bleeding. Because of the proximity of several large vessels to the oropharyngeal area, including the internal carotid artery, traumatic injury may result in heavy bleeding. With severe bleeding, the airway must be protected; if immediate control of the hemorrhage is not possible, intubation or tracheotomy should precede aggressive packing of the pharynx. Whenever possible, the patient should be stabilized with fluid replacement prior to definitive operative control of the bleeding site.

C. Follow-up for possible complications. The most dreaded complication of "pencil injury" is thrombosis of the internal carotid artery and its intracranial branches. Neurologic deficits and even death have been reported following what first appeared to be minor trauma to the palate or tonsillar region, secondary to this injury. For this reason, some physicians recommend hospitalization of a patient with injuries caused by sharp objects for a period of 48–72 hours of close observation. If neurologic deficits become apparent or if the injury is in the immediate area of the carotid artery, arteriography should be performed.

III. Caustic ingestion followed by corrosive esophagitis
remains one of the more serious and controversial problems facing physicians who deal with the aerodigestive tract. Because of the controversies in management, the section that follows should be used only as a general guide and not as a definitive course of treatment. Caustic ingestion followed by corrosive esophagitis occurs most frequently in children under the age of 10 years. Safety caps and public education have done much to reduce the incidence in children, yet these mea-

sures have not served the adult population similarly. A history of attempted suicide and alcoholism are frequent associations in the adult group.

A. **Types of corrosive esophagitis injuries.** Corrosive esophagitis is a burn of variable depth within the esophageal wall. Ingestion of acids produces an injury that differs from that produced by bases. Caustics such as sodium hydroxide and potassium hydroxide produce liquefaction necrosis and may penetrate deeply, causing full-thickness burns, with acute perforation. Acids produce coagulation necrosis. This type of burn is generally not as deep as that produced by an equivalent concentration of base. Acid ingestions are, however, more prone to secondary perforation and stricture formation. Chlorates (bleaches) constitute a third category of caustics with the potential to cause a burn resulting in stricture. They generally cause much milder injury than do strong alkalis and acids. Ammonia usually produces burns that are equivalent in severity to those of the chlorates. The aforementioned are the most frequently ingested caustics.

B. **Stages of injury.** There are three stages in the esophageal reaction to a caustic injury.

1. **The acute or inflammatory phase** begins immediately and lasts for approximately 2 weeks.

2. **The intermediate phase** follows the acute phase and lasts for 8 weeks. During this phase, cicatrix with organization takes place. Eighty percent of esophageal strictures are evidenced within 8 weeks after caustic ingestion.

3. **The third phase** of injury is that of chronic obstruction secondary to stricture.

C. **Signs and symptoms.** The history may indicate the ingestion of a caustic. Suspected cases should be treated until more definitive clinical data are obtained. If possible, the known or suspected caustic agent and container revealing the chemical composition should be brought to the hospital for examination.

D. **Examination.** Normal findings on physical examination, including inspection of oropharyngeal mucosa, do not rule out serious esophageal damage, thus the need to initially treat and further evaluate all suspected cases. Patients with significant caustic ingestion often present with burns of the lips, oral cavity, hands, and "dribble" burns of clothing and skin. They may be drooling and refuse anything by mouth. More severe cases may manifest signs or symptoms of an acute complication such as laryngeal involvement, mediastinal perforation, cardiovascular collapse, and gastric damage.

E. **Diagnosis.** In suspected cases of corrosive esophagitis, esophagoscopy should be performed between 24 and 48 hours when the patient's general condition is stable. The esophagoscope must not be passed further than the upper limit of the first burn for fear of perforation. The visualized area of burn should be described, and the presence or absence of circumferential lesions noted. As an initial procedure, a barium swallow is not indicated. Esophoscopy should not be performed after 48 hours because of the risk of perforation.

F. Treatment

1. Initial measures

   a. **Neutralizing substances.** There is good reason to consider keeping the patient without oral intake and to avoid the following measures inasmuch as there is usually a considerable time lapse prior to obtaining management by a physician. The induction of vomiting should be avoided. Gastric lavage is controversial. If the patient will accept liquids by mouth, various neutralizing agents for alkali caustics have been suggested, including milk, water, citrus fruit juices diluted with vinegar, egg whites, butter, and olive or mineral oil. For acids, substances to consider include milk, water, milk of magnesia (1 tsp in 1 cup of water), aluminum hydroxide gel followed by egg whites, butter, and mineral oil. For bleaches, warm water or milk may be used. In instances of severe burn, when there is a danger of perforation, oral intake must be withheld.

   b. **Nasogastric intubation.** If severe burns are identified on esophagoscopy, passage of a nasogastric tube risks perforation and is somewhat controversial. Swallowing a heavy gauze string, weighted or unweighted, has been recommended to provide localization of the lumen for further dilatation, should it prove necessary.

   c. **Antibiotics.** Penicillin (1,000,000 units q4–6h IV) is considered by most to be the initial antibiotic of choice. It should be started immediately in a suspected burn. If esophagoscopy reveals burns, antibiotics—either IV or PO—should be continued until mucosal healing is complete.

   d. **Steroids.** If burns are seen on esophagoscopy, steroids (e.g., prednisone 40–60 mg initially and tapered over weeks) should be added to the antibiotic regimen. If used initially, they are continued until mucosal healing is complete. There is no general agreement as to whether steroids are clinically beneficial in decreasing the granulomatous response and subsequent stricture formation. When strictures do form while the patient is on steroids, they are generally more pliable and readily dilated, as contrasted with strictures in untreated patients. To be effective, steroids should be started immediately following identification of burns or within 24–48 hours after ingestion of the caustic. The usefulness of steroids is questionable if there is evidence of complications such as perforation and mediastinitis. An extra measure of caution must be taken when endoscoping a patient on steroids.

   e. **Oral intake** of liquids initially is permitted when the patient is swallowing saliva and when there is little risk of perforation. Solids should probably be avoided until healing is complete.

2. **Subacute and chronic measures**

a. **Esophagoscopy** should be performed 2–3 weeks after antibiotic therapy is begun. At this time steroids and antibiotics may be discontinued only if mucosal healing is complete.

b. **Barium swallow** is not a substitute for esophagoscopy. Since most strictures form within 8 weeks, patients should be evaluated at 2- to 3-week intervals with barium studies that may have to be repeated during the next 2 months.

c. **Bouginage.** If the barium study suggests narrowing, esophagoscopy should again be performed to assess the lumen size. If there is evidence of stricture formation, bouginage with dilatation of the esophagus can safely be performed 2–3 weeks after steroids are discontinued. Bougies should be passed carefully to avoid false passages and a perforation. The frequency of dilatation depends on the ability of the esophageal lumen to retain patency after bouginage. Difficult strictures and some strictures in children may require a retrograde dilatation following gastrostomy.

3. **Surgical intervention**

a. **Acute measures.** Acute surgical removal of an extensively burned esophagus may be required. Segments of colon, stomach, or jejunum can be used to effect a conduit from the pharynx to small bowel, as needed. In selected cases, free tissue transfer of intestine with microvascular anastomosis is most efficacious.

b. **Chronic measures.** When chronic dilatation fails to achieve an adequate food passage or when it runs a high risk of perforation, esophageal removal and replacement has to be considered.

Selected Readings

Anderson, K. O., Rouse, T. R., and Randolph, J. G. A controlled trial of corticosteroids in children with corrosive injury of the esophagus. *N. Engl. J. Med.* 323:637–670, 1990.

Baugh, R., and Gilmore, B. B., Jr. Infectious croup: A critical review. *Otolaryngol. Head Neck Surg.* 95:40–46, 1986.

Bergstrom, L., and Owens, O. Posterior choanal atresia: A syndesmal disorder. *Laryngoscope* 94:1273–1276, 1984.

Crockett, D. M., McGill, T. J., Healy, G. B., and Friedman, E. M. Airway management of acute supraglottitis at the Children's Hospital, Boston; 1980–1985. *Ann. Otol. Rhinol. Laryngol.* 97:114–119, 1988.

Dingham, R. D., and Natvig, P. *Surgery of Facial Fractures.* Philadelphia: Saunders, 1976. Pp. 267–294.

English, G. M. *Otolaryngology.* New York: Harper & Row, 1990.

Fairbanks, D. N. F. *Pocket Guide to Antimicrobial Therapy in Otolaryngology—Head and Neck Surgery* (5th ed.). Washington, D.C.: American Academy of Otolaryngology—Head and Neck Surgery Foundation, 1989.

Ferguson, C. P. Congenital abnormalities of the infant larynx. *Otolaryngol. Clin. North Am.* 3:185, 1970.

Fineman, S. M. Urticaria and angioedema. In G. J. Lawlor Jr. and T. J. Fischer (eds.), *Manual of Allergy and Immunology* (2nd ed.). Boston: Little, Brown, 1988. Pp. 214–224.

Frank, M. D., Gelfand, J. A., and Atkinson, J. P. Hereditary angioedema: The clinical syndrome and its management. *Ann. Intern. Med.* 84:580, 1976.

Fried, M. P. Controversies in the management of supraglottitis and croup. *Pediatr. Clin. North Am.* 26:931, 1979.

Fried, M. P. *The Larynx: A Multidisciplinary Approach*. Boston: Little, Brown, 1988.

Friedberg, S. A., and Bluestone, C. D. Foreign body accidents involving air and food passages in children. *Otolaryngol. Clin. North Am.* 3:395, 1970.

Gross, C. W. Medical management, nasotracheal intubation, and tracheotomy in the treatment of upper airway obstruction in children. *Otolaryngol. Clin. North Am.* 10:157, 1977.

Heimlich, H. J., and Uhley, M. H. The Heimlich maneuver. *Clin. Symp.* 31:3, 1979.

Hengerer, A. S., and Strome, M. Choanal atresia: A new embryologic theory and its influence on surgical management. *Laryngoscope* 92:913–921.

Holinger, L. D. Foreign bodies of the larynx, trachea and bronchi. In C. D. Bluestone and S. E. Stool (eds.), *Pediatric Otolaryngology* (2nd ed.). Philadelphia: Saunders, 1990. Pp. 1205–1214.

Levitt, G. W. Cervical fascia and deep neck infections. *Otolaryngol. Clin. North Am.* 93:703, 1976.

Liston, S. L., Gehrz, R. C., and Jarvis, C. N. Bacterial tracheitis. *Arch. Otolaryngol.* 107:561, 1981.

May, M., Tucker, H. M., and Dillard, B. M. Penetrating wounds of the neck in civilians. *Otolaryngol. Clin. North Am.* 9:361, 1976.

Montgomery, W. W. *Surgery of the Upper Respiratory Tract* (vol. I) (1st ed.). Philadelphia: Lea & Febiger, 1983.

Mustoe, T., and Strome, M. Adult epiglottis. *Am. J. Otolaryngol.* 4:393, 1983.

Rood, S. R., Parnes, S. M., and Myers, E. N. *The Management of Epistaxis: Self-Instructional Package*. American Academy of Otolaryngology, 1977.

Shanon, E., et al. Penetrating injuries of the parapharyngeal space. *Arch. Otolaryngol.* 96:256, 1972.

Sheffer, A. L., Fearon, D. T., and Austin, K. F. Clinical and biochemical effects of Stanazol therapy for hereditary angioedema. *J. Clin. Immunol.* 68:181, 1981.

Shumrick, K. A., and Sheft, S. A. Deep neck infections. In M. M. Paparella, D. A. Shumrick, J. L. Gluchman, and W. L. Megahoff (eds.), *Otolaryngology* (vol. III). Philadelphia: Saunders, 1991. Pp 2545–2564.

Sprinkle, P. M., Veltri, R. W., and Kantor, C. M. Abscesses of the head and neck. *Laryngoscope* 84:1142, 1974.

Strome, M. Choanal atresia: An updated approach. *Trans. Am. Acad. Ophthalmol. Otolaryngol.* 82:499, 1976.

Strome, M. Tracheobronchial foreign bodies: An updated approach. *Ann. Otol. Rhinol. Laryngol.* 86:649, 1977.

Trone, T. H., Schaefer, S. D., and Carden, H. M. Blunt and penetrating laryngeal trauma: A 13-year review. *Otolaryngol. Head Neck Surg.* 88:257–261, 1980.

Tucker, J. A., and Yarington, C. T., Jr. The treatment of caustic ingestion. *Otolaryngol. Clin. North Am.* 12:343, 1979.

Weber, A. L. Radiology of the larynx. *Otolaryngol. Clin. North Am.* 17:13, 1984.

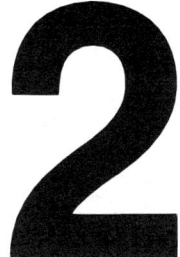

Ear

I. Introduction

A. Anatomy of the ear (Fig. 2-1)

1. The **auricle,** or **pinna,** is the projecting cupped appendage that, along with the external canal, constitutes the external ear. It is composed of skin, subcutaneous tissue, fat, rudimentary muscles, and cartilage. The cup shape assists in the capture of sound waves. Although normal variations occur, certain components are common to the auricle:

   a. **Helix**—the rolled edge of the periphery

   b. **Antihelix**—shaped like a "Y"; within confines of the helix

   c. **Concha**—bowl-shaped depression in center

   d. **Meatus**—entrance to the external auditory canal

   e. **Tragus**—also called "goat's beard" because hair often projects from the cartilaginous prominence located anterior to the meatus

   f. **Lobule**—fleshy inferior portion of auricle

2. **External auditory canal.** The external auditory canal is a tubular conduit connecting the sound-filled environment to the tympanic membrane. It is lined by skin. In the outer one-third, the skin is cushioned with fat, cartilage, connective tissue, and muscle. In the medial two-thirds, the skin is very thin and adherent to the bony canal. The lateral canal often has hair and normally contains cerumen glands. The canal augments hearing by functioning as an air conduit for sound. The canal is often convoluted, requiring manipulation for cleansing or for viewing the tympanic membrane.

3. The **tympanic membrane** is the receptive diaphragm for auditory impulses and is the "window" to the middle ear. The pars tensa is a cone with its apex at the umbo (see **C**) and is composed of three layers: outer (squamous), middle (two fibrous layers, one with concentric and one with radial orientation), and inner (mucous membrane). The pars flaccida (see **D**) lacks the middle (fibrous) layer. The tympanic membrane collects sound waves in a complex fashion. Its large size, compared to the size of the stapes foot plate, allows for a pressure gradient of 17-fold. Certain landmarks should be noted:

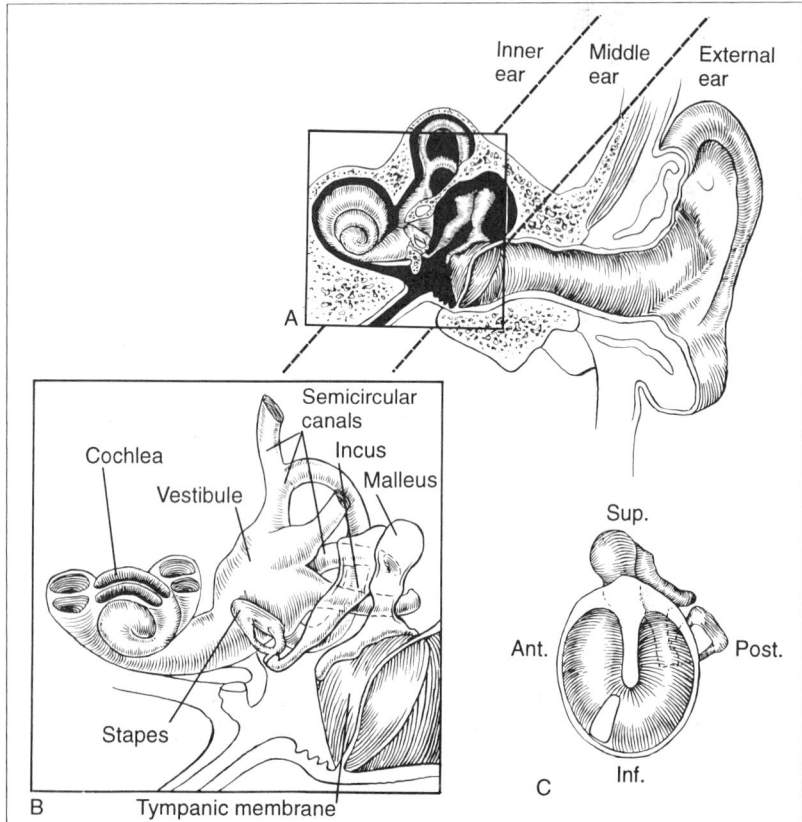

Fig. 2-1. Anatomy of the ear. A. External, middle, and inner ear. B. Middle ear, relationship of ossicles to tympanic membrane and inner ear. C. Tympanic membrane with light reflex and ossicles as seen through it.

     a. Annulus—rolled edge at periphery

     b. Manubrium—handle-shaped process of the malleus in apex of tympanic cone

     c. Umbo—end of manubrium in center of the tympanic membrane

     d. Pars flaccida—Shrapnell's membrane

     e. Incus—vertical bone in superoposterior quadrant seen through tympanic membrane

  4. Middle ear. The contents of the **middle ear space** are the malleus, incus, stapes, middle ear muscles (stapedius and tensor tympani), chorda tympani nerve, various smaller blood vessels, nerves, and mucosa. The middle ear or tympanic cleft is a mucosal-lined cavity containing the ossicles and their related tendons and muscles. It extends anterior and posterior, inferior and superior to the tympanic membrane. The superior portion of the tympanic cavity located above the pars tensa portion of the tympanic membrane is known as the epitympanum, or attic, and opens into the mastoid antrum through the additus. The additus extends posteriorly between the epitympanum and the mastoid antrum.

The middle ear cavity is entered in its anterior portion by the eustachian tube, which provides ventilation and pressure equalization of the middle ear and mastoid. In addition, it prevents reflux of nasopharyngeal contents into the middle ear cleft. At birth, the mastoid consists only of the antrum, a superior cavity that opens into the additus.

Beginning at birth and continuing for several years, the mastoid cells form as outgrowths of the antrum that extend to all portions of the temporal bone and to the zygoma, in extensively pneumatized bones. There is great variability in individual mastoid dimensions. These cells are lined with mucosa and are subject to the same disease processes as the middle ear mucosa.

The primary function of the middle ear is to conduct sound from the external environment to the fluids of the inner ear. The function of the mastoid air cells is unknown, but they are thought to participate in the pressure-regulating mechanism.

5. **Inner ear**

   a. **Anatomy.** The inner ear consists of a bony labyrinth filled with perilymph surrounding a membranous labyrinth filled with endolymph. The labyrinth is composed of three semicircular canals, a vestibule, and a cochlea. The three semicircular canals are at right angles to each other. Each canal contains a crista, or sense organ. When fluid moves in these canals, the sense organs are stimulated and send electrical impulses through the vestibular nerve. The cochlea makes two and one-half turns and contains the inner and outer hair cells within the organ of Corti, which connect to fibers of the cochlear division of the eighth cranial nerve. The vestibule contains the oval window, in which the stapes is situated and also the utricle, a sensory receptor responsive to positional change, and the saccule, whose function is unknown.

   b. **Physiology**

      (1) **Hearing.** The auricle acts as a sound-localizing device, although it probably is not as effective in humans as it is in animals with larger, more mobile appendages. The external ear acts as a conduit to transmit sound waves to the tympanic membrane. Vibration of the tympanic membrane initiates ossicular motion, which transmits sound via the oval window to the perilymphatic fluid, which in turn displaces endolymph fluid and the basilar membrane, activating auditory receptors (auditory hair cells). Hair-cell motion initiates activity in the auditory nerve

(eighth cranial nerve) that, via complex neural pathways, arrives in the auditory cortex and is perceived as sound.

(2) Equilibrium. The three semicircular canals each contain a crista, or sense organ. These sense organs are responsive to fluid movement in the endolymph caused by rotational acceleration. Each crista has a resting potential that is either increased or decreased, depending on the direction of fluid motion. Each canal is located in a plane that is approximately 90 degrees in relation to the others and is maximally stimulated by rotation in the plane in which the canal lies. This location enables the body to sense the direction of rotation. The sense organ of the macula responds to linear acceleration.

Through reflex connections to the extraocular muscles, the eyes attempt to provide visual fixation when the head rotates. Reflex connections to muscles produce a "righting" reflex and other postural adjustments. The visual system and peripheral sensors also contribute independently to the balance mechanism. Aberrations in these areas can similarly be responsible for imbalance or disequilibrium.

6. The **facial nerve** is encased in the temporal bone for a distance of 37–45 mm. This is the longest bony enclosure of a nerve in the human body, and makes the facial nerve subject to injury from swelling or trauma to the temporal bone. The nerve enters the internal auditory meatus superior to the cochlear nerve and travels through the internal auditory canal, passing next through the labyrinthine portion of the temporal bone for a short distance to reach the geniculate ganglion. Here the nerve turns sharply posterior (first genu) and passes superior to the oval window (tympanic segment). It then turns inferiorly (second genu), traveling vertically through the mastoid (mastoid segment), and exits through the stylomastoid foramen. The nerve has three primary branches in the temporal bone:

   a. The **greater superficial petrosal nerve** branches at the level of the geniculate ganglion and controls lacrimation.

   b. The **stapedial branch** exits in the mastoid segment and controls the stapedius muscle.

   c. The **chorda tympani nerve,** which branches just above the stylomastoid foramen, carries taste to the anterior two-thirds of the tongue.

7. The **carotid artery** is located in the petrous apex. Rarely is it involved in diseases of the ear, but it can be involved in severe temporal bone injuries involving the petrous apex or in extensive resection of the temporal bone.

8. The **jugular bulb,** located on the floor of the middle ear space, usually lies inferior to the tympanic membrane. Occasionally, the jugular bulb is positioned more superiorly and may be

noted on examination of the tympanic membrane as a bluish discoloration below the umbo.

9. The **sigmoid sinus** is the S-shaped portion of the lateral sinus that is responsible for the majority of the venous drainage from the head to the jugular vein. It passes through the posterior wall of the mastoid and may be injured in a surgical procedure or involved in extensive infection of the mastoid cells, producing **sigmoid sinus thrombosis.**

10. The **dura** of the middle cranial fossa is closely related both to the mastoid cells and to the middle ear cleft, being separated by a thin layer of bone, the tegmen tympani. The tegmen tympani is penetrated by small veins and arteries that can transmit an infection from the middle ear or mastoid to the meninges and brain.

B. General signs and symptoms of ear disease

1. **Otalgia.** Ear pain can be caused by pathology directly related to the ear, the periauricular area, or distant sites (referred otalgia). With otalgia, it is imperative that, before treatment is initiated, a definitive diagnosis be established. Below are areas to be considered, other than the ear and periauricular area, that can cause otalgia. The ear receives innervation from cranial nerves V, VII, IX, X, XI, and from cervical nerves C2 and C3. Any of the other areas innervated by these nerves can refer pain to the ear.

   a. Oral cavity

      (1) Dental infection

      (2) Glossitis and stomatitis (particularly herpes)

      (3) Neoplasia

   b. Pharynx (naso-, oro-, and hypopharynx)

      (1) Malignancy, especially in the pyriform sinus

      (2) Pharyngitis

      (3) Retropharyngeal or peritonsillar abscess

      (4) Tonsillitis

      (5) Posttonsillectomy, adenoidectomy

   c. Esophagus

      (1) Foreign body

      (2) Tumor

      (3) Esophagitis

   d. Larynx

      (1) Tumor

      (2) Mucosal ulceration

      (3) Cricoarytenoid arthritis

       (4) Laryngitis

       (5) Epiglottitis

    e. Neuralgia

       (1) Trigeminal

       (2) Geniculate

       (3) Glossopharyngeal

       (4) Sphenopalatine

   f. Other

       (1) Thyroiditis

       (2) Temporomandibular joint

       (3) Lung and bronchial disease

       (4) Great vessel aneurysm

       (5) Migraine

2. Otorrhea. Drainage from the ear is a common complaint. Depending on the associated history and physical examination, this symptom may indicate serious disease. It is important to document the nature of otorrhea, related symptoms, and events such as trauma that may have been precursors. The following types of otorrhea warrant consideration:

   a. Cerumen is the most common cause of otorrhea. The color varies from brown to pale yellow. The consistency varies from liquid to solid. Water in the ear or otic drops can increase the discharge.

   b. Blood. Although the primary cause is trauma (slap, instrumentation), acute perforations, external otitis, and tumors can also cause bleeding. Except in severe trauma and with clotting disorders, bleeding is rarely severe.

   c. Serum is seen occasionally with the rupture of a bleb from bullous myringitis; however, serum usually indicates a dermatitis affecting the external canal.

   d. Pus in acute otitis media is usually viscous, yellow or white. In chronic otitis media, the color changes to yellow gray or greenish and is thinner. "Pus" from external otitis is usually cheesy in nature.

   e. Cerebrospinal fluid (CSF) is usually clear and may be profuse. A sample should be taken for laboratory analysis (sugar, sodium, protein, and cells). A history of trauma, surgery, or tumor is often present. A prior history of meningitis may be obtained.

3. Hearing loss. As opposed to otalgia, hearing loss always indicates a disease process somewhere in the acoustic pathway (external ear to cerebral cortex). Hearing loss is usually described as conductive, sensorineural, or mixed (a combination of sensorineural and conductive). A hearing loss is often difficult for the patient to describe and, indeed, is frequently brought to the physician's attention by a family member or friend. The patient often denies a hearing loss, saying that people are speaking unclearly.

a. **Conductive hearing loss** results in the interference of transmission of sound energy from the outside environment to the receptor organ (cochlear hair cells). Interference can occur anywhere from the auricle to the organ of Corti. Conductive hearing loss is frequently a temporary or correctable condition.

b. **Sensorineural hearing loss** results from defects both in the transmission of sound energy into electrical impulses and in the transfer of these impulses to the auditory cortex. This hearing loss results from a variety of causes, including trauma, viral diseases, ear infection, and the aging process (presbycusis) (see **IX.A.8.**).

c. **Mixed hearing loss** indicates an additive effect of a conductive and sensorineural hearing loss. In a mixed hearing loss, it is important to differentiate whether the loss is primarily conductive (i.e., correctable) or sensorineural.

4. **Vertigo** may best be described as a sensation of motion of either the patient or the environment. Severe vertigo with nystagmus and vomiting almost always indicates a disease process involving the peripheral vestibular apparatus. Vertigo may be the only symptom of ear disease, or it may be combined with other symptoms, such as hearing loss, otalgia, or otorrhea. Severe vertigo, particularly when acute, must be regarded as a significant symptom of ear pathology, and a thorough evaluation performed. Vertigo should be distinguished from dizziness (Figs. 2-2 and 2-3).

5. **Tinnitus** is an altered sound perception not associated with an external stimulus. It can be correlated with systemic considerations; e.g., sensorineural hearing loss, medications, temperature elevation, headache syndromes, vertigo, etc. It can also occur as an independent entity. Subjective and objective tinnitus have been defined:

a. **Signs and symptoms**

(1) Subjective tinnitus is perceptible only to the affected individual.

(2) Objective tinnitus can be identified by others.

b. **Diagnostic tests**

(1) **Audiologic**—many patients have an associated high frequency sensorineural hearing loss.

(2) **Auditory brainstem response (ABR)**—appropriate for all unilateral tinnitus.

(3) **MRI** (enhanced)—indicated for abnormal ABR or other suggestive audiometric data for acoustic neuroma.

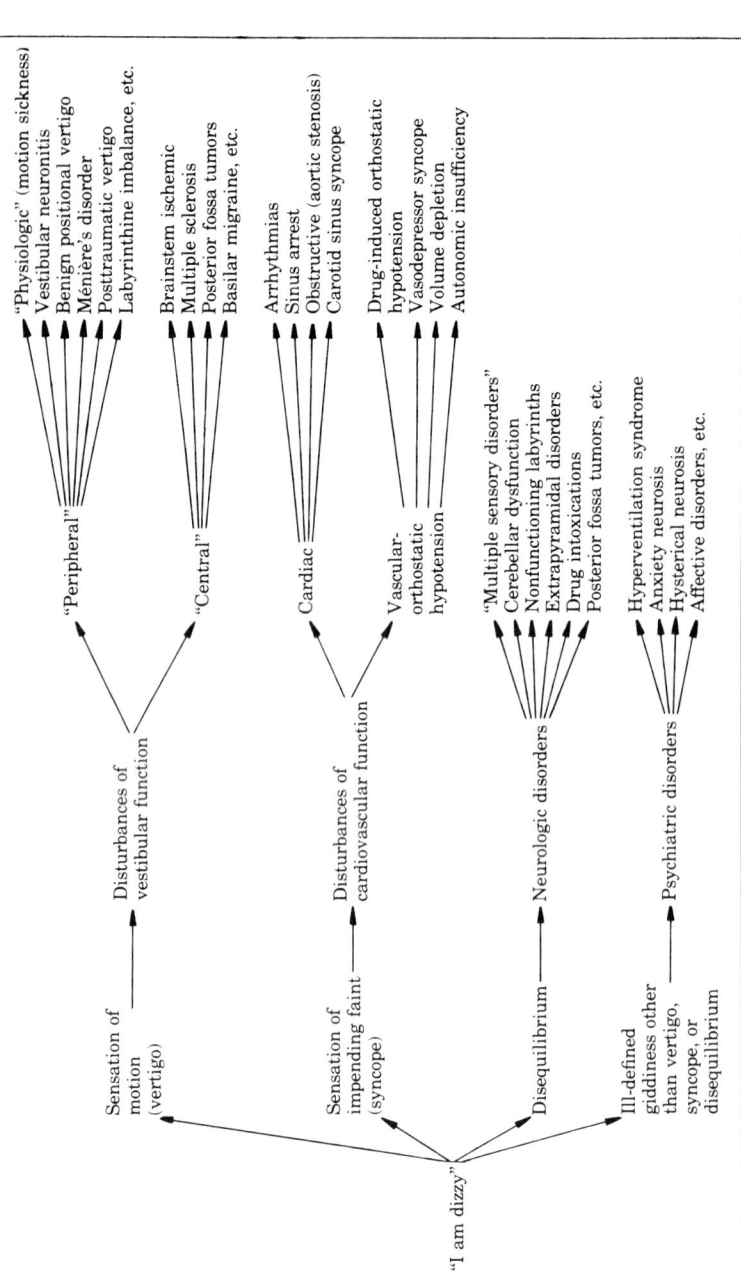

Fig. 2-2. Clinical spectrum of dizziness. (From M. A. Samuels, *Manual of Neurology: Diagnosis and Therapy.* 4th ed. Boston: Little, Brown, 1991.)

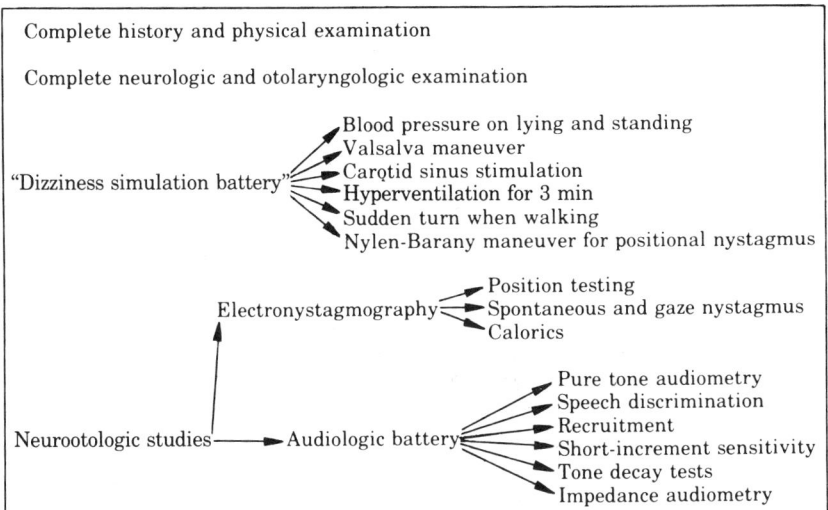

Complete history and physical examination

Complete neurologic and otolaryngologic examination

"Dizziness simulation battery"
- Blood pressure on lying and standing
- Valsalva maneuver
- Carotid sinus stimulation
- Hyperventilation for 3 min
- Sudden turn when walking
- Nylen-Barany maneuver for positional nystagmus

Electronystagmography
- Position testing
- Spontaneous and gaze nystagmus
- Calorics

Neurootologic studies → Audiologic battery
- Pure tone audiometry
- Speech discrimination
- Recruitment
- Short-increment sensitivity
- Tone decay tests
- Impedance audiometry

Fig. 2-3. Clinical evaluation of the dizzy patient. (From M. A. Samuels, *Manual of Neurology: Diagnosis and Therapy.* 4th ed. Boston: Little, Brown, 1991.)

(4) Hematology screen—appropriate in all instances—can define multiple medical precursors; e.g., hyperlipidemia, diabetes, Paget's disease.

c. Treatment—The object is symptom control; however, cure is rarely effected.

(1) Identify and control medical correlates, temporomandibular joint (TMJ), hypertension, etc.

(2) Reduce environmental noise exposure—provide ear defenders as indicated.

(3) Avoid exposure to aminoglycosides and other medications known to cause tinnitus.

(4) Resolve if possible all remediable otologic pathology; e.g., chronic suppuration, effusion, negative middle ear pressure.

(5) Tinnitus maskers—popular but do not meet most patient's expectations. These devices provide external noise and, via residual inhibition, can decrease awareness for some patients.

(6) Electrical stimulation—investigatory; the short-lived response is not infrequently associated with tissue damage.

(7) Biofeedback or relaxation techniques—of occasional benefit, best performed by competent professional.

(8) Medications—generally directed toward controlling the affect—none with clear superiority.

(9) Cognitive therapy—an affect-control modality.

II. Physical examination

A. External evaluation

1. Auricle

a. **Position.** The top of the auricle should not fall caudal to a line drawn from the occiput to the lateral canthus of the eye. Such "low-set" ears can signal other congenital anomalies. The angle that the auricle makes with the side of the head varies. The condition of "lop-ear" from excessive protrusion is correctable.

b. **Consistency.** The ears of neonates are almost alarmingly soft and can maintain an iatrogenic crease for an extended period. Adult ears take on the normal "springy" consistency associated with cartilage.

c. **Size and shape.** A great deal of variation occurs. The auricles should be symmetric. Congenital anomalies that can occur are multiple and range from insignificant to complete absence of pinnae.

2. The mastoid, postauricular sulcus, squamosal, and zygomatic areas should be checked routinely for pathology of skin or underlying bone. A postauricular scar may be present—an indication of prior otologic surgery that the patient may have forgotten.

3. Seventh cranial nerve function. The nerve can be injured anywhere in its tortuous course through the temporal bone. All branches should be checked by raising eyebrows, lid closure, whistle or pucker, smile, scowl, and neck muscle tightening. Testing taste, lacrimation, and stapedial muscle function can pinpoint the site of injury.

B. Otoscopy. Several methods are available to illuminate the external canal and tympanic membrane. With use of any method, however, two principles should be kept in mind: (1) the bony external canal is tender when manipulated, and must be instrumented gently. (2) Patients should be advised in advance of any instrumentation to prevent a startle and sudden head movement.

The **pinna** should be positioned to open the meatus, to straighten the canal, and to provide a direct visual path to the tympanic membrane (Fig. 2-4). In the child or adult, the pinna should be pulled posteriorly and superiorly. In the neonate, the lobule may require a tug directly caudad. One method of examination is the head mirror with reflected light. This method allows two-handed manipulation and is well suited for cerumen removal, wick placement, and other manipulation. In common practice, the conventional electric otoscope is an all-purpose instrument. It should have several features:

Small handle ("C" batteries)
Intense light (halogen is preferred)

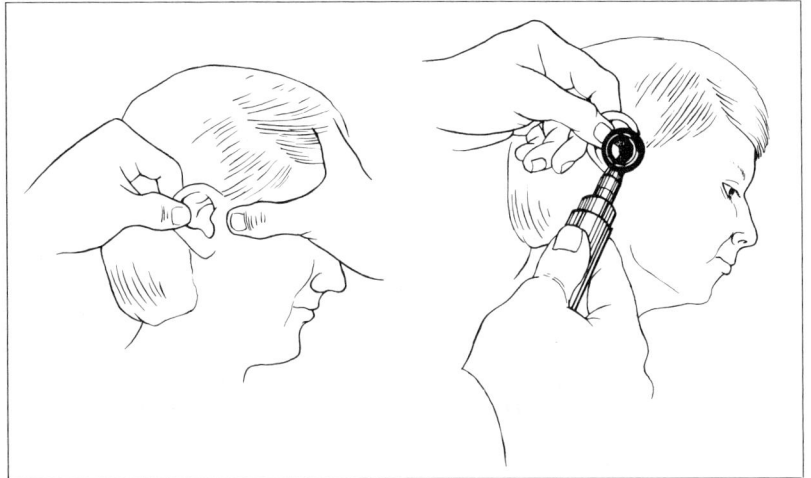

Fig. 2-4. Otoscopy. Pinnae pulled laterally and head positioned at 15–20 degree angle toward opposite shoulder.

Air seal head (for pneumatic otoscopy)
Open head (for instrumentation)
Rubber tubing and bulb (for pneumatic otoscopy)

Other methods such as loupes, headlight, and the suspension microscope are available to the otologist. Micro-otoscopic telescopes are also available.

After removal of cerumen and after good visualization of the canal and tympanic membrane are achieved, the anatomy is evaluated and a drawing made. Osteomas and exostoses of the canal wall should be included in the drawing. The following manipulations can then be performed.

C. **Pneumatic otoscopy** is performed routinely on all patients. A handheld bulb is used for changing pressure in the external canal. A tight seal is essential. The tympanic membrane should be observed to move actively and crisply in both directions. The examiner can be misled and assume normal mobility (e.g., a retracted tympanic membrane will move out with negative pressure, then passively return, without the need of positive pressure). Immobility or sluggish movement can be detected. The patient can perform his or her own pneumatic otoscopy. A Valsalva maneuver with a pinched nose and closed mouth can autoinflate the middle ear with tympanic membrane motion. This is a reasonable measure of eustachian tube function. An alternative method is to swallow with an occluded nose and mouth.

D. **Palpation.** Occasionally, the canal or tympanic membrane requires manipulation. A small suction tip (No. 20) can be used to check for mobility, for the presence of a perforation, or for other pathology. Although the drum is sensitive, gentle palpation is tolerated by most patients.

E. **Examination of the child.** The child often sets the tone of the examination. The examiner must be prepared to kneel on the floor, to sit in the chair while the child stands, or to place the child on a lap. Games are useful such as watching the painless "Tinkerbell" otoscope light on the child's hand, blowing out the light, and looking for bunnies in the ears. Children like to squeeze the bulb for the "wind" in their ears.

Should care and cleverness prove unsuccessful, the child should be "papoosed" by the parent. The parent sits on the chair, the child is on the lap. The child's legs are placed between the parent's clamped legs. The head of the child is snuggled sideways on the upper chest, and the parent hugs the patient. An assistant then controls the head.

F. **Tuning fork testing** helps to define normal from abnormal hearing, conductive loss versus a sensorineural loss, and the frequency range of the loss. These tests provide a gross estimate, but are not a substitute for an audiogram. Tuning fork tests are usually unsuccessful under the age of 5 years.

1. **Rinne. Positive** if air conduction is greater than bone conduction (a rare label for the normal to be "positive"). The tuning fork, preferably 512 Hertz (Hz), is placed on the mastoid tip firmly (almost to the point of discomfort) and then placed near the meatus so that the two prongs of the fork are aligned with the direction of the ear canal. (Rotate a tuning fork near your ear and note the change of loudness.) The patient states which position sounds louder.

   Air>Bone (Rinne is positive)   Normal or sensorineural loss of that ear
   Bone>Air (Rinne is negative)   Conductive loss of that ear

2. **Weber.** Tests for symmetry of hearing. The tuning fork is placed on the forehead or on the central incisor. The patient reports subjectively in which ear the tone is loudest. The test is fraught with error, because the patients may "not hear anything" or, in the case of a conductive loss, are afraid to report that the "bad" ear hears "better."

   a. **Symmetric** can be interpreted as normal hearing or symmetric hearing loss (either conductive or sensorineural).

   b. **Lateralization** toward the poorer-hearing ear usually indicates a conductive component (try this with a finger in one of your ears). Lateralization toward the better-hearing ear may indicate a sensorineural component in the opposite ear.

G. **Clinical speech testing.** Clinical speech testing may be performed by whispering simple words into an ear. The opposite ear should be "masked" by producing a noise in it. The otologist commonly uses a Baronay Box, which produces 100–110 decibels 0 (dB) of sound at ear level. Other noisemakers may also be used, such as a partially occluded suction tubing (producing a hissing noise). It is helpful to practice this technique on normal patients, always keeping the same distance from the ear and varying the intensity

Table 2-1. Audiologic evaluation of cochlear and retrocochlear disorders

Test	Cochlear lesions	Retrocochlear (eighth nerve) lesions
Pure tone audiometry	Sensorineural hearing loss	Sensorineural hearing loss
Speech discrimination	Good	Poor
Recruitment	Yes	No
Stapedial reflex	Normal	Impaired
Tone decay	No	Yes
Clinical examples	Ménière's syndrome	Acoustic schwannoma

Source: M. A. Samuels, *Manual of Neurology: Diagnosis and Therapy.* 4th ed. Boston: Little, Brown, 1991.

of the noise. The hand should be held in such a way as to prevent the patient from lip reading. This whispered voice test is much more accurate than having the patient listen to a watch tick. Bi-syllabic words of equal stress (spondaic words) should be used when testing. (Examples are *baseball, airplane, cowboy, railroad, eardrum, ice cream, hotdog.*)

Results should be expressed as normal hearing or as mild, moderate, or severe hearing loss. A person skilled in this method can estimate the hearing loss (in decibels) with surprising accuracy.

H. **Audiometry** should be considered as an extension of the physical examination. The audiometric tests cannot diagnose a disease process but should be used in conjunction with the history, physical examination, and other testing to arrive at a diagnosis (Table 2-1).

1. **Pure tone testing** presents a single-frequency tone to the patient through a headphone. The intensity of this tone is then varied until the tester determines the lowest intensity (in dB) that is audible. This testing is repeated in each ear at various frequencies, usually 250, 500, 1000, 2000, 4000, 6000, and 8000 cycles per second (cps). The test is then repeated using a bone conduction vibrator placed over the mastoid bone (usually in this test only 250–4000 cps are tested). In sensorineural hearing losses and in normals, bone conduction and air conduction (headphones) are equal. With conductive hearing losses, bone conduction scores are better than air conduction scores. Air conduction scores can never be better than bone conduction scores. The results are expressed as decibels of hearing loss with a range of 0–100 dB (the smaller the number, the better the hearing). The normal adult range is approximately 0–20 dB, and the children's range is 0–15 dB.

2. **Speech reception threshold (SRT)** is found by giving the patient a list of spondaic words (see **G**) at a frequency equal to a 1000-cps signal. The intensity of the stimulus (words) is then varied until a level is reached at which the patient can repeat half of the test items. This level is known as the speech reception threshold and is expressed in decibels. This test estimates the patient's handicap in connected conversation. The SRT for each ear should approximate (±10 dB) the average for the pure tones

at 500, 1000, and 2000 cps in each ear. (The range from 500–2000 cps is often called the speech frequency.)

3. **Speech discrimination tests** are used to test the clarity of articulated speech. A list of monosyllabic words that represent the phonetic balance of spoken English is used. The words are given at a comfortable intensity above the speech reception threshold (usually about 40 dB). The results are reported as a percentage of the words of the list that are repeated correctly. Normal discrimination is 90% or above, with most normal-hearing individuals scoring 96–100%. For the non-English-speaking, separate word lists must be used that approximate the phonetic balance of their native tongue. Unfortunately, such lists are not available for all languages.

4. **Audiometric testing to identify the site of a lesion** is frequently performed to determine if a hearing loss is caused by a cochlear or retrocochlear lesion (eighth nerve to auditory cortex). Some of these tests are listed below; however, their usefulness has greatly diminished now that auditory evoked response testing is available.

   a. SISI (short-increment sensitivity index)

   b. Tone decay

   c. Bekesey

   d. Recruitment testing

III. **Radiographic evaluation** of the temporal bone is extremely difficult because of the small size of the structures being evaluated and the numerous overlying shadows. The routine use of x rays on an emergency basis (except in ideal circumstances) should be avoided.

A. **Plain films** usually consist of three to four views of the ear. The size and aeration of the mastoid can be determined, as can (sometimes) breakdown of the cell partitions caused by acute mastoiditis. In addition, large erosive lesions can be identified.

B. **Computed tomography (CT),** usually with iodinated intravenous contrast, gives the best bony definition of the temporal bone. Assessment of congenital abnormalities as well as bone destruction by tumor is best done by scanning. Soft tissue definition is acceptable.

C. **Magnetic resonance imaging (MRI)** with gadolinium gives excellent soft tissue definition of structures in and around the temporal bone. Inflammatory lesions and tumors are well defined.

D. **Angiography** of temporal bone lesions—especially glomus tumors—may help in defining their extent and blood supply. Newer noninvasive MRI-angio techniques may replace this modality.

IV. **Special testing**

A. **Calorics.** Nystagmus can be elicited by instilling water of a temperature different from the body temperature into the external ear canal. This condition is produced by a change in temperature in the **lateral** semicircular canal, causing endolymphatic flow in the canal and stimulation of the sense organ (crista). Nystagmus is described according to the direction of the **fast** component. Cold water produces a quick component away from the ear tested; conversely, warm water produces a quick component toward the ear tested (COWS: cold—opposite; warm—same). By comparing the length and intensity of nystagmus in each ear, a gross measurement of vestibular function can be made. Ice water (2 ml) can be used; however, it may stimulate severe vertigo with vegetative symptoms of nausea, vomiting, and diaphoresis. Water calorics are **contraindicated** in tympanic membrane perforations, temporal bone fracture, and CSF leaks.

B. **Electronystagmogram (ENG)** is based on the principle that the eye is a dipole, with a positive charge at the cornea and a negative charge at the retina. By placing recording electrodes around the eye, movements, including nystagmus, will cause a deflection in current that can be recorded. Caloric stimulation (30 and 44°C), positional testing, optokinetic testing, pendulum tracking, and spontaneous nystagmus are all recorded as part of the ENG report.

Currently, the ENG is the preferred method of vestibular testing because it gives a permanent record. The intensity (slow-phase velocity) of the nystagmus can be measured accurately. The electronystagmogram can give a better overall functional picture of the entire balance system.

C. **Brainstem auditory-evoked response (BSER), or auditory brainstem response (ABR),** is a development that uses a computer to average random cortical electrical activity (EEG). A series of stimuli (clicks) is presented to the ear to be tested, and scalp electrodes monitor the response. By analyzing the wave thus produced, a "map" of the auditory pathways can be produced. Because no patient response is necessary, this method is invaluable in testing neonates, young children, and others in whom an accurate response to conventional audiometry is questionable. Site of lesion testing, including the diagnosis of acoustic neuromas, is another important application of the ABR. Because patient movement can affect the outcome of the ABR, sedation may be required in some patients. The waveforms produced (I–V) are currently thought to represent synaptic connections in the auditory and other nuclei in the brainstem.

D. **Tympanometry, acoustic impedance, acoustic reflex.** Tympanometry is accomplished by using a probe that seals the ear canal. Varying pressure is then introduced into the canal, and the compliance of the eardrum is recorded on a graph. The normal ear shows a smooth, bell-shaped "peak" of compliance; fluid or other mass effects in the middle ear produces a flattened curve. Clues to various other ear pathology (eustachian tube dysfunction, ossicular discontinuity) can be gained by analysis of this graph.

Using the same equipment, high intensity ($\geq$85 dB) sound can be introduced into the ear to produce a notch on the graph caused by contraction of the stapedius muscle. Since this muscle is innervated by a branch of the seventh cranial nerve, this test can be used for topographic testing. Decay of this reflex is often seen with acoustic neuromas. Because this reflex occurs at about 80 dB above threshold, a rough estimate of hearing sensitivity can be obtained in some patients. About 5% of the population have absent stapedial reflexes with otherwise normal ears.

E. **Posturography and rotation testing** have recently been added to the vestibular test armamentarium. They help to further evaluate vestibular reflex responses. Their limitations, however, are the same as with any reflex test. They do not actually measure vestibular output, and thus many factors can interfere with their validity.

V. Diseases of the auricle

A. **Preauricular appendages (accessory auricles).** Preauricular appendages are small, skin-covered tags that appear in the preauricular area on a line drawn from the tragus to the corner of the mouth. They may contain small pieces of cartilage.

1. **Signs and symptoms.** Except for their appearance, preauricular appendages are usually asymptomatic, but the examiner should be cautioned to look for other anomalies.

2. **Management.** Removal is not indicated unless the appendages are cosmetically undesirable.

B. **Preauricular pits.** Preauricular pits commonly occur at the root of the helix, although they may occur in other locations. They can descend down to the lower border of the tragus and can contain glandular structures.

1. **Signs and symptoms.** Purulent drainage with swelling and pain can occur when the pits become infected.

2. **Management.** When these tracts become repeatedly infected, surgical excision is necessary.

C. **Auricular atresia (aplasia).** Auricular atresia may be unilateral or bilateral, and can range from mild malformations to complete absence of the auricle. It is frequently associated with anomalies of the external canal, middle ear, and temporal bone. Hearing loss is frequent. Atresia can be inherited, associated with embryopathies (rubella, thalidomide), or chromosomal abnormalities. For this reason, careful evaluation for other anomalies is mandatory, particularly in regard to derivatives of the first and second branchial arch.

1. **Signs and symptoms** are purely cosmetic unless a hearing loss is present.

2. **Management.** Restoration of hearing must take precedence, but surgical management must be carefully coordinated between the otologic and reconstructive surgeon.

D. **Trauma to the auricle**

1. **Lacerations** can range from simple lacerations to complete avulsion and are often associated with multiple trauma.

a. Management

   (1) Careful cleansing of the wound with removal of foreign debris is necessary. In extensive injuries, general anesthesia may be required. Local blocks may also be used in the cooperative patient. Except in simple lacerations, local infiltration should be avoided because it distorts the anatomy and may disrupt the blood supply to the cartilage. The cartilage should be sutured only if necessary to reform the contour of the ear. If cartilaginous suturing is necessary, fine (5-0 or 6-0), noncolored suture should be used to prevent its showing through the skin. If possible, the perichondrium should be closed using fine, absorbable suture. Knots should be buried and the skin approximated with interrupted 6-0 monofilament nylon. A sterile pressure dressing (mastoid type) should then be applied.

   (2) Avulsion of the auricle must be repaired in the operating room with a team well versed in reconstructive techniques. The auricle can be preserved in sterile, iced saline until reconstruction can be accomplished.

   (3) With lacerations to the auricle, prophylactic antibiotics are not indicated except in dirty wounds (e.g., human bite). Penicillin is the drug of choice in these instances.

2. Hematoma or seroma usually occurs with trauma to the auricle that produces hemorrhage under the perichondrium or skin.

   a. Signs and symptoms. The hematoma or seroma is often blue, round, and smooth. Pain may be present. Because it disrupts the blood supply to the cartilage, prompt treatment is required to prevent aseptic necrosis and deformity (cauliflower ear).

   b. Management. If hematomas or seromas are seen early in their course, before clot formation has occurred, aspiration with an 18-gauge needle and application of a pressure dressing may be sufficient. Careful follow-up is necessary to assess reaccumulation of the fluid. If the fluid reaccumulates or if aspiration is unsuccessful, incision and drainage, with the placement of drains, is indicated and should be performed in the operating room. Particularly resistant cases may require the placement of through-and-through mattress sutures over a bolus of cotton to ensure a good result. Fluid removal from the area should be Gram stained, cultured, and appropriate antibiotics begun. If there is evidence of infection (e.g., purulent aspirate or cellulitis), intravenous antibiotic coverage should be started immediately to cover *Staphylococcus* and *Streptococcus* until culture results are obtained.

3. Burns. As with burns to other areas of the body, severe deformity is usually due to secondary infection and cartilaginous necrosis.

a. **Signs and symptoms.** The ear may be reddened, have vesicles, or be shiny white, depending on the degree of the burn. First- and second-degree burns are usually painful, whereas third-degree burns are not. A large number of patients will develop suppuration and chondritis, regardless of the depth of the burn.

b. **Management.** The burned area should be cleansed, an antibiotic ointment applied, and a light sterile dressing placed over the ear. Pressure should be avoided to prevent further embarrassment of the blood supply. Antibiotics should be used only when there is evidence of infection. Any debridement should be delayed to allow the devitalized areas to demarcate.

4. **Frostbite** occurs frequently to the auricle due to its protrusion and relatively poor blood supply.

a. **Signs and symptoms.** The auricle becomes white, with a slightly shiny appearance. There is loss of sensation to the affected area. Bullae may be present.

b. **Management.** Gradual rewarming is advisable using tepid compresses. Thereafter, the ear is treated like a burn. Antibiotic cream is applied to breaks in the skin, and a light sterile dressing is placed over the ear. Pressure is to be avoided. No debridement should be performed until viability is determined.

E. **Auricular chondritis (auriculitis).** Auricular chondritis may be caused by a spreading external otitis, trauma, or insect bite, but is often idiopathic.

1. **Signs and symptoms.** The entire ear is red and tense, including the lobule. Tenderness is usually present, but may not be severe. The periauricular soft tissues may be involved. *Streptococcus pyogenes* is often the causative organism.

2. **Management** consists of IV semisynthetic penicillin in high dosages and treatment of any underlying causes such as external otitis. Bacitracin or other antibiotic ointment should be used on skin breaks.

3. **Complications.** Lack of prompt and effective treatment results in loss of cartilage and in auricular deformity.

F. **Polychondritis (relapsing).** Relapsing polychondritis involves the ear as well as other cartilages (septal, costal). In contrast to auriculitis, the lobule is spared. Systemic steroids in high doses is the treatment of choice.

G. **Tumors.** Both basal cell and squamous cell carcinomas often involve the pinna since it is exposed to sunlight. Biopsy is necessary to determine the proper treatment. Squamous cell tumors may involve local nodes (mastoid, high cervical parotid). Nodal disease must be resected in block or irradiated.

VI. Diseases of the external canal

A. **Cerumen impaction.** Cerumen is a normal finding in ear canals. It acts as a protection from maceration and lubricates the skin. Normally, cerumen migrates laterally and is discharged from the canals. In certain patients, however, this mechanism is less efficient. This problem can be aggravated by the use of cotton-tipped applicators, which tend to pack the wax into the canal.

1. **Signs and symptoms** consist of hearing loss, pressure sensation, or otalgia.

2. **Diagnosis** is made by the appearance of the wax, which varies from almost white to dark black-brown.

3. **Management** consists of removal with instrumentation (e.g., curette, suction) or by irrigation. Removal can often be facilitated by the use of softening drops (glycerol peroxide, liquid dioctyl sodium [Colace]). Good illumination and exposure are necessary for this procedure. Irrigation should be avoided in patients who give a history of infection, bleeding, or perforated tympanic membrane. In some patients with recurrent impactions, self-administration of softening drops and gentle irrigation with a bulb syringe can avoid numerous trips to the doctor.

B. **Trauma.** Most trauma to the external canal is caused by instrumentation of the ear canal, either by the patient or by the physician. Cotton-tipped applicators are a common offender.

1. **Signs and symptoms.** The appearance of a laceration or hematoma in the skin of the canal makes the diagnosis.

2. **Treatment** consists of antibiotic drops and water precautions in simple lacerations and hematomas. More complex lacerations, particularly circumferential lacerations, should be treated by packing the external canal with a Merocel wick and using antibiotic ear drops to prevent canal stenosis.

C. **Foreign bodies** are extremely common in younger children, but may be seen in any age group. The foreign body may consist of anything that is small enough to enter the canal.

1. **Signs and symptoms.** The history, particularly in young children, is often not helpful in establishing the diagnosis. Symptoms consist of hearing loss, pain, or drainage.

2. **Management.** In an adult or cooperative patient, gentle removal with a foreign body curette, suction, or forceps (alligator-type) is often possible. In less cooperative patients and in those patients in whom the foreign body is wedged into the canal, operative removal under anesthesia with magnification is indicated.

Vegetable foreign bodies (e.g., dried beans) swell after insertion and often require operative intervention. Extreme caution and gentleness must be exercised in foreign body removal. Imprudent attempts at removal have resulted in severe lacerations of the canal, tympanic membrane perforations, ossicular disruptions, and facial nerve injury. Proper equipment and expertise are essential.

D. Furuncle. Single or multiple furuncles are common in the external portion of the ear canal.

   1. Signs and symptoms. Furuncles appear as localized swellings that may be fluctuant. Tenderness to palpation or insertion of an ear speculum is often marked.

   2. Management consists of drainage of fluctuant areas, heat, and the use of a topical antibiotic (e.g., Bacitrocin). Systemic antibiotics are necessary only with cellulitis or systemic symptoms (e.g., fever) and should consist of antistaphylococcal drugs. Narcotics may be necessary for 24–48 hours for pain control.

E. External otitis (diffuse) also known as "swimmers ear." This condition is very common, particularly during the summer months. Water maceration or trauma (or both) are often etiologic.

   1. Signs and symptoms consist of itching, pain (often severe), a plugged sensation in the ear, and a discharge, which is often cheesy.

   2. Diagnosis. Physical examination elicits pain on auricular movement or tragal pressure. The canal is diffusely swollen and tender and may be completely closed. Desquamated debris is usually present in the canal. The tympanic membrane may be obscured by debris or swelling. Cultures usually grow *Pseudomonas, Proteus* or, less frequently, *Staphylococcus* and *Streptococcus.*

   3. Management consists of gentle cleaning of the canal and topical antibiotic drops containing a steroid such as polymyxin B–neomycin-hydrocortisone (Cortisporin Otic Suspension) to reduce swelling. With marked swelling of the canal, a Merocel wick should be inserted to allow the drops to be delivered to the entire length of the canal. A wick of sufficient length should be inserted so that the patient may remove it in 48 hours. Drops are placed on the wick 4 times/day, and thereafter in the canal for a total of 7–10 days. Instructions to observe strict water precautions are of importance (i.e., no swimming, and inserting a vaseline-coated plug in the canal before showering or washing hair). Cotton-tipped applicators or other manipulation by the patient should be avoided. Pain often lasts for 3–4 days after beginning treatment, and should be controlled with sufficient pain medication. Systemic antibiotics are necessary only for cellulitis extending outside the canal, in diabetics or immunosuppressed patients. Systemic antibiotics alone are never sufficient treatment for external otitis. If symptoms persist after 1 week of medical treatment, reexamination is essential. If adequate visualization of the tympanic membrane is not possible initially, a follow-up examination should be performed. It may be necessary to remove debris from the canal on several occasions during the course of treatment.

F. Necrotizing external otitis (sometimes confusingly referred to as malignant external otitis). This condition is an external otitis that has spread outside the confines of the external canal to involve bone, mastoid cells, and periaural soft tissue. It is usually diagnosed in diabetics or those immunosuppressed (including a few reported cases in newborns). Early reports cited a 50–80% mortality, but this rate has been improved with adequate and prompt therapy. Marked reduction in the incidence of necrotizing otitis externa can be achieved with prompt initiation of oral antipseudonomal drug therapy (ciprofloxacin) in those patients at risk for the disease with symptoms of early otitis externa.

1. **Signs and symptoms.** Pain is usually more severe than with simple external otitis and is often described as "deep" or "boring." The disease process usually begins with an external otitis, but tends to progress on standard medication.

2. **Diagnosis**

   a. **Physical examination** reveals granulation tissue at the junction of the bony and cartilaginous canal. There may be exposed bone in the canal. Facial nerve paralysis may be present.

   b. **Computerized axial tomography** (CAT scan) can aid in the diagnosis by showing destruction of bone.

   c. **Cultures** should be obtained. *Pseudomonas* or *Proteus* are most often the causative organisms.

3. **Management** consists of high doses of tobramycin and ticarcillin intravenously (often for weeks), topical aminoglycoside drops, and judicious debridement of devitalized bone or areas of accumulated pus. Oral antipseudomonal drugs such as ciprofloxacin may replace IV antibiotics in early cases, and may also allow for early cessation of IV medication. In the diabetic, careful control of the diabetes aids in recovery. The immunosuppressed patient needs aggressive medical intervention.

G. Exostoses. Exostoses are seen as smooth subcutaneous swellings of the bony external canal and are usually asymptomatic unless they entrap water, causing external otitis. In rare cases, exostoses completely close the ear canal, causing a conductive hearing loss, wherein surgical removal is indicated.

H. Dermatitis. As a skin-lined tube, the external canal is subject to dermatitis. Since it is a closed pouch and thereby more prone to maceration by moisture, dermatitis may affect the canals alone. Seborrhea, atopic dermatitis, and psoriasis are common and may predispose to recurrent suppuration. **Management** involves specific measures for the underlying etiology, as well as topical treatment of any associated external otitis.

I. Tumors. Although rarer than those of the auricle, basal cell and squamous cell carcinomas can involve the external canal. Neoplasia should be suspected when otitis externa is refractory to therapy. Persistent granular or necrotic tissue should be biopsied. An adequate biopsy will establish the diagnosis. Radical surgery is usually required.

VII. Diseases of the tympanic membrane

A. **Bullous myringitis.** Bullous myringitis may be of viral etiology, although some reported cases have been caused by *Mycoplasma* infections. *Haemophilus influenzae* infection can present with tympanic membrane bullae in a child.

1. **Signs and symptoms.** Pain and a full feeling in the ear are common. The blebs can rupture spontaneously, causing a small amount of serous or serosanguineous drainage. Sensorineural hearing loss has been found in up to one-third of affected patients.

2. **Diagnosis** is made by the appearance of one or more "blebs" that are thin walled and involve only the squamous layer of the tympanic membrane. There may be an associated effusion in the middle ear. Unless there is a secondary infection, the pain subsides in 24 to 48 hours. The fullness may persist for several weeks.

3. **Management** consists of symptomatic treatment. An audiogram should be performed. If a new sensorineural component is identified, viral titers should be obtained (i.e., EBV and CMV) and adjunctive steroid therapy considered. Narcotic agents may be required for pain control. Puncture of the blebs with a fine needle or myringotomy knife may provide pain relief, but is not usually recommended. Since only the squamous layer of the tympanic membrane is involved, careful puncture of the blebs will not produce a perforation. Antibiotics (e.g., ampicillin) are of value when a concomitant otitis media is present.

B. **Granular myringitis** is an unusual disease of unknown etiology.

1. **Signs and symptoms.** Symptoms consist of itching, mild pain, and otorrhea. The otorrhea is usually sparse. Symptoms have often been present for many months before the diagnosis is made. The tympanic membrane is covered with granulation tissue that is often obscured by the discharge.

2. **Management** consists of long-term antibiotic steroid drops (4–6 weeks) and weekly cleaning. Broad-spectrum systemic antibiotics, culture-directed, are sometimes beneficial. In resistant cases, operative curetting of the granulation tissue and coverage with split-thickness grafts become a consideration.

3. **Complications.** Untreated cases can give symptoms for years and ultimately may heal by squamous overgrowth, producing a markedly thickened tympanic membrane and mild conductive hearing loss.

C. **Perforations (traumatic)** result from either direct trauma (e.g., cotton-tipped swabs) or pressure transmitted to the closed canal (slap, explosion).

1. **Signs and symptoms** consist of pain, bleeding, a hollow feeling in the ear, and hearing loss. The appearance varies but usually

consists of an irregularly shaped perforation with hemorrhage at the edges. Ossicles and other middle ear structures may be visible through the perforation.

2. **Diagnostic tests.** The initial evaluation must include an audiogram to rule out an associated ossicular discontinuity or sensorineural hearing loss. Associated vertigo warrants immediate attention by a specialist. Temporal bone x rays may be necessary to exclude a temporal bone fracture.

3. **Management.** The uncomplicated traumatic perforation usually heals spontaneously. The rate of healing depends on the size of the perforation. Perforations can heal in a few days or may take weeks to months. Perforations that have not healed after 6 months of observation can be repaired. Antibiotic drops are indicated only if there is contamination of the perforation by water or debris. Systemic antibiotics are not indicated. Pain medication may be necessary for the first few days following a perforation. The patient must observe water precautions (vaseline-impregnated cotton plug) until the perforation has healed and should be followed at regular intervals until healing is complete. An audiogram should be obtained at the beginning and end of treatment. With vertigo and a hearing loss—either sensorineural or conductive—an ossicular disruption or perilymphatic fistula is suspect. Emergent surgery may be necessary in this setting.

D. **Slag burns** are a unique type of traumatic perforation caused by hot metal (slag) burning through the tympanic membrane. These burns are usually seen in welders.

Management. Early operative intervention is indicated to remove the slag from the middle ear and to close the perforation. These perforations rarely heal spontaneously.

E. **Tympanosclerosis.** Tympanosclerosis is a pathologic condition of the tympanic membrane (and occasionally of the middle ear) consisting of chalky white, plaquelike patches occurring at any site within the membrane. The patches consist of hyaline degeneration of the membrane with calcium deposition and usually result from repeated bouts of inflammation. When localized to the eardrum, tympanosclerosis represents a benign condition.

1. **Signs and symptoms.** Hearing loss is not evident unless extensive involvement of the entire tympanic membrane is present. It is differentiated from cholesteatoma by its chalky white, plaquelike appearance as compared to the pearly white, cheesy appearance of cholesteatoma.

2. **Management.** Treatment is not indicated.

VIII. **Diseases of the middle ear and mastoid**

A. **Acute otitis media (suppurative)** is an acute infection involving the middle ear (and mastoid) that is seen in all age groups. It is particularly prevalent in children during the winter months. Acute otitis media often follows or coincides with a viral upper respiratory infection (URI). Children with AIDS (acquired immunodeficiency syndrome) often have recurrent acute otitis media (AOM) as their initial presenting symptom.

1. **Signs and symptoms** consist of an acute onset with variable ear pain, pressure sensation, or hearing loss. Drainage may be present depending on the stage of infection, and the process may be unilateral or bilateral. The stages consist of:

   a. **Hyperemia,** a reddened, thickened tympanic membrane.

   b. **Exudation** with serous fluid in the middle ear space.

   c. **Suppuration** in which the fluid becomes purulent and the tympanic membrane may perforate.

   d. **Resolution** in the uncomplicated case in which the tympanic membrane heals, the fluid becomes thin and serous, finally resolving. Physical findings depend on the stage of disease in which the ear is inspected. Resolution can occur at any stage depending on the virulence of the organism, the host resistance, and antibiotic usage.

2. **Bacteriology.** The most prevalent organisms cultured in acute otitis media are *Streptococcus pneumoniae,* nontypable *Haemophilus influenzae* and, to some extent, *Moraxella catarrhalis. H. influenzae* type B, group A streptococcus, *Staphyloccus aureus,* gram-negative enteric bacillae and anaerobic bacteria are far less prevalent. In infants and neonates, group B streptococcus and *Escherichia coli* assume more import.

3. **Management**

   a. **Antibiotics.** Amoxicillin (30–40 mg/kg/day) is the drug of choice in children under 12 years of age. It has better absorption and fewer side effects than ampicillin, and can be given 3 times/day instead of 4. Treatment should be continued for 10 days at least. In adults, amoxicillin is also the drug of choice. Penicillin-allergic patients should receive trimethoprim-sulfamethoxazole (TMP-SMZ). Up to a 10% failure rate is anticipated for the above medications due to resistant organisms. Frequent examinations are essential, and alternative drug treatment must be considered. These include amoxicillin-clavulanate and oral cefalosporins.

   b. **Myringotomy** is indicated to establish a bacteriologic diagnosis in patients not responding to conventional medication, in those immunosuppressed, in the neonate, and if complications ensue. Pain control should be obtained via medication, narcotics if necessary.

   c. **Topical antibiotics.** Drops may be indicated if there is a perforation or if drainage has produced a secondary external otitis. Decongestant preparations that include antihistamines do not shorten the course of the disease. Vasoconstriction (pseudoephedrine) may alleviate associated symptoms of pressure or the nasal congestion of an upper respiratory infection (URI).

B. **Mastoiditis (acute coalescent).** Mastoiditis is an unusual entity since the advent of antibiotics. Untreated, about 1–5% of cases of acute otitis media progress to mastoiditis. Treated, the incidence is much lower. The pathogenesis involves a blockage of the additus with granulation tissue or swollen mucosa so that free drainage of purulent material cannot occur. This complication leads to pressure in the mastoid cells with breakdown of cell partitions.

1. **Signs and symptoms** include continued pain, low-grade fever, malaise, and hearing loss. Drainage is inconsistently present, but when present has been noted to change from thick, mucopurulent secretions to thinner, foul-smelling secretions. Physical examination reveals a thickened, sometimes bulging tympanic membrane. There is thickening of the mastoid cortex with a somewhat doughy feel, a sagging of the posterosuperior canal wall, and later a protrusion of the ear.

2. **Laboratory data** include an elevated white blood count (WBC) with a left shift. X rays show breakdown of the normal cell partitions of the mastoid, best demonstrated on CT. (It should be noted that in acute otitis media with effusion, x rays will show **clouding** of the mastoid. This clouding should not be confused with acute mastoiditis, because it represents fluid in the mastoid cells, not cell breakdown.)

3. **Management.** Unless an abscess is present, the management includes a myringotomy to decompress the middle ear and provide for culture and sensitivity. Pending culture-directed specificity, an acceptable initial choice of antibiotic for intravenous usage is ceftriaxone, which covers most pathogens. If the process does not resolve, a complete (cortical, simple) mastoidectomy should be performed.

C. **Complications of acute otitis media.** With the exception of mastoiditis, complications can occur at any stage of acute otitis media. Whether or not complications occur depends on the virulence of the organism, the resistance of the host, anatomic abnormalities, and the institution of appropriate antibacterial therapy. The complications can be divided into:

1. **Otologic complications.** Petrositis, labyrinthitis, and facial paralysis.

2. **Intracranial complications.** Meningitis, epidural abscess, subdural abscess, brain abscess, and sigmoid sinus thrombosis. It should be noted that otitis media is still the most common cause of meningitis (excluding meningococcus) and is the most common cause of brain abscess.

3. **Treatment** consists of managing the complication and directing attention to the otitis media. A myringotomy is indicated to establish bacteriologic specificity. Facial nerve paralysis usually resolves spontaneously after adequate treatment of the otitis media. All of these complications, of course, constitute medical emergencies.

D. Acute necrotizing otitis media. This unusual form of otitis media occurs most frequently in children with severe systemic disease (e.g., measles).

1. **Signs and symptoms.** In a few hours, a large perforation develops and may be associated with destruction of the ossicles. The perforation is frequently kidney shaped. The organism involved is most often beta-hemolytic streptococcus, although *S. pneumonia* has been cultured.

2. **Treatment** consists of high doses of a semisynthetic penicillin. Secondary operative repair of the perforation must await the appropriate age in children (>10 years).

E. Eustachian tube dysfunction. Eustachian tube dysfunction has a wide clinical spectrum from very mild to chronic otitis media, as described below.

1. **Signs and symptoms.** The mildest symptoms consist of a blocked or hollow feeling, pressure, mild otalgia, and occasional crackling or popping noises in the ear. These often accompany a URI or allergy.

2. **Diagnosis.** Otologic examination is normal except that the drum moves sluggishly or not at all during a Valsalva maneuver. Tympanometry may reveal a flattened curve or negative pressure. Audiologic examination is normal.

3. **Management.** These mild symptoms are self-limiting in most patients. Antihistamines and decongestants may help in lessening the symptoms but not their duration. If the symptoms are allergy-related, the underlying cause should be treated. Repeated Valsalva maneuvers may alleviate the symptoms.

F. Hyperpatent (patulous) eustachian tube is usually seen in patients who have undergone a rapid weight loss or suffer from disorders of muscle wasting. Estrogen has also been associated with the syndrome.

1. **Signs and symptoms** may be much the same as with eustachian tube dysfunction—a "hollow" or "stopped-up" sensation and pressure. Patients often state that they can hear their own breathing. Short periods of recumbency relieve the symptoms temporarily.

2. **Diagnosis** is made by observing the tympanic membrane while the patient occludes one nostril and breathes with the mouth closed. The drum will move with respiration.

3. **Management** consists of treating (or removing) the underlying cause (such as birth control medications). With persistent symptoms, tympanotomy tube insertion may give relief. Teflon injections near the eustachian tube orifice are now used infrequently. Rarely, however, is this disorder a persistent problem.

G. Otitis media with effusion (OME). OME describes a nonpurulent effusion in the middle ear space. The fluid varies from thin to mucoid. Mucoid fluid usually signifies a more chronic process. The fluid is secondary to obstruction of the eustachian tube. Defining the cause of the obstruction is indicated prior to initiating therapy whenever possible. The varied etiologies include inflammation (bacterial, viral, allergic), congenital malformation, polyps or tumors of the nasopharynx, hypertrophied adenoids, cleft palate, radiation, endocrine, or iatrogenic. Serous fluid is commonly seen in the resolution stage of acute otitis media. OME is the most common cause of hearing loss in children. It is less frequent in the adult and, when seen, the nasopharynx should be carefully evaluated for malignancy.

1. **Signs and symptoms.** The tympanic membrane may appear normal. Usually it is slightly retracted even in early onset. Fluid, with or without bubbles, may be seen and may be amber in color. With thicker fluid, the amber color is not prevalent, and the drum is dull. Prominence of the vessels is not infrequent, but in contrast to acute otitis media, the margins are distinct.

2. **Diagnostic tests.** Pneumatic otoscopy reveals diminished or no movement of the tympanic membrane. Tuning fork tests and audiometry usually reveal a conductive hearing loss. Conductive loss on audiometry should not exceed 30–40 dB with serous otitis media.

3. **Management**

   a. In older children autoinflation and politzerization of the eustachian tube are possible, sometimes effecting resolution. If the fluid results from a resolving otitis media, the process is usually self-limiting, 90% in 3 months. Decongestants and antihistamines have not proved to be effective management for OME. Recognizing that a small percentage of serous effusions contain bacteria or may be associated with nasopharyngeal or eustachian tube infection, often a 6- to 8-week therapeutic trial of an antibiotic (amoxicillin or TMP-SMZ) is warranted. Pressure-equalizing (PE) tubes (ventilation tubes) are indicated in refractory cases to alleviate hearing loss and arrest development of permanent tympanic membrane and ossicle malfunction. Adenoidectomy is probably beneficial in selected instances of recurrent OME and acute otitis media.

   b. For adults an underlying cause should be determined if possible. CT scans of the nasopharynx and sinuses are indicated to rule out infection or tumor. With a suggestive history, an allergy evaluation is indicated. Myringotomy with or without tube insertion may be indicated in selected instances.

H. **Barotrauma (aerotitis).** Barotrauma results from a change in atmospheric pressure with an occluded eustachian tube. This usually occurs during scuba diving or during descent when flying.

   1. **Signs and symptoms** include pressure, pain (often severe), and hearing loss. Often, there is a concurrent URI or other cause of eustachian tube congestion. Examination reveals a dull drum

with fluid behind it. The fluid may be bloody. Hemorrhagic areas in the tympanic membrane are frequent. Tuning fork tests and audiometric evaluation usually define a conductive hearing loss.

2. **Management.** The fluid can take several weeks to clear. Simple decongestants may alleviate the pressure sensation. Mild analgesia may be necessary in the acute phase. Instruction in pressure-equalizing techniques (Valsalva; gum chewing; prophylactic vasoconstrictors, both oral and nasal) is warranted to prevent further episodes. Pressure change with severe nasal congestion should be avoided.

I. **Chronic otitis media.** As opposed to acute otitis media, chronic otitis media is a surgical disease in most instances. While the name suggests a lengthy process, it would be more accurate to say that irreversible changes in the middle ear or mastoid have taken place. Depending on the process, the disease can be either **dangerous** (implying an extending process) or **benign.** A chronic perforation that is dry and noninflamed is an example of a benign process, as is chronic adhesive otitis media, in which fibrous tissue has replaced a chronic inflammatory process. Cholesteatoma, on the other hand, is an example of a potentially dangerous process. In this disease, squamous epithelium enters the middle ear and mastoid and expands, causing bony erosion. This entrapped skin may become infected, which hastens the erosive process and can spread to surrounding structures (labyrinth, meninges, sigmoid sinus, brain, facial nerve).

1. **Signs and symptoms** may be noticeably absent in chronic ear disease. Pain is unusual, except when there is active acute infection. Discharge may be present and intermittent. Hearing loss is inconsistent. The presenting complaint may be a complication (e.g., vertigo or facial nerve paralysis) without any noted prior history of ear disease. Physical examination may reveal a perforation or cholesteatoma. A cholesteatoma in this setting is most often identified in the pars flaccida (attic) and may be obscured by a crust. There may be an associated discharge, which must be removed for the correct diagnosis to be made.

2. **Diagnostic tests**

   a. **Audiometry** can identify a mild to marked hearing loss, usually conductive or mixed, depending on the extent of destruction.

   b. **CT scanning** of the temporal bone can identify bony destruction in the attic and mastoid area.

3. **Management** consists initially of treatment of any associated acute infection with both systemic antibiotics (culture appropriate) and topical antibiotic drops. Subsequent surgery is often required. Evidence of a complication such as vertigo, facial nerve paralysis, or brain abscess requires immediate intervention by an otolaryngologist.

J. Tuberculous otitis media is more frequent in children, but may occur in any age group. It can occur with or without evidence of pulmonary or other site involvement.

1. **Signs and symptoms** consist of drainage from the ear and occasional lymphadenopathy. Pain is not common, but hearing loss is frequent. Early in the disease, the tympanic membrane appears grayish-yellow. Tuberculous otitis media usually progresses to **multiple perforations.**

2. **Diagnosis** is made by acid-fast smear and culture.

3. **Management** is first medical, with antituberculous drugs; and second, surgery with repair of the tympanic membrane and ossicular chain after the infection has been completely eradicated. HIV infection should be excluded.

K. Syphilis can mimic tuberculosis in the clinical appearance of the ear.

1. **Signs and symptoms.** In addition to the signs and symptoms in **J.1.**, a fluctuating sensorineural hearing loss and vertigo may be present in both the tertiary and congenital forms (see **IX.A.3.c.**). An osteitis of the ossicles is present.

2. **Diagnostic tests.** Diagnosis is made either by darkfield examination of the exudate or by serologic tests.

3. **Management** consists of treatment of the syphilis with penicillin or steroids or both.

L. Conductive hearing loss. In addition to the processes mentioned in **VI–VIII,** certain disease entities cause conductive hearing losses. The remainder of the examination is usually normal.

1. **Otosclerosis** involves fixation of the stapes by the otosclerotic process and is most often bilateral.

   a. **Signs and symptoms.** This entity presents as a progressive hearing loss, conductive in nature. A family history of hearing loss is often present. Females are more frequently affected than males (2.5 : 1.0). The remainder of the examination is normal.

   b. **Treatment** consists of surgical replacement of the fixed stapes or the use of a hearing aid.

2. **Other ossicular fixations** can occur as congenital aberrations from inflammation or trauma. The diagnosis is made at the time of surgical exploration.

M. Tumors

1. **Malignant.** As with the auricle, squamous cell carcinoma and basal cell carcinoma can involve the middle ear, either primarily or by extension from surrounding structures. Malignant parotid tumors can likewise involve the temporal bone. Metastatic disease to the temporal bone has been reported.

   a. **Signs and symptoms** include pain and drainage (from secondary infection) that is sometimes bloody. Since these tumors are often associated with chronically draining ears, pain in these patients should raise the suspicion of malignancy and lead to biopsy.

   b. **Other malignant tumors, lymphomas, and rhabdomyosarcomas** infrequently involve the ear, and then usually in a younger age group.

2. **Benign tumors**

   a. **Polyps** can protrude through a perforation and imply a chronically infected area.

     (1) **Symptoms** are usually those of a draining ear.

     (2) **Treatment** consists of topical antibiotic and steroid drops. Polyps should not be pulled out, because they can be attached to middle ear structures. However, judicious surgical removal may aid in the diagnosis and also can enhance drainage and, thereby, treatment. A polyp frequently results from an underlying chronic otitis media and should be evaluated as noted above (see **I.**).

   b. **Glomus tympanicum and jugulare (chemodectomas).** These tumors usually arise from paraganglionic cells in the tympanic plexus of the middle ear. Glomus jugulare tumors are chemodectomas arising from the jugular bulb.

     (1) **Signs and symptoms** are that of a stuffy feeling, hearing loss, and typically a pulsating tinnitus. On physical examination, a bluish mass is visible behind an intact tympanic membrane.

     (2) **Diagnostic tests.** Plain radiographs may reveal bony destruction. Angiography, contrast study CT scans, or MRI scans can demonstrate the lesion.

     (3) **Management** primarily consists of surgical extirpation. Biopsy is usually contraindicated since the tumors are very vascular. Radiation therapy or embolization should be considered in large tumors.

   c. **Congenital cholesteatoma** is a misnomer, in that these "tumors" are formed from embryonic cell rests of ectoderm and may involve any area of the temporal bone.

     (1) **Signs and symptoms** depend on the size of the lesion and the area involved. Usually, a white mass is identified behind an intact tympanic membrane in children. In adults, congenital petrous apex cholesteatomas can present with hearing loss or facial paralysis.

     (2) **Management** is surgical.

IX. Diseases of the inner ear. Diseases of the inner ear may involve the cochlea, producing sensorineural hearing loss, or the vestibule, producing vertigo, or both. Some disease processes described below are assigned arbitrarily to one system or another, even though both systems may be involved.

A. Diseases of the cochlea

1. **Sudden hearing loss (idiopathic sudden deafness).** The syndrome known as sudden hearing loss (SHL) can be defined as the sudden onset of a sensorineural hearing loss without preexisting ear pathology or another accountable etiology. To establish a diagnosis of SHL, known etiologies for acute sensorineural deafness must be excluded. The more common etiologies are listed below.

   a. **Infection.** Mumps, herpes zoster, CMV, meningitis, encephalitis, syphilis, otitis media.

   b. **Trauma.** Head injury (with or without fracture), noise trauma, barotrauma.

   c. **Vascular.** Embolism, coagulopathy, cerebrovascular accident.

   d. **Otologic.** Ménière's disease, acoustic neuroma, perilymph fistula, cholesteatoma.

   e. **Other.** Multiple sclerosis, malignant tumor (metastatic or primary), drug toxicity, Cogan's syndrome (hearing loss associated with nonsyphilitic interstitial keratitis), diabetes, autoimmune disorders. Idiopathic SHL is most often unilateral, but may be bilateral in a small number of cases. Controversy exists as to its etiology, but viruses and vascular syndromes are most often postulated.

      (1) **Signs and symptoms.** The patient typically gives a history of an abrupt onset of hearing loss over a period of minutes to hours. Depending on the severity and rapidity of onset, associated symptoms may be vague. Tinnitus often accompanies the loss. Pain is virtually never present. Vertigo, usually brief in duration, occurs in a significant number of patients. The otologic examination is negative except for the hearing loss.

      (2) **Diagnostic tests.** Audiometric testing typically shows a sensory loss, cochlear in origin, that ranges from mild to severe. Calorics and ENG may reveal a canal paresis but may also be normal. ABR confirms the cochlear nature of the hearing loss. Radiographs are helpful in excluding other causes of hearing loss (cholesteatoma, acoustic neuroma), but are normal in SHL. Other laboratory data may be normal. The sedimentation rate can be elevated.

      (3) **Management.** Recovery typically occurs in 50–60% of patients. Young patients with mild hearing loss, particularly in those who have less loss in the higher frequencies (upward sloping loss), have a better prognosis. Recent evidence indicates that if the patient is seen within 24 hours of the onset of SHL, high-dose steroids (60 mg prednisone/day), tapered over a 2-week period, can improve the recovery rate.

2. **Noise-induced hearing loss.** Exposure to extreme noise can diminish the ear's capacity to detect pure tones. This change can be temporary or permanent.

   a. **Temporary threshold shifts**

   (1) **Short-term masking** lasts a fraction of a second. It is thought to be due to the refractory period of nerve fibers after discharge. The tone most affected is the tone of the "noise," up to a level of input of 70 dB. Above 90 dB, a tone half an octave above the noise is the tone that is most affected. Recovery is swift, being exponential in time, and is independent of the length of the inducing noise.

   (2) **Ordinary temporary threshold shifts** last usually more than 2 minutes, but less than 16 hours. The threshold shift increases linearly with intensity above a level of 70–75 dB. Below 70–75 dB no threshold shift is seen, even with indefinite exposure. High frequencies produce a greater response than low frequencies, with the greatest sensitivity at 3000 Hz. Maximum shift is seen at a frequency half an octave above the present noise. Therefore, the greatest effects to broad-band noise will be seen at frequencies between 4000 and 6000 Hz.

   If exposure is intermittent, the effect is the same as that seen for the mean exposure level over that time period. As the quiet intervals between noise exposure lengthen, partial recovery occurs and may lead to an underestimation of the noise effects that are actually seen. The above reasoning does not hold well for impulse noise either. These effects seem to be poorly predicted at present due to difficulty in quantifying the impulse parameters.

   (3) **Prolonged temporary threshold shifts.** If a threshold shift of greater than 40 dB is produced, recovery is neither complete in 16 hours nor exponential. Instead, recovery is linear and may require days to weeks before full recovery occurs.

   (4) **Permanent threshold shift.** When noise exposure is loud and long enough, complete recovery does not occur, leaving a permanent threshold shift in pure tone perception. Whether this is due to a buildup of minor traumas or to a few major events is still debatable. In one of the few studies attempting to deal with this complex problem, Passchies and Vermeer have shown that exposure for 8 hours/day for 5 days/week for 10 years, at levels of 80–90 dB, results in a permanent shift in hearing thresholds, the effect being greatest at 4000 Hz and proportional to the level of exposure. This finding correlates with the 4000-Hz notch typically associated with noise-induced hearing loss. Recruitment and paracusia, signs of cochlear injury, often accompany the losses and worsen the disability. More annoying to many is the tinnitus that also occurs.

b. **Pathology.** Noise trauma is associated with outer hair cell injury (see **I.A.5.**). This injury can range from simple disruption of the stereocilia to total hair cell loss or disruption of the organ of Corti. The exact mechanism of injury is still unsettled, with the line between temporary and permanent shifts far from clear. With exposure to a sudden loud noise, the response seems to be mechanical; however, with long-term exposure, two theories have been proposed.

(1) **Mechanical theory.** Long-term exposure is accompanied by episodes of occasional loud noise leading to intermittent loss of hair cells. The loss gradually accumulates to a significant level.

(2) **Chemical theory.** Long-term exposure is accompanied by gradual buildup of toxic metabolites or depletion of required chemicals necessary for maintenance of cell function and viability. Ischemia may be a contributing factor. Hyperlipidemia both in children and adults increases the cumulative negative effect of noise exposure. The triad of hyperlipidemia, hypertension, and noise exposure has an additive deleterious effect, which is probably vascular in origin.

Regardless of which theory is used, the focal point is the hair cell, with the outer hair cells being affected before the inner hair cells.

c. **Management.** Treatment necessitates reduction in noise exposure below the level that causes permanent threshold shifts. This reduction may be difficult to attain. Commercial earplugs may be of value if a noisy environment cannot be avoided. Specially designed acoustic plugs for musicians, which give better balance to the sound reduction, are available. Patients must be made aware of the negative impact of hyperlipidemia and hypertension with continued noise exposure. Treatment of these associated conditions should be instituted. As for treatment of an already existing hearing loss, little except hearing aid amplification and lip reading is of benefit.

3. **Inflammation**

a. **Bacterial.** Sensorineural hearing loss due to bacterial infections can be the result of either direct bacterial invasion or of diffusion of bacterial toxins into the inner ear. Bacteria can invade via the bloodstream, CSF, cochlear aqueduct (channel connecting CSF to perilymphatic space), internal auditory canal, or directly through the middle ear. This invasion can produce a serous or suppurative labyrinthitis.

(1) **Serous labyrinthitis** is caused by a diffusion of bacterial toxins into the inner ear, producing an inflammatory response.

(a) **Signs and symptoms** are those of a sensorineural hearing loss and vertigo. A marked nystagmus and sensorineural loss are found on physical examination. Serous labyrinthitis is usually associated with an acute otitis media or chronic otitis media with acute infection.

(b) **Management** should include IV antibiotics such as ampicillin in high doses, myringotomy to promote drainage and to obtain culture, surgical removal of chronically infected tissue, or all three, when appropriate. A partial to full recovery of the inner ear function is possible if treatment is prompt.

(2) Suppurative labyrinthitis

(a) **Signs and symptoms.** The symptoms and physical findings are the same as with serous labyrinthitis, except that the patient is more toxic and the hearing loss is profound. WBC is elevated with a left shift.

(b) **Treatment** is the same as with serous labyrinthitis and is directed to prevent the spread of infection to adjacent structures (meninges, brain). An antibiotic with less bacterial resistance than ampicillin, such as ceftizomine, should be considered in this setting. Recovery of hearing does not occur.

(3) Chronic otitis media. Mild to moderate sensorineural hearing loss can occur with low-grade infection due to diffusion of bacterial toxins through the round, or oval, window into the cochlea. The vestibule is not involved.

(a) **Signs and symptoms** are a slowly progressive sensorineural hearing loss (with or without a superimposed conductive loss due to destruction of the ossicles).

(b) **Treatment** is as for chronic otitis media, to produce a safe, dry ear (see **VIII.I.**).

b. Viral. Mumps, rubella, rubeola, varicella, influenza, herpes zoster, cytomegalovirus, adenovirus, and others have been shown to produce a sensorineural hearing loss through invasion of the inner ear. Effective management is through vaccination programs; however, steroids may have efficacy in the acute situation. Several of the viruses are important enough to deserve special mention.

(1) Mumps is the most common cause of unilateral sensorineural hearing loss in children. Rarely does it cause bilateral loss.

(2) Rubella produces a symmetric, bilateral loss, greatest in the higher frequencies.

(3) Herpes zoster (Ramsay Hunt syndrome) produces burning aural pain, vesicular eruptions in the external canal and concha, and sensorineural hearing loss. Vertigo and facial paralysis are often associated with the infection. Early treatment of patients with acyclovir and prednisone has markedly improved the prognosis for return of facial nerve function.

c. **Granulomatous diseases. Syphilis** can cause sensorineural hearing loss in either the congenital or acquired form. In either case, there is a mononuclear cell infiltration of the inner ear, leading to an obliterative endarteritis. A progressive endolymphatic hydrops is also seen.

   (1) **Signs and symptoms** include a fluctuating hearing loss and episodic vertigo. Tinnitus is also present. The symptoms, therefore, mimic Ménière's disease. In the congenital form, pathologies such as Hutchinson's teeth and saber shins may be present. A conductive component of the hearing loss may be present if there is an associated osteitis.

   (2) **Diagnosis.** Examination of the ear may be normal. The diagnosis is confirmed by a positive FTA-ABS serology. (A negative VDRL or RPR card test cannot exclude the diagnosis.)

   (3) **Management** is long-term therapy with penicillin and systemic steroids. The length of treatment is debatable. Treatment can stop the progression of the hearing loss and, in some cases, afford partial recovery. Vertigo may continue despite therapy and should be treated with meclizine, Dramamine, or similar medications.

4. **Trauma**

   a. **Temporal bone fractures** can be classified as longitudinal, transverse, or mixed, depending on their angle to the axis of the temporal bone.

      (1) **Longitudinal** fractures produce a conductive hearing loss and are discussed in Chapter 1.

      (2) **Transverse** fractures occur in about 15% of temporal bone fractures and are usually caused by a blow to the occiput. The fracture line extends from the foramen magnum across the petrous apex and through the internal auditory canal. The eustachian tube or jugular foramen is often involved.

         (a) **Signs and symptoms.** A direct fracture of the inner ear is common, producing a profound sensorineural hearing loss and vertigo. The tympanic membrane is often intact. Facial nerve paralysis occurs in about 50% of these injuries.

         (b) **Management** consists of decompression and, if necessary, reapproximation of the facial nerve. The hearing loss is irreversible. Vertigo is treated by bed rest, meclizine, Dramamine, or diazepam.

      (3) **Mixed** fractures are the most frequent types of injury and can produce any symptoms noted previously as well as other neurologic abnormalities.

         Management depends on the extent of injuries.

(4) Labyrinthine concussion. Closed head injuries can cause sensorineural hearing loss by sudden deceleration and rapid alteration of the hydrodynamics of the inner ear. In rare cases, the seventh cranial nerve may be sheared. Vertigo may be present along with the hearing loss.

Management is directed at control of vertigo through anti-vertiginous drugs (meclizine, Dramamine, or diazepam).

5. **Nonorganic hearing loss.** A decrease in hearing not associated with organic changes may be deliberate (malingering) or not. The ability to verify this type of hearing loss is directly correlated with the audiologist's suspicions and ingenuity in testing the subject. Several types of testing are available.

   a. **Stenger.** A tone is presented to the better ear at a level 10 dB above threshold, so that the subject responds 100% of the time. A tone is then simultaneously presented to the poorer ear, starting at 0 dB and gradually increasing. The level at which the patient ceases to respond or notes a change to the better hearing ear should be 10–20 dB above the measured threshold of the poorer ear.

   b. **Delayed feedback.** The patient reads a paragraph. His voice is played back with a short delay (0.15–0.18 seconds) at a decibel level below the measured threshold. He will become confused or slow down his reading if the actual threshold is below the level of the playback.

   c. **Swinging voice test.** A story is read to the patient with key words entering only one ear at a time. The patient is then tested for comprehension.

   d. **Auditory brainstem response (ABR).** This test is an objective recording of auditory-evoked brainstem responses. The accuracy of this test in determining hearing thresholds is well established and it should be considered definitive in diagnosing a nonorganic loss.

   e. **Management** in malingering consists only of establishing normal thresholds with ABR. When a nonorganic loss lacks a conscious component, psychiatric evaluation is necessary to determine and to treat the underlying cause.

6. **Endocrine**

   a. **Diabetes** causes diffuse vascular changes throughout the body, and the inner ear is no exception.

      (1) Signs and symptoms. A bilateral progressive sensorineural hearing loss greater in the higher frequencies often accompanies diabetes. Sudden hearing loss has also been reported. Vertigo may be present. No correlation exists between the duration or severity of the diabetes and the severity of the hearing loss. It is not known if better control of the blood sugar levels decreases progression of the hearing loss.

(2) Management consists of amplification when necessary.

b. Thyroid

Myxedema. Hypothyroidism causes an increase in acid mucopolysaccharide accumulation. Hyperthyroidism has not been associated with hearing loss.

(1) Signs and symptoms. If acid mucopolysaccharide deposition occurs in the eustachian tube or middle ear, a serous otitis with a conductive hearing loss ensues. The evolution of the sensorineural component remains unclear.

(2) Management consists of thyroid hormone replacement, which in some instances partially reverses the hearing loss.

7. Congenital

a. Hereditary. Genetic causes of sensorineural hearing loss can be grouped in many ways to emphasize associated organ systems involved, mode of inheritance, or pathologic changes.

(1) Mode of inheritance. Defects are either dominant, recessive, X-linked, or involve quantitative changes in chromosomal material. The type of hearing loss seems to show some relationship to the mode of inheritance.

(a) Dominant syndromes usually show flat hearing losses and may be progressive throughout one's life. Their penetrance is variable, leading to a large range of disabilities. Examples are Waardenburg's disease, Schäfer's syndrome, Huntington's chorea, and von Recklinghausen's disease.

(b) Recessive syndromes tend to show loss of hearing greater in high frequencies with some retention of low-frequency hearing. They tend not to be associated with other congenital lesions and not to be progressive throughout life. Examples are Hurler's syndrome, Morquio's syndrome, Tay-Sachs disease, Wilson's disease, and Usher's syndrome.

(c) X-linked syndromes are less common. There seems to be retention of hearing at all frequencies (Hunter's and orofacial digital I syndrome).

(d) Quantitative changes in chromosomal material are evident in the **trisomy syndromes.** These syndromes tend to have severe hearing loss associated with multiple organ defects, such as trisomy 13 and trisomy 18.

(2) Associated organ system. See *Genetic and Metabolic Deafness* by Konigsmark and Gorlin.

(3) **Pathologic changes.** Temporal bone studies show that the pathologic correlates in congenital hearing loss can range from submicroscopic lesions not visible by present methods of study to total agenesis. Several abnormal patterns of developments seem to occur more frequently.

(a) **Scheibe's deformity.** There is a normal bony labyrinth, a normal utricle and semicircular canals, and a limited development of the stria vascularis with few hair cells and support cells in the organ of Corti. Reissner's membrane is collapsed on the stria and organ of Corti.

(b) **Mondini deformity.** Vestibular structures may be underdeveloped. Only the basal coil of the cochlea is developed with the mid- and apical turns incomplete, making the cochlea only about one and one-half turns. The saccule and endolymphatic sac are dilated.

(c) **Michel's deformity.** There is a total lack of development of the inner ear.

b. **Acquired.** There are many causes of congenital hearing loss that are not genetic in origin. Below is a list of the most common.

(1) **Rubella (German measles).** When contracted by the mother during the first trimester of pregnancy, rubella causes a group of defects. Temporal bone studies show anything from complete agenesis to the more common Mondini deformity. There is degeneration of the membranous portion of the cochlea and saccule. The hearing loss is usually asymmetric between ears, with a flat audiogram. Other associated anomalies include mental retardation, microcephaly, cardiac defects (usually patent ductus arteriosis), dental defects, and congenital cataracts.

(2) **Erythroblastosis fetalis.** Lesions in this condition are thought to be due to a high bilirubin level and can be prevented by keeping the level low with exchange transfusions and ultraviolet lighting. The loss often occurs in higher frequencies and may relate to changes in the cochlea. Mental retardation and cerebral palsy are also associated with this condition.

(3) **Thyroid disease (cretinism).** A mixed sensorineural and conductive loss is present in cretin children. The middle ear can be quite deformed, without significant change in the inner ear. Mental and physical growth are also retarded.

(4) **Birth injury.** Birth injury includes prematurity, hypoxia, prolonged labor, toxemia of pregnancy, and anesthesia.

The hearing loss, when present, is usually bilateral, symmetric, and mainly in the higher frequencies.

(5) Drugs. The effects of most ototoxic drugs given to the pregnant mother are not known; however, two drugs— thalidomide and quinine—have had unfortunate clinical trials. Thalidomide can produce any type of inner ear lesion, and quinine usually produces a bilateral deafness.

(6) Meningitis can produce a mild to profound hearing loss due to spread of infection to the labyrinth, producing a labyrinthitis.

(7) Management should be directed at early diagnosis and appropriate amplification and education. Evoked response audiometry can establish a diagnosis early in life and enhance the chances for a child attaining full potential. Cochlear implantation appears to hold promise for children 2 years of age and older with profound sensorineural hearing loss.

8. Presbycusis is a loss of the ability to perceive or discriminate sounds due to the aging process. It is the most common cause of hearing loss in humans. The audiometric pattern is dependent on the type or combination of types of presbycusis present.

Discrimination may or may not be significantly impaired. The diagnosis is based on purely clinical grounds, mainly by the exclusion of all other possible causes of hearing loss. Positive proof of the diagnosis is found only at autopsy with temporal bone sections. Changes in the middle ear are known to occur with aging. The tympanic membrane thickens and the ossicular joints can undergo arthritic changes. There is no evidence, however, that these alterations have a significant effect on hearing. There are at least four histologic variants in the inner ear and its neuronal connections that alone or in combination seem to explain the audiometric findings of presbycusis.

a. Sensory. Characterized by atrophy of the organ of Corti in the basal end of the cochlea with loss of hair cells and support cells. There is also neural degeneration, which is thought to be secondary to hair cell loss. The audiogram shows a loss of hearing in the high frequencies—4000–8000 Hz.

b. Neural. Due to loss of neurons in the cochlear nerve, especially in the basal turn. Minimum loss in the pure tones is noted, but marked loss of discrimination is present.

c. Strial atrophy caused by atrophy of the stria vascularis. While this atrophy is greatest at the apical end, the loss is equal for all frequencies because the endolymph is distributed throughout the cochlea.

d. Cochlear conductive. Atrophy of the spiral ligament alters the shape of the cochlear duct, leading to loss of hearing. This degeneration is greatest at the basal end and progresses to the apical end. The audiogram shows a straight line loss greatest at the higher frequencies.

e. **Management** consists of careful evaluation and appropriate amplification.

9. **Ototoxicity.** Toxic effects on the inner ear have been observed with a wide variety of therapeutic and chemical agents. Aminoglycoside antibiotics, chloramphenicol, erythromycin, ethacrynic acid, furosemide, salicylates, and quinine are but a few drugs in common usage that produce ototoxicity. In addition, chemotherapeutic agents used in the treatment of cancer (e.g., nitrogen mustard and cisplatinum) can be toxic to the inner ear. The toxicity usually includes both the cochlea and vestibule, but in some drugs one effect may precede the other. The effects may be temporary (salicylates, ethacrynic acid) or permanent (aminoglycosides) and, in most patients, are directly related to the blood levels of the agent. In some instances, two agents given together may produce more severe ototoxicity than blood levels of either agent might suggest (e.g., aminoglycoside and furosemide).

a. **Signs and symptoms** are usually that of tinnitus, vertigo, or unsteadiness and hearing loss. Since most of these agents are used in the extremely ill, the symptoms can be easily overlooked.

b. **Diagnosis.** Examination reveals normal canals and drums. Nystagmus may be present. Tuning fork testing is consistent with a sensorineural hearing loss. The diagnosis can be confirmed by serial audiograms and vestibular testing that shows progression of the loss.

c. **Management.** Prevention is the only management. Serum levels of ototoxic drugs should be carefully monitored, when appropriate, and the patient questioned frequently about ototoxic symptoms. Ototoxic drugs, particularly aminoglycosides, should not be used if another less toxic agent will produce similar therapeutic results.

10. **Autoimmune hearing loss.** Progressive sensorineural hearing loss that occurs over a period of months may have an autoimmune etiology.

a. **Signs and symptoms.** The pattern of loss is that of bilateral progressive sensorineural hearing loss. The loss is commonly asymmetric and may fluctuate. The trend, however, is a fairly rapid loss unassociated with any obvious etiology.

b. **Associated symptoms** may include those found in many autoimmune disorders, including myalgias, arthralgias, dry eyes, and dry mouth, to name a few.

c. **Diagnostic tests.** An autoimmune hearing loss is considered when faced with a progressive sensorineural hearing loss. An elevated sedimentation rate, positive antinuclear antibodies, positive rheumatoid factor, and positive lupus erythematosus (LE) prep all give supportive evidence for the entity, but are not specific or sensitive. More sophisticated laboratory tests are being developed to bridge the diagnostic gap.

    d. Treatment for autoimmune hearing loss involves the use of high-dose steroids. The exact dosage and duration of treatment are still being evaluated. Treatment for 1–3 months is not uncommon. Chemotherapeutic agents are also being evaluated to prevent deafness in patients who cannot tolerate long-term steroid therapy or who fail to respond to steroids.

  11. For profound hearing losses, traditional management has always centered on hearing aids and rehabilitation utilizing the other senses. Cochlear implants have now added to this rehabilitation armamentarium. Cochlear implants can give patients environmental awareness and, at times, an understanding of sounds. They are presently approved for children over 2 years of age and for adults. Future developments may allow for their use in less severely handicapping losses and for younger children.

B. Diseases of the vestibular system (vertigo)

  1. Signs and symptoms. Dizziness is an extremely frequent complaint. In evaluating this symptom, it is first necessary to identify those patients in whom dizziness is a symptom of a vestibular disorder. Careful questioning is often necessary. Vertigo is defined as a sensation of motion when no motion is present and almost always indicates disease of the vestibular system. The motion may be described as the patient moving or his or her environment moving. When motion is not noted by the patient, both vestibular and nonvestibular causes of dizziness may be accountable. Some of the more common nonvestibular causes of dizziness are listed below:

    a. Eye disorders (refractive, muscle imbalance)

    b. Hypotension (postural and nonpostural)

    c. Anemia

    d. Syncope

    e. Hypoglycemia

    f. Paroxysmal atrial tachycardia

    g. Heart block

    h. Drug-induced causes (barbiturates, tranquilizers)

    i. Psychogenic

    j. Hyperventilation

  2. Peripheral versus central vertigo. The history can be very helpful in distinguishing peripheral vertigo (diseases of the end organ) from central vertigo (e.g., eighth cranial nerve, brainstem vestibular nuclei, medial longitudinal fasciculus, cerebellum, vestibulospinal tract). Although not completely foolproof, the characteristics outlined below are helpful:

	Peripheral	**Central**
Severity	Most often very severe with associated nausea and vomiting	Less severe, usually no nausea or vomiting
Hearing loss	Often present	Seldom present (except with acoustic neuromas)
Tinnitus	Often present	Seldom present (except with acoustic neuromas)
Nystagmus	Horizontal (if present)	Horizontal or vertical (if present)

3. History

a. Distinguish true vertigo (the illusion or sensation of whirling or falling) from syncope, disequilibrium, or lightheadedness. Does the patient have a sensation of motion or of objects moving about him or her? Associated illness or incident (e.g., URI, otitis media, during airplane descent or exertion).

b. Characteristics of attacks:

(1) Episodic or continuous

(2) Onset and duration (minutes, hours, days)

(3) Severity (nausea, vomiting, ataxia)

(4) Vertigo with nausea and vomiting is most likely end organ disease in the absence of acute central nervous system (CNS) problems.

(5) Aura or prodroma (e.g., tinnitus, fullness, hearing loss)

(6) Course (subsiding, unchanged, worsening)

c. Associated symptoms

(1) Hearing loss or fluctuation

(2) Tinnitus

(3) Otalgia or otorrhea

(4) Facial palsy

d. Presence or absence of symptoms of central nervous system diseases, including loss of consciousness, sensory deficits, convulsions, confusion, memory loss, dysphagia, paralysis, or history of head trauma.

e. Drugs. A number of agents, such as anticonvulsants, alcohol, salicylates, sedatives, tranquilizers, and certain antibiotics, can induce vestibular toxicity.

4. Physical examination

a. Complete head and neck examination, including the nose, paranasal sinuses, pharynx, oral structures, and larynx. The neck, orbits, mastoids, and temporal squamae are sim-

Table 2-2. Common disorders producing acute attacks of vertigo

Vestibular etiology
   "Physiologic" (e.g., motion sickness, height vertigo)
   Vestibular neuronitis (acute peripheral vestibulopathy)
   Labyrinthitis
   Ménière's syndrome
   Labyrinthine imbalance
   Posttraumatic vertigo
   Perilymphatic fistula
Central etiology
   Brainstem transient ischemic attacks
   Multiple sclerosis
   Basilar artery migraine
   Posterior fossa tumors

Source: M. A. Samuels, *Manual of Neurology.* 4th ed. Boston: Little, Brown, 1991.

ilarly auscultated for bruits. The postauricular area, auricle, external auditory canal, and tympanic membrane are carefully inspected. Cerumen is removed to adequately examine the external canal and tympanic membrane. Discharging ears should be appropriately cultured.

Pneumatic otoscopy aids in identifying perforations, granulomas, and middle ear pathology. If there is evidence of a perforation, previous surgery, head trauma, or barotrauma, a **fistula test** is performed. This test is best performed by insufflation with a rubber bulb fitted with an olive tip; however, a pneumatic otoscope (Seigle) will suffice, provided a good seal in the canal is achieved. When positive pressure is applied, the eyes are carefully examined for any nystagmic movement. If a fistula is present, the eyes will beat to the opposite side, and the patient will report intense vertigo similar to his or her complaint.

The use of +20-diopter Frenzel lenses enhances the examiner's perception of the nystagmus. **Weber** and **Rinne** tuning fork tests are performed with a 512-cps tuning fork. A clinical estimate of the patient's **speech reception threshold** is obtained.

b. **Neurologic examination**

(1) **Cranial nerves**

(a) **First cranial nerve. Olfactory nerve.** Smell—test patient with scents of coffee, tobacco, cloves, and mint. Standardized tests of olfaction are also available.

(b) **Second cranial nerve. Optic nerve.**

Assess degree of spontaneous nystagmus
Vision
Pupillary responses
Light reflex, consensual reflex, accommodation
Fundoscopic examination

(c) Third, fourth, and sixth cranial nerves. Oculomotor, trochlear, and abducent nerves. Eye motion and conjugate motion.

(d) Fifth cranial nerve. Trigeminal nerve.

Open mouth against resistance
Corneal reflex
Facial sensation

(e) Seventh cranial nerve. Facial nerve.

Facial motion
Taste
Hitselburger's sign. Sensation of posterosuperior EACs (external auditory canals).

(f) Eighth cranial nerve. Vestibulocochlear nerve. Tuning forks; masked speech testing.

(g) Ninth cranial nerve. Glossopharyngeal nerve. Palatal and pharyngeal reflex; position of soft palate.

(h) Tenth cranial nerve. Vagus nerve.

Vocal cord examination
Motion of soft palate

(i) Eleventh cranial nerve. Accessory nerve. Forced motion of head; shoulder shrug.

(j) Twelfth cranial nerve. Hypoglossal nerve. Motion and strength of tongue.

(2) Cerebellum function tests

(a) Finger-to-nose test

(b) Adiodochokinesia (ability to perform rapid alternating movements)

(c) Romberg test

(d) Tandem studies

(e) Deep tendon reflexes

c. Nystagmus refers to eye movements that are sustained, involuntary, and rhythmic with a speed that is different in the two directions of motion (fast and slow components). Traditionally, nystagmus is described by the direction of the fast component. As described by this method, nystagmus can be horizontal (right to left beating), vertical (upward or downward beating), or rotary (clockwise or counterclockwise beating). Spontaneous nystagmus indicates a vestibular system disorder (either central or peripheral), with the exception of congenital-familial nystagmus and the nystagmus observed with blindness.

(1) Examination for spontaneous nystagmus. The patient is seated or supine with the head immobile. The patient's eyes must not move except to follow the examiner's finger. The finger should not be closer than 18 in. from the patient and is moved from left to right, superiorly to inferiorly, and vice versa in sweeps no greater than 30 degrees from the neutral gaze. End-point nystagmus at the extremes of lateral gaze is not uncommon and not considered pathologic. Again, the use of a Frenzel lens enhances the examiner's ability to detect nystagmus by magnification and by interfering with the patient's ability to "fixate" and suppress the nystagmus (a known characteristic of peripheral lesion–induced nystagmus).

(2) Examination for positional nystagmus. Patients often complain that their vertigo is related to head position or changes in position. Positional vertigo can occur in disorders of the labyrinth or of the central nervous system. The Nylen-Bárány test is performed by moving the patient from the sitting position to a lying position with the head extended 45 degrees backward. The test is performed with the head extended, turned to the right, then to the left. Symptoms of nystagmus and vertigo are noted. A Frenzel lens should be used. The latency, duration, direction, and fatigability of the nystagmus are recorded.

d. Diagnostic tests. In addition to the clinical tests mentioned above, patients with vestibular system disorders may require one or more of the following tests to establish the diagnosis.

(1) Audiometry, including site of lesion testing

(2) Electronystagmography

(3) Auditory brainstem response (ABR)

(4) CT scan, MRI scan

(5) Spinal tap, especially if tumor or subarachnoid bleeding is suspected as a cause for vertigo

(6) Electroencephalography (EEG)

(7) More sophisticated vestibular testing may be indicated in patients with persistent symptoms of dysequilibrium or in whom a diagnosis has not been made. These include harmonic acceleration testing, head autorotational testing, dynamic posturography, and tracking testing.

5. Specific disorders of the vestibular system. The disorders characterized below are not meant to be a complete treatment of vestibular pathology, but only to represent some of the more common or classic disorders. Other disorders of the inner ear described previously can also present with vertigo as the primary symptom. For a more thorough discussion of vestibular disorders, the reader is referred to the bibliography at the end of this section.

a. Ménière's disease (endolymphatic hydrops) is the classic and probably most common disorder of the peripheral vestibular system.

(1) Signs and symptoms. The classic triad of Ménière's disease is vertigo, tinnitus, and sensorineural hearing loss. The vertiginous episodes are usually sudden in onset and severe with nausea and vomiting. They last minutes to hours with lingering symptoms of unsteadiness for days. These episodes are usually preceded by a fullness in the ear or increasing tinnitus. Hearing loss usually fluctuates, becoming worse near the time of the attacks and then initially returning to or near to normal. The loss is of the sensorineural variety, greater for low frequencies early, later changing to a flat configuration. The hearing loss tends to be progressive and can lead to profound hearing loss, but rarely to total deafness. Discrimination decreases and recovers with the pure tones. Recruitment is also present. Nystagmus is evident, usually away from the involved ear during the attack. Caloric response may be normal early but decreases as the disease progresses. The frequency of attacks is variable. Ten to thirty percent of people with Ménière's are affected bilaterally.

Three isolated variants exist:

(a) Cochlear Ménière's syndrome has two components—fluctuating sensorineural hearing loss and tinnitus.

(b) Vestibular Ménière's syndrome has a sense of aural pressure or fullness and vertigo.

(c) Tomarkins crisis (drop attacks) has a sudden violent episode of vertigo, during which the patient falls to the ground. The attack is characteristically brief, and the patient is always alert.

(2) Pathologic studies show endolymphatic hydrops with few changes in the sensory and neural structures. It is postulated that attacks are due to rupture of the membranous labyrinth, with mixing of endolymph and perilymph.

(3) Management. No completely effective medical treatment exists that will halt the attacks and prevent progressive hearing loss. Since the attacks vary widely as to severity and frequency, the management should be individualized. A patient with mild, infrequent episodes can reasonably be managed with reassurance. Conversely, those with frequent severe attacks must be considered for a more aggressive medical or surgical approach. Management of acute attacks consists of treatment with antivertiginous medication (Dramamine, meclizine, diazepam, scopolamine) and correction of any fluid and electrolyte imbalance that might occur from vomiting. Bed rest, sedation, and hydration are the mainstays of severe attacks, and hospitalization is sometimes necessary. Long-term medical management to reduce the number of attacks or to halt the progression of the hearing loss (or both) is more controversial. However, smoking must be stopped and caffeine consumption decreased. Salt intake should be decreased as well. Although several surgical procedures are promising in this respect, evaluation by a competent otologic surgeon is necessary to choose the procedure that will best benefit the patient.

b. Vestibular neuronitis

   (1) Signs and symptoms. Vestibular neuronitis is a disease characterized by severe vertigo, sudden in onset, with no associated hearing loss. The attack is usually protracted and may last from a few days to several weeks. Relapses in the first 6 months are not unusual. A viral cause is suspected.

   Nystagmus is usually evident and is horizontal. Other neuropathies are not present. The otologic examination is normal.

   (2) Diagnostic tests. The audiogram is normal. Calorics and ENG show a depressed vestibular response in the affected ear.

   (3) Management of the acute attack is similar to Ménière's disease (antivertiginous drugs, hydration). The disease is usually self-limiting, but can become chronic and disabling. In this rare instance, vestibular nerve section can be beneficial.

c. Benign paroxysmal vertigo (positional). Patients with numerous disease processes may be subject to postural vertigo (cerebellar-pontine angle tumor, multiple sclerosis, vascular insufficiency). Some peripheral diseases such as Ménière's disease may be exacerbated by changes in position. Benign positional vertigo may be brought on by head trauma, ear infection, or may occur spontaneously.

   (1) Signs and symptoms consist of vertigo with the head in a certain position. Other head positions do not precipitate the attack. No hearing loss or other neurologic symptoms are noted. The nystagmus created is usually rotary and is produced by placing the head in a hanging position with the affected ear down. There is a latent period of 2–20 seconds prior to the onset of nystagmus, and the nystagmus is of short duration (usually less than 1 minute). Repeated positioning of the patient produces decreasing nystagmus and symptoms (fatigue).

   (2) Management. The disease is usually self-limiting, lasting 6 months or less. Avoidance of the precipitating head position usually suffices. Vestibular rehabilitation exercises can be helpful. Disease lasting longer than 6 months, particularly in the younger patient, should be reevaluated for central causes. Operative section of the nerve to the posterior semicircular canal (singular nerve) has been advocated for persistent cases, but this therapy is controversial.

Table 2-3. Drugs useful in the symptomatic treatment of vertigo

Generic name	Trade name	Duration of activity (hr)	Usual oral adult dose	Relative levels of sedation	Other modes of administration
Cyclizine	Marezine	4–6	50 mg q6h	+	IM
Dimenhydrinate	Dramamine	4–6	25–50 mg q6h	+ +	Rectal, IM, IV
Diphenhydramine	Benadryl	4–6	25–50 mg q6h	+ +	IM, IV
Meclizine	Bonine, Antivert	12–24	12.5–25.0 mg q8–12h	+	
Promethazine	Phenergan	4–6	25 mg q6h	+ +	Rectal, IM, IV
Scopolamine	Transderm Scōp	72 (transdermal)	0.5 mg	+	PO, SC, IV
Hydroxyzine	Vistaril	4–6	25–100 mg tid	+ +	IM
Ephedrine		4–6	25 mg q6h	0	IM

Source: M. A. Samuels, *Manual of Neurology.* 4th ed. Boston: Little, Brown, 1991.

d. Motion sickness. Motion sickness is produced by a mismatch of vestibular, visual, and somatosensory inputs, such as induced in a ship or automobile. The vertigo is variable, depending on the intensity of the mismatched stimuli and the patient's response. It is diminished by providing improved visual input of the surroundings and often responds to symptomatic medical treatment such as with transdermal scopolamine, Dramamine, or meclizine. Prophylactic usage of medication often eliminates or greatly diminishes the dizziness in patients prone to motion intolerance.

e. Perilymph fistula. Even mild trauma such as sneezing, coughing, or vigorous nose blowing can produce a leak of perilymph in the areas of the oval or round windows. More commonly, a history of implosive trauma, such as diving or plane flight, or vigorous exertion is elicited.

(1) Signs and symptoms are episodic vertigo, especially with motion or straining, aural fullness, tinnitus, and mild or fluctuating hearing loss.

(2) Diagnosis is history-dependent, but confirmed by a "fistula test" in which the patient strains while holding the nose, inducing increased middle ear pressure. This reproduces the symptoms and can be documented subjectively or objectively by simultaneous ENG. Often, caloric weakness is also found.

(3) Treatment may require exploratory tympanotomy to find and seal the fistula; however, most perilymphatic fistulas heal spontaneously. Disabling vertigo, progressive hearing loss, or persistent symptoms necessitate surgical intervention.

6. Central vestibular disorders

a. Acoustic neuroma. Better named **vestibular schwannoma,** the acoustic neuroma is a tumor of Schwann cell origin, usually occurring on the vestibular nerve. It comprises 8% of all brain tumors and about 80% of all cerebellar-pontine angle (CPA) tumors. Although the tumor is benign, it can be very destructive due to its location. The tumor occurs with about equal frequency on both the superior and inferior divisions of the vestibular nerve. It can occur anywhere along the length of the nerve, and thus symptoms can be those of a lesion in the cochlea, in the internal auditory canal, or in the cerebellopontine angle.

(1) Signs and symptoms are usually unilateral sensorineural hearing loss, unilateral tinnitus, or unexplained vertigo. Progression of symptoms is usually slow, but hemorrhage into the tumor may produce a sudden exacerbation. Fifty percent of patients notice hearing loss as a first symptom, with it being sudden in onset 5–10% of the time. Tinnitus can be the only symptom, or it can be associated with the hearing loss. Vertigo rarely is the initial complaint but is frequently present at the time of diagnosis. The description of the vertigo is usually a vague sensation of motion. In the past, trigeminal symptoms of facial pain or numbness were seen in up to three-fourths of people with neuromas, but now with earlier diagnosis, this figure is decreasing. Facial weakness is uncommon, with less than 10% of patients showing this symptom.

(2) Diagnostic tests

(a) ENG (electronystagmogram). Approximately 70–80% of patients show spontaneous nystagmus. Calorics are decreased in 50% of patients with small tumors and 90% of those with large tumors.

(b) Audiology. Approximately 96% of patients have a hearing loss. It is a high tone loss in 64%, a flat loss in 20%, a low tone loss in 8%, and a trough-shaped loss in 8%. There is a marked decrease in discrimination greater than expected for the given hearing loss. Testing to differentiate cochlear from retrocochlear lesions is only suggestive, since 20% of acoustic neuromas affect the cochlea. Evidence of retrocochlear alterations is noted by absent stapedial reflexes and presence of tone decay (adaptation). Cochlear signs of involvement showing recruitment may also be positive.

(c) Auditory brainstem response (ABR) is one of the most accurate noninvasive studies. A delay in wave V (the presumed inferior colliculus wave) on one side of greater than 0.4 msec over the opposite side is highly suggestive of a lesion impinging on the eighth cranial nerve.

(d) X rays can show widening and shortening of the internal auditory canal, seen in 55% of acoustic neuromas on plain x rays.

(e) CT scan. With improved techniques, CT scans are one of the more accurate noninvasive tests available.

(f) MRI scan with gadolinium is the *most* accurate test for detecting acoustic neuromas. Three- to four-mm tumors can consistently be imaged.

(g) Cerebrospinal fluid. Lumbar puncture may show an increase in CSF pressure and usually shows a CSF protein greater than 50 dl.

(h) Posterior fossa myelogram. Although this test can detect 95% of all acoustic tumors with virtually no false-negatives and only 5% false-positives, MRI with gadolinium enhancement is the imaging study of choice.

(3) Management. Surgery is the major form of therapy, with the approach dependent on the size and location of the tumor. Proton beam and "gamma knife" radiation have been recently added to the treatment regimen. Long-term results with these modalities, as well as a lack of known incidence of complications, make their treatment role unclear at present.

b. **Multiple sclerosis** is a demyelinating disease that primarily affects white matter in the CNS in young patients (less than 40 years of age).

(1) Signs and symptoms. Charcot's triad of nystagmus, scanning speech, and intention tremor make the diagnosis easy when all are present; however, this is not the case early in the disease. Vertigo is present in about 30% of patients with multiple sclerosis. Nystagmus is present in 40–70% and can be of any type, but dissociated nystagmus is pathognomonic of the disease. Hearing loss, when present, is usually unilateral, high frequency, and sudden with recovery after a variable time. The diagnosis must often wait for a more typical syndrome to appear, although ENG and evoked response audiometry may help to localize the lesions.

(2) Management. There is no uniformly beneficial treatment. Currently, several experimental regimens are being investigated. The patient should be under the care of a neurologist.

c. **Vascular disorders.** Dysequilibrium can be induced by vascular insufficiency and is usually seen in elderly patients.

(1) Signs and symptoms depend on the anatomic area affected by the diminished blood flow.

(a) Vertebrobasilar insufficiency symptoms include vertigo, hemiparesis, visual disturbances, dysarthria, facial numbness, ataxia, and headache. These result from transient episodes of ischemia. Decrease in hearing is rare because the posterior inferior cerebellar artery is involved; however, if the anterior inferior cerebellar artery is occluded, decreased perfusion of the inner ear will also occur.

(b) Wallenberg syndrome (lateral medullary syndrome) produces symptoms due to infarction of the lateral portion of the medulla. These include vertigo, nausea, vomiting, nystagmus, ataxia, diminished sense of pain and temperature on the ipsilateral face and contralateral body, dysphagia with ipsilateral palatal and vocal cord paralysis and Horner's syndrome.

(c) Occlusion of the internal auditory artery or anterior vestibular artery can produce sudden vertigo with nausea and vomiting, often without deafness.

(d) Subclavian steal syndrome symptoms are vertigo, occipital headache, diplopia, blurring of vision, and pain in the upper extremity. A difference of 20 mmHg in the systolic blood pressure between the two arms with a diminished radial pulse is diagnostic.

(e) Cervical vertigo is due to cervical spondylosis and intervertebral disc degeneration. Symptoms are produced due to lack of proprioception of the neck musculature, as well as vascular compression or spasm of the vertebrobasilar system. Symptoms include vertigo, syncope, headache, visual disturbances, tinnitus and, occasionally, hearing loss.

(f) Migraine due to constriction and subsequent dilatation of the vertebrobasilar vessels produces vertigo, dysarthria, ataxia, visual disturbances, and intense unilateral pulsatile headache.

(g) Cardiovascular abnormalities can cause dizziness or lightheadedness. Presyncopal symptoms also include nausea, pallor, diaphoresis, and blurred vision. True vertigo is not common. Some causes are cardiac arrhythmias, cardiac sinus arrest, aortic stenosis, and cardiac sinus syncope. Vascular hemodynamic disorders include such entities as orthostatic hypotension, vasovagal episodes, hypoglycemia, and atherosclerosis.

(2) Diagnosis is most often based on a thorough history and physical examination, often with neurological consultation. Angiography may be needed.

(3) It is critical to identify patients with **vascular etiology of dizziness** before the serious sequelae of brainstem stroke ensues.

(4) Treatment is both medical and surgical, requiring appropriate neurological and vascular surgical consultation.

d. Epilepsy. Temporal lobe epilepsy can produce variable degrees of dysequilibrium.

(1) Signs and symptoms can be true vertigo, mimicking Ménière's disease, or mild dysequilibrium. Often "absences" with repetitive movements such as chewing, facial grimacing, or lip smacking are seen, as well as auditory hallucinations.

(2) Treatment is directed to the seizure disorder, using such medications as phenytoin or carbamazepine.

e. Hyperventilation. Lightheadedness is often associated with episodes of hyperventilation due to anxiety or emotional upset.

(1) Signs and symptoms are lightheadedness, circumoral or digital paresthesias, diaphoresis, trembling, acute anxiety, and palpitations.

(2) **Diagnosis** is made by having the patient recreate the attack by hyperventilation for 3 minutes or more.

(3) **Treatment** is by reassurance or a method of rebreathing (into a bag), which prevents hypocapnia and alkalosis due to inhalation of expired carbon dioxide.

7. **Facial nerve paralysis.** Although not technically an otologic disorder, the course of the facial nerve through the temporal bone and its frequent association with diseases and trauma to the ear make it appropriate to discuss. Disorders of the facial nerve outside the temporal bone are discussed in Chapter 6. Attention should also be directed to the description of the anatomic course of the nerve described in this chapter.

a. **Topognostic testing.** Location of the point of damage to the nerve by various techniques has historic value, but little prognostic value. Most lesions of the facial nerve in Bell's palsy are at the geniculate ganglion, where the facial canal is the narrowest. Loss of function of the stapedius reflex, salivary flow, lacrimation, and taste probably have more to do with differential response of various size nerve fibers carrying these responses, rather than location of the lesion.

b. **Electroneurography (ENG)** is presently the best clinical test for monitoring facial nerve function. It involves stimulation of the facial nerve near the stylomastoid foramen with recording responses on the face. Comparison of the electrical response with the other side gives an estimate of the degree of degeneration of the facial nerve. Degeneration of greater than 95% leads to poor expected recovery. Less than 90% degeneration usually bodes well for a good recovery. Test results are a reflection of injury 2–3 days prior to testing, because it takes that long for the neural elements to degenerate.

c. **Electromyography.** This procedure is used to test the musculoelectrical activity. An electrode must be placed within the substance of the muscle and its potential recorded. If total interruption of the nerve has occurred, no motor unit activity will be seen approximately 2–3 weeks after the injury. If degeneration occurs but the lesion is not complete, fibrillation potentials will be recorded.

d. **Etiology.** It is important to assess not only the site of injury to the facial nerve, but also the etiology so that appropriate therapy can be instituted. Only after all possible causes have been ruled out can a diagnosis of idiopathic facial paralysis be considered (Bell's palsy).

e. **Trauma**

(1) **Trauma at birth.** The extratemporal portion of the facial nerve may be injured during delivery, especially when the forceps are inappropriately applied. Unless a specific laceration occurs, facial paralysis is transient. Facial

paralysis may also occur as a congenital neurologic deficit, but is most frequently associated with multiple neuropathies.

(2) Intratemporal. Injury to the facial nerve **within the temporal bone** most often is a result of surgical trauma. This occurs most frequently in the vertical segment of the facial nerve during mastoid surgery, although dehiscence of the bony covering of the facial nerve in the horizontal segment may allow for injury to occur during middle ear procedures, such as stapedectomy. Surgical removal of an acoustic neuroma may also result in transient or permanent facial paralysis.

Temporal bone fractures may result in loss of facial nerve function. Facial nerve paralysis may occur with both transverse and longitudinal fractures. Although up to 90% of all temporal bone fractures are longitudinal, approximately 15% of these fractures have concomitant facial nerve injury. Up to one-half of transverse temporal bone fractures may occur with a facial nerve paralysis that may be immediate, due to transection or bony impingement on the nerve. These fractures often require immediate surgical intervention for repair. Delayed paralysis is most often due to posttraumatic edema. The question of immediate or delayed surgery must be based on the individual patient, as well as the evidence of progressive degeneration.

(3) Extratemporal. Injury to the facial nerve *distal to the stylomastoid foramen* most often occurs during parotid surgery. Prevention entails identification of the nerve at the outset of the procedure. Extratemporal injury may also occur following trauma to the face. Attempts at reanastomosis or nerve grafting should be done as soon as the appropriate diagnosis is made in order to allow the maximum return of function. (See Chap. 6, **III.A.**)

f. Infection

(1) Acute infection (bacterial). Otitis media, whether acute or chronic, is the most common cause of facial nerve paralysis from bacterial origin, especially in the young child.

Signs and symptoms consist of an acute otitis media, often with a bulging drum and a relatively rapid onset of facial nerve paralysis. Chronic disease often implicates a cholesteatoma with either an infectious neuritis or compression from an enlarging cholesteatoma.

Management. Myringotomy to decompress the middle ear and mastoid and appropriate antibiotics usually result in recovery of the nerve in acute otitis media. Cholesteatomas with facial paralysis require emergent surgery.

Acute necrotizing (malignant) otitis externa is an infectious process originating within the external auditory canal that spreads to the contiguous cartilage and bone. The most common organism is *Pseudomonas aeruginosa*. The facial nerve may be involved either within the soft tissue of the parotid at the stylomastoid foramen or within the fallopian canal (canal of the facial nerve) (see **VI.F.**).

Management consists of the topical and IV antibiotics with judicious debridement.

(2) **Viral. Herpes zoster oticus (Ramsay Hunt syndrome)** is a viral disorder involving the facial nerve and associated with hearing loss, vertigo, and herpetic rash around the pinna. Although it is known that this is a viral disorder, assessment of surgical intervention and appropriate therapy is often similar to that of Bell's palsy.

Management. Early treatment with acyclovir and prednisone offers the best chance for recovery of facial function. Surgical decompression of the facial nerve is of limited value.

Guillain-Barré syndrome may represent a central nervous system viral disorder, often accompanied by facial paralysis. The therapy in these situations is supportive.

(3) **Chronic infection** most often entails a chronic otitis media with an associated cholesteatoma. Facial nerve paralysis is not usually sudden unless an acute process intervenes. **Therapy** should be directed at removal of the infectious process with careful surgical identification of the facial nerve. The presence of facial paralysis with a purulent otorrhea should be viewed as a significant problem and as an indication for immediate hospitalization.

(4) **Idiopathic (Bell's palsy).** The term *Bell's palsy* should be used only for those situations when the etiology of the facial paralysis cannot otherwise be ascertained. It is perhaps the most common of all the groupings of facial paralysis. Current theories as to the etiology of this disorder have not been proved or confirmed; however, Bell's palsy may represent an isolated viral neuritis or a single manifestation of a polyneuritis. Vascular ischemia may also play a role, causing the facial nerve to swell within its bony canal.

Diagnosis. The diagnosis is made by exclusion of all other etiologies of facial paralysis. Enhanced MRI scanning may show increased activity around the geniculate ganglion region.

Management remains controversial; however, if corticosteroids are used, they should be limited to those in whom the facial paralysis is diagnosed early (within 1–7 days). Facial nerve decompression is probably not beneficial.

(5) Miscellaneous causes

Neoplastic. Any neoplasm of the temporal bone can involve the facial nerve secondarily; however, a neuroma of the facial nerve must be a prime consideration. Other possible lesions are glomus tumors, squamous cell carcinomas primarily arising from the external auditory canal, congenital cholesteatoma, meningioma, and acoustic neuroma. Eosinophilic granuloma must be considered in children with multiple punched-out lesions of the squamous portion of the temporal bone. Biopsy of the lesion is diagnostic.

Metabolic. Facial paralysis is occasionally associated with sarcoidosis (Heerfordt's syndrome), Wegener's granulomatosis, periarteritis nodosa, and diabetes. **Therapy** is directed at the underlying disorder. Facial nerve decompression is rarely indicated in such a situation.

Selected Readings

Adams, D. A., et al. Congenital syphilitic deafness: Further review *J. Laryngol. Otol.* 97:399, 1983.

Bardsley, A. F., and Mercer, D. M. The injured ear: A review of 50 cases. *Br. J. Plast. Surg.* 36:466, 1983.

English, G. *Otolaryngology* (vol. I) (rev. ed.). Hagerstown, Md.: Harper & Row, 1984.

Gates, G. A., Avery, C. A., Prihoda, T. J., and Cooper, J. C., Jr. Effectiveness of adenoidectomy and tympanostomy tubes in the treatment of chronic otitis media with effusion. *N. Engl. J. Med.* 317:1444, 1987.

Glasscock, M. Sensorineural deafness. *Otolaryngol. Clin. North Am.* 11:1, 1978.

Goodhill, V. *Ear Diseases, Deafness and Dizziness.* Hagerstown, Md.: Harper & Row, 1979.

Gower, D., and McGuirt, W. F. Intracranial complications of acute and chronic infectious ear disease: Problem still with us. *Laryngoscope* 93:1028, 1983.

Hamid, M. A. New tests of vestibular function. In E. N. Myers, C. D. Bluestone, D. E. Brackmann, and C. J. Krause, (eds.), *Advances in Otolaryngology—Head and Neck Surgery.* St. Louis: Mosby Yearbook, 1990. Pp. 15–38.

Healey, G. B. Hearing loss and vertigo secondary to head injury. *N. Engl. J. Med.* 306:1029, 1982.

Hoffman, R. A., and Shepsman, D. Bullous myringitis and sensorineural hearing loss. *Laryngoscope* 93:1544, 1983.

Katz, J. *Handbook of Clinical Audiology* (2nd ed.). Baltimore: William & Wilkins, 1978.

Klein, J. O. Recent advances in antibacterial therapy for pediatric otolaryngology. In E. N. Myers, C. D. Bluestone, D. E. Brackmann, and C. J. Krause, (eds.), *Advances in Otolaryngology—Head and Neck Surgery.* St. Louis: Mosby Yearbook, 1990. Pp. 183–198.

Konigsmark, B. W., and Gorlin, R. J. *Genetic and Metabolic Deafness.* Philadelphia: Saunders, 1976.

Lewis, J. S. Surgical management of tumors of the middle ear and mastoid. *J. Laryngol. Otol.* 97:299, 1983.

Paparella, M., and Shumick, D. *Otolaryngology* (vol. II). Philadelphia: W. B. Saunders, 1980.

Parkin, J. L. Antimicrobial treatment of otitis media: Penicillins, cephalosporins, sulfonamides. *Otolaryngol. Head Neck Surg.* 89:376, 1981.

Pillsbury, H. Hypertension, hyperlipoproteinemia, chronic noise exposure: Is there synergism in cochlear pathology? *Laryngoscope* 96:1112–1138, 1986.

Rughes, R., and DelaCruz, A. *Otologic Radiology.* New York: Macmillan, 1986.

Schuknecht, H. F., and Gulya, A. J. Endolymphatic hydrops: An overview and classification. *Ann. Otol. Rhinol. Laryngol.* 92 [Suppl. 106]:1, 1983.

Schuknecht, H. F. *Pathology of the Ear.* Cambridge, Mass.: Harvard University Press, 1974.

Shambaugh, G. E., Jr., and Glascock, M. E., III. *Surgery of the Ear* (3rd ed.). Philadelphia: Saunders, 1980.

Shulman, A. *A Strategy for Tinnitus Treatment Control—Insights in Otolaryngology.* St. Louis: Mosby Yearbook, 1990.

Shumrick, D. *Otolaryngology* (vols. I and II) (2nd ed.). Philadelphia: Saunders, 1980.

Veldman, J. E., and McCase, B. E. *Otoimmunology.* Berkeley: Kugler Publishers, 1987.

Weiss, H. D. Dizziness. In Samuels, M. A. (ed.), *Manual of Neurology: Diagnosis and Therapy* (4th ed.). Boston: Little, Brown, 1991. Pp. 53–70.

Wolfson, R. J. Vertigo. *Otolaryngol. Clin. North Am.* 6:1, 1973.

Wolfson, R. J., et al. Vertigo. *Ciba. Fond. Symp.* 33:6, 1981.

3

Nose and Paranasal Sinuses

I. Introduction

A. Anatomy of the nose

1. **Structure and support.** The external nose has a bony and cartilaginous framework. The bony portion consists of the paired nasal bones, the ascending or frontal processes of the maxilla, and the bony septum. The cartilaginous framework consists of the alar (lower lateral) cartilages, the upper lateral cartilages, and the cartilaginous septum.

   The inferior, middle, and superior turbinates are located on the lateral nasal wall. Below each turbinate is its corresponding meatus. The nasolacrimal duct opens into the inferior meatus. The frontal sinus, maxillary sinus, and anterior ethmoid cells open into the middle meatus. The posterior ethmoid cells open into the superior meatus, with the sphenoid sinus opening into the sphenoidal recess (Fig. 3-1). The concept of the osteomeatal complex (OMC) is important anatomically, physiologically, and surgically. It incorporates the anterior ethmoid cells, maxillary sinus ostia, and anterior middle meatus. Mucosal swelling, infection, or anatomic variation can narrow this unit, adversely affecting ventilation and mucociliary clearance, the net result of which is recurrent acute or chronic sinusitis.

2. **Blood supply.** The nasal blood supply is provided by branches of both the internal and the external carotid arteries. The sphenopalatine, the descending palatine, and the superior labial arteries are branches of the external carotid artery. The anterior and posterior ethmoid arteries are derived from the internal carotid artery.

   Anteriorly, the nasal septum is supplied by the sphenopalatine, greater palatine, superior labial, and anterior ethmoid arteries. The anastomoses of these vessels are called **Kiesselbach's plexus.** The posterior septum receives its blood supply from the posterior ethmoid and sphenopalatine arteries. The blood supply to the lateral nasal wall is from the anterior ethmoid, posterior ethmoid, and sphenopalatine arteries.

B. Examination of the nose and sinuses

1. **Physical examination.** A nasal speculum and focused light, such as a head mirror, should be used. The nasal speculum is held in the palm of one hand with the forefinger on the ala, and

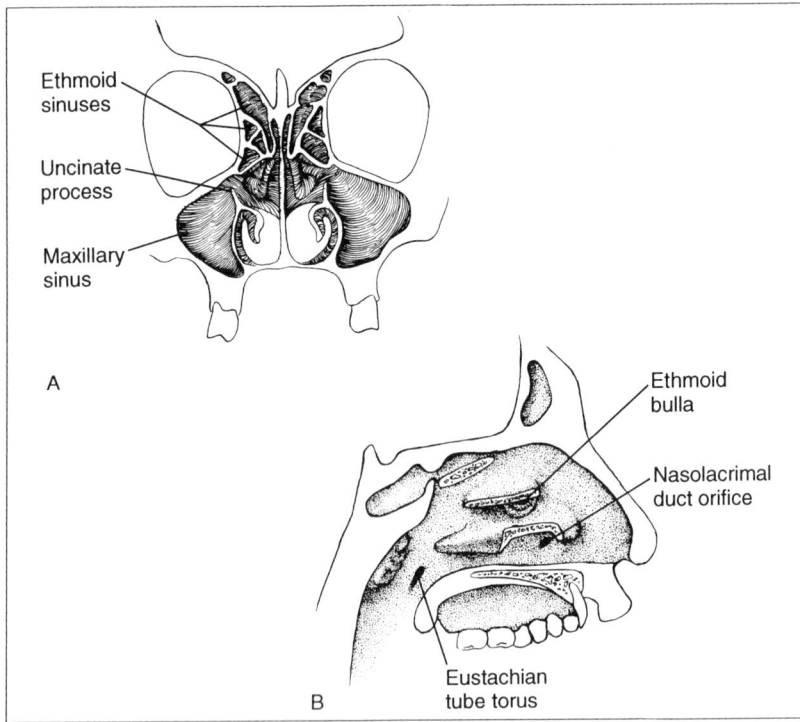

Fig. 3-1. Sinus anatomy and ostial regions. A. Axial view of sinuses and nasal chambers. B. Lateral nasal wall—partial turbinate removal.

the blades are opened vertically. The other hand is used for positioning the patient's head.

a. **Topical vasoconstrictors** are useful adjuncts.

(1) **Topical phenylephrine** is used in 0.25–0.50% concentration. An atomizer can be used for application. Phenylephrine should be avoided in patients with arteriosclerotic cardiovascular disease or glaucoma.

(2) **Topical epinephrine,** 1:1000 concentration, can be applied using cotton pledgets, giving maximum vasoconstriction. Epinephrine is contraindicated in the presence of arteriosclerotic cardiovascular disease.

(3) **Topical cocaine,** a vasoconstrictor and topical anesthetic, is discussed under topical anesthesia (see **b.2.**).

b. **Topical intranasal anesthesia** can be obtained by application of lidocaine or cocaine. The anesthetic of choice is placed on cotton strips and inserted. All excess medication must be removed before placement to avert excessive absorption.

(1) **Lidocaine.** If 4% lidocaine is applied, it has a 15-minute duration of action. The total dose should not exceed 200 mg. The first signs of lidocaine toxicity are CNS hyperactivity followed by cardiovascular depression.

(2) Cocaine. Topical cocaine is used in a 4 or 5% solution. It has a 45-minute duration of action and also causes local vasoconstriction. The maximum topical dose should be approximately 200 mg.

Toxicity. Toxic effects have occurred with as little as 20 mg of cocaine applied topically. Early signs of cocaine toxicity are stimulation, garrulousness, restlessness, increased respiratory rate, increased blood pressure, tremors, convulsive movements, bradycardia, and then tachycardia. A patient can pass through this intial stage without its being recognized and progress to the depressive effects: hypotension, decreased respiratory rate, and convulsions leading to cardiorespiratory collapse.

Therapy of a toxic reaction includes cardiopulmonary support and short-acting barbiturate.

c. **Combined vasoconstrictors and topical anesthesia.** A combination of 1% phenylephrine and 4% xylocaine mixed in equal aliquots, administered via a nasal insufflator, is particularly efficacious for office nasal endoscopy.

2. **Diagnostic techniques**

a. **Transillumination** of the sinuses can be performed with a bright penlight in a darkened room. Maxillary sinus transillumination is performed by placing the light over each maxillary sinus and observing the transmission through the palate. Frontal sinus transillumination is performed by placing the light below the midportion of each eyebrow. In each instance, the light transmission through the sinuses is compared. If equal, usually opacification can be ruled out. It is of limited value today.

b. **Nasal culture.** The correlation between nasal cultures and sinus cultures taken at surgery is low. Although nasal cultures are of questionable reliability, they may have some validity when a purulent discharge is cultured at the sinus ostia. An antral aspirate is of greater value than nasal culture in cases when culture documentation is essential.

c. **Antral puncture.** Antral puncture is most often performed by placing a nasal antral trocar or 18-gauge spinal needle into the inferior meatus and by directing the trocar in a posterior and lateral direction through the thin bony plate separating the turbinate from the maxillary sinus. This procedure can be performed for drainage or irrigation of a maxillary sinus when an air-fluid level is seen on x ray and a response has not been observed to a conservative medical regimen (see sec. **IV.B.3.**). Aspiration can be used for culture documentation when specific identification of the pathogen is mandatory, as in immunosuppressed patients. The complications of antral puncture include hemorrhage, osteomyelitis, air embolism, injury to the globe, and injury to the optic nerve.

3. **Radiology of the nose and paranasal sinuses.** Radiography is often essential for the accurate diagnosis of sinus disease.

Routine sinus x rays include the Caldwell, Waters, lateral, and submental vertex (base) views. The frontal and ethmoid sinuses are seen on the Caldwell view. This view best demonstrates air-fluid levels in the frontal sinus. The maxillary sinuses are best seen on the Waters' view. The lateral view demonstrates the sphenoid and frontal sinuses, along with the nasopharynx and sella turcica. The sphenoid sinuses, nasopharynx, nasal cavity, and the medial and lateral antral walls are seen on the submental vertex view.

Computed tomography (CT) scans add a new dimension. Polytomography is now less applicable; more reliable than plain films, it gives less definition than CT and is associated with more radiation exposure. CT can precisely pinpoint minor alterations in the osteomeatal complex (OMC). It is an invaluable adjunct for selecting surgical candidates for functional endoscopic sinus surgery (ESS), *yet it cannot and should not be used as the principal determinant for surgery.* Clinical correlation is essential. Both axial and coronal views should be performed, although information obtained by coronal views is far more applicable to surgical correlation.

II. Trauma to the nose and sinuses

A. Traumatic paranasal sinus fractures

1. **Frontal sinus.** A frontal sinus fracture usually results from direct force to the region, the area of impact being superior to the nasofrontal suture.

   a. **Examination** usually reveals a depression of the anterior frontal sinus wall. The fracture may also involve the posterior wall and cribriform plate. The nasofrontal duct and dura are subject to injury as well. Dural tears may result from a fracture of the posterior frontal sinus wall, fracture of the roof of the ethmoid coexisting with a frontal sinus injury, or fracture of the cribriform plate following telescoping of the perpendicular plate of the ethmoid. Subsequent cerebrospinal fluid (CSF) rhinorrhea, as well as laceration of the anterior ethmoidal arteries, may be present. Usually there is only slight, if any, displacement of the nasal bones with forehead trauma.

   b. **Diagnosis.** Fractures of the frontal sinus usually involve the anterior wall. These fractures can be diagnosed either by direct inspection and palpation or by radiography. In areas of question (e.g., the posterior wall), polytomography or CT should be performed.

   c. **Treatment.** If only the anterior wall is involved, the area can be explored through a laceration or brow incision. The fragments should be elevated and stabilized whenever possible. The sinus should be drained only if the integrity of the duct is questioned. In nondisplaced posterior wall fractures, no specific therapy is usually necessary. Displaced posterior wall fractures require a neurosurgical consultation. Similarly, displacement of the posterior wall is an indication to explore the sinus and, in most instances, obliteration should be considered. Antibiotics may be necessary to prevent retrograde meningitis.

Late realignment of fracture deformities is difficult because of bony fixation. These defects are often repaired with implantable material.

d. **Complications** of frontal sinus fractures include osteomyelitis and secondary abscess formation. Intracranial complications can occur, including meningitis as well as epidural and subdural abscesses. Orbital cellulitis can develop from an extension of the infection to the contiguous orbit. Mucoceles and pyoceles within the sinus may evolve if the nasofrontal duct is injured and not recognized. A headache may be the only indication of an impending complication.

(1) **Injury to the nasofrontal duct** with edema and hematoma formation may cause secondary obstruction. Pain can develop secondary to the vacuum within the sinus (aerosinusitis). The therapeutic goal is to ensure a physiologic conduit. Minor injury is treated expectantly with topical and systemic vasoconstrictors. With severe injury and ductal disruption, attempts can be made to reconstruct the duct. If unsuccessful, obliteration of the sinus may be necessary. Obliteration is mandatory when there is a persistent CSF leak via the posterior sinus wall.

(2) **CSF rhinorrhea.** It is estimated that as many as 25% of frontoethmoid sinus fractures are associated with a CSF leak. Most leaks occur within 48 hours, with a late onset secondary to liquefaction of blood within the sinus. Usually, CSF rhinorrhea stops within several days after injury. The CSF leak is associated with dural tears as noted in **1.a.** The site of origin can often be delineated by CT scan, with evidence of a fracture of the posterior frontal sinus wall, roof of the ethmoid, cribriform plate, or fluid within the sphenoid sinus. Air in the subdural space is often associated with a CSF leak. The leak can be confirmed by obtaining a glucose level on fluid collected. Clinistix and test tape measurements are often not accurate; however, they can be of some assistance early in the diagnostic spectrum. A definitive diagnosis can be made by injecting fluorescein, radioactive serum albumin, or indium into the subarachnoid space by lumbar puncture and subsequently testing for their presence on cottonoid pledgets appropriately inserted intranasally.

Routine packing is discouraged if a CSF leak is suspected. The head should be elevated. Antibiotics may be recommended in an effort to prevent meningitis. Surgical intervention is usually withheld for several weeks, as most often leaks subside spontaneously. When indicated, an osteoplastic flap approach to the frontal sinus can be used. The repair of a cribriform plate or roof of ethmoid fracture has been traditionally performed through an external ethmoidectomy approach. ESS is currently being evaluated for repair of these injuries.

2. **Ethmoid sinus** fractures often occur in association with other injuries, especially with injuries to the frontal sinus. These fractures result most often from an impact over the nasal bones with retrodisplacement of the interorbital structures. Often there are associated orbital rim fractures as well as telescoping of the ethmoidal plate, with lateral displacement of the medial orbital walls. Associated injuries include obliteration of the nasofrontal duct, laceration of the anterior ethmoidal artery, and disruption of the trochlea.

   a. **Signs and symptoms.** Diagnostically, there is flattening of the midface and lateral displacement of the palpebral fissures. Pseudohypertelorism may occur secondary to tearing of the medial palpebral ligament. Extraocular muscle motion may be limited, especially of the medial rectus. The trochlea suspends the superior oblique muscle on the superior medial corner of the orbit, acting as a pulley. Displacement can be associated with diplopia on downward gaze. An associated CSF leak may be present.

   b. **Diagnosis.** Radiographs are essential, and the complexity of the bony structures in this region necessitates axial and coronal CT scans.

   c. **Therapy.** Antibiotics are almost always indicated. Nasal packing should be avoided because packing allows for an avenue of secondary infection. Depressed fractures of the nasal bones may require wiring with external stenting. External traction is rarely necessary. Septal reduction should precede nasal repair; however, excessive force during manipulation is contraindicated because movement of the perpendicular plate of the ethmoid, in association with septal mobility, may induce a CSF leak.

   d. **Complications.** Epistaxis may occur and is usually secondary to a laceration of the anterior ethmoidal artery. Ligating the vessel via an external ethmoidectomy approach may be necessary. Other complications of ethmoid fractures include persistent visual disturbances, chronic frontal sinusitis secondary to injury of the nasofrontal duct, meningitis, and midface deformity.

3. **Maxillary sinus** fractures can occur with zygomaticomaxillary complex (ZMC) or orbital floor fractures.

   a. **Signs and symptoms.** Occlusal changes are not infrequent with these fractures, and an open-bite deformity may occur. Often there is hypesthesia or anesthesia of the cheek secondary to edema or transection of the infraorbital nerve. Whenever the orbit is involved in a fracture, retinal artery occlusion may occur secondary to edema and/or hematoma. Vision must be assessed, and any changes merit ophthalmologic consultation.

b. **Diagnosis.** Orbital floor fractures can cause inferior rectus entrapment and upward gaze diplopia. A red glass cover test is the best means of evaluating diplopia. A red glass is placed in front of one eye, and the patient is asked to look at a light in all positions of gaze. If diplopia is present, the patient will see two separate, partially overlapping lights, and ophthalmologic consultation should be obtained.

Radiographically, posttraumatic clouding suggests a fracture, providing sinusitis was not present before the injury. CT scans are also valuable in assessing the degree of injury.

c. **Therapy.** The use of antibiotics is controversial in simple maxillary sinus fracture. If an open wound exists, antibiotics should be considered. Displacement requires reduction with fixation.

4. **Sphenoid fracture.** Sphenoid fracture usually occurs in association with massive head trauma. Vital signs should be checked regularly until stable. The head and neck are immobilized until a cervical spine fracture is ruled out radiographically. A rapid but thorough neurologic and physical examination is performed, followed by repeat neurologic examinations. The sphenoid sinus is evaluated radiographically by CT scans, and an air-fluid level may be found. Frequently, CSF rhinorrhea develops. Intracerebral injury may be present; subdural and epidural hematoma can develop. The patient is also at risk for developing cerebral edema. A neurosurgical consultation should be obtained if the patient has signs of an intracranial injury.

5. **Orbital complications of sinus fractures**

a. The **trochlea** of the superior oblique muscle may be **lacerated,** causing diplopia on downward gaze.

b. The **medial palpebral ligament** may be torn. This ligament anchors the tarsal plate and passes anterior to the lacrimal canaliculi and sac. The therapy of medial palpebral ligament tears is directed toward their reattachment to either the nasal bones or lacrimal crests.

c. **Injury** to the **lacrimal apparatus** may be diagnosed by introducing fluorescein into the conjunctival sac and documenting its presence or absence within the nose. Probing and irrigation may open the ductal system. Often, patency can occur after many months, without surgical intervention. An immediate dacryocystorhinostomy is rarely indicated. This operation can be performed at a later date, after ophthalmologic consultation is obtained.

d. **Entrapment** of the medial rectus or inferior rectus muscles can occur with injuries to the ethmoid complex or maxillary sinus. Entrapment can be diagnosed by demonstrating diplopia on lateral gaze with medial rectus injuries, or on upward gaze with inferior rectus injuries. The forced-duction test is valuable in assessing inferior rectus entrapment. In this test, the eye is anesthetized, and the muscle in question is grasped with a forceps near the globe. Passive attempts at movement are made, and limitation suggests entrapment.

   e. Orbital cellulitis can occur with infection spreading from the contiguous sinus. Characteristics of orbital cellulitis include lid edema, exophthalmos, and chemosis of the conjunctiva, along with progressive immobility of the eye, which is associated with severe pain. Hospitalization is mandatory, and intravenous antibiotics are essential. Frequent eye exams with assessment of vision and eye motion must be performed. Incision and drainage of an abscess in the infected region is necessary if resolution is not effected with medical therapy. After initial drainage with quiescence, an external ethmoidectomy is often performed.

   f. Retinal artery occlusion may also occur.

B. Nasal trauma

   1. Nasal fractures (See Chap. 1, Nasal Fractures.)

     a. Nasal trauma during delivery. During delivery, nasal trauma can result in external nasal deformity, septal deviation, and obstruction. At birth the nasal supporting structure is cartilaginous; once the stress is removed, minor aberrations gradually resume their pretraumatic configuration. Major septal deformities are readily reduced in the nursery. In the rare instance of significant nasal vault trauma with an attendant obstruction, total rapid reduction of displaced segments is essential (see Chap. 1, Nasal Fractures).

   2. Septal injuries. After trauma, a nasal septal deviation must be evaluated as to whether the deviation antedated or resulted from the most recent injury.

     a. Signs and symptoms. The history can be helpful but may not be reliable. Most patients never carefully inspect their nose until a traumatic episode. On examination, mucosal lacerations, mucosal ecchymoses, and mobility usually signify an acute injury. The septum is deflected off the midline and obstructs the airway.

     b. Diagnostic aids. X rays are not always essential since the diagnosis is primarily a clinical one. At times, x rays may assist in confirming a difficult diagnosis.

     c. Therapy. Posttraumatic septal deviations should be corrected whenever possible within 5 days of injury. Asch forceps or a nasal elevator is used for the reduction. If an adequate reduction is not obtained, a septoplasty can be performed approximately 6 months after the acute injury.

d. Complications. Nasal septal hematoma is a complication of nasal trauma. Blood collects beneath the mucoperichondrium or -periosteum. On intranasal examination, there is a markedly swollen, sometimes fluctuant area. This area is best palpated with a cotton-tipped applicator, and the diagnosis confirmed by aspiration with an 18-gauge needle. If blood is obtained, a vertical incision through the mucoperichondrium is made to provide adequate drainage. Then packing is usually necessary to oppose the mucosa to the underlying cartilage. Untreated, a nasal septal abscess is often a sequela. Hospital admission for this condition is warranted if systemic signs of infection (e.g., fever) are present. Antibiotics must include therapy directed toward *Staphylococcus* as well as gram-negative organisms.

A nasal saddle deformity can result from an inadequately treated nasal septal hematoma or abscess.

III. Nasal obstruction

A. Infection: nasal furunculosis and cellulitis

1. **Signs and symptoms.** A nasal furuncle usually presents as an erythematous, indurated, raised, firm lesion of the nasal tip. It can have a surrounding area of cellulitis and is usually caused by a staphylococcal infection of the nasal vibrissae.

2. **Therapy.** The venous drainage of the nasal tip region is into the cavernous sinus. Thrombosis of the cavernous sinus infrequently results from staphylococcal infection.

   The infection must be treated aggressively with an antibiotic that provides staphylococcal coverage, such as dicloxacillin, 500 mg PO qid. A topical antibiotic ointment (2% mupirocin [Bactroban] or neomycin-polymyxin-bacitracin) may be of value. Warm soaks are applied locally. Incision and drainage should not be performed until there is adequate antibiotic coverage, since this can result in bacterial seeding to the cavernous sinus. The patient is observed daily until the infection begins to resolve. If spreading cellulitis occurs or if systemic symptoms develop, hospitalization for intravenous therapy is appropriate.

B. Nasal and sinus foreign bodies result from penetrating trauma, childhood insertion, or iatrogenic causes.

1. **Signs and symptoms.** Adults present either with a chief complaint of a foreign body or with chronic or recurring unilateral sinus infection following facial injury. Children present with unilateral rhinorrhea or unilateral infection. Whenever a child presents with unilateral rhinorrhea, a foreign body should be suspected.

   During the extraction of a maxillary tooth, a portion of the root or tooth restoration can be forced into the antrum. This problem can go undetected until recurrent sinus infection occurs.

2. **Therapy.** In adults, nasal foreign body removal can be effected after application of topical cocaine 4%. The object can then be

removed by suction or manipulation with appropriate instruments. Surgery is obviously required to remove a foreign body within the sinus. In children, general anesthesia is frequently necessary to remove the object. In a coooperative child, the foreign body can occasionally be retrieved as an office procedure.

3. **Sequelae.** Rhinoliths and maxillary sinus antroliths develop around a chronic foreign body nidus that has been in place for prolonged periods of time.

C. Mucosal aberrations

1. **Common cold.** The common cold is the most frequent infectious process involving the nasal mucosa.

    a. **Signs and symptoms.** The well-known presenting symptoms include a sensation of nasal congestion, watery rhinorrhea, and sneezing, often accompanied by malaise and myalgia. On physcial examination, there is marked edema of the nasal mucosa. The edema can cause obstruction of the sinus ostia. Within a few days of the onset of symptoms, some patients develop a secondary bacterial sinusitis.

    b. **Therapy.** The common cold is treated symptomatically with analgesics, mucolytics, and vasoconstrictors. There is no known cure or proved method of consistently preventing this malady.

2. **Allergic rhinitis** can be seasonal or perennial. It presents with nasal obstruction, nasal pruritus, rhinorrhea, and sneezing. Patients often describe their symptoms as "sinus trouble" or a common cold.

    a. **Signs and symptoms.** The diagnosis of allergic rhinitis is based on a history of seasonal symptoms, including sneezing, pruritus, and rhinorrhea. On physical examination, swollen turbinates covered with edematous blue or pale mucosa are frequently observed. Nasal polyps are often found in association with allergic rhinitis, but can also be caused by chronic infectious sinusitis.

    b. **Diagnostic tests.** An elevated immunoglobulin E (IgE) level, total eosinophil count, positive skin tests, or a radioallergosorbent test (RAST) confirms the history. The presence of eosinophils on nasal smear is also suggestive of allergic rhinitis.

    c. **Therapy.** If possible, affected patients should avoid the responsible allergen. Symptomatic relief can be achieved with oral antihistamines and decongestants.

        (1) **Antihistamines.** Chlorpheniramine, an alkylamine, can be given in an adult dose such as 4 mg qid. If patients do not respond, an antihistamine of a different class, such as tripelennamine, an ethylenediamine, should be given (see Chapter Appendix). The usual adult dose of tripelennamine is 25 mg qid. Often one class of antihistamine may be effective when another fails. The newer, "nonse-

dating" antihistamines are far more frequently pre-scribed—astemizole, terfenadine. Terfenadine has a relatively rapid onset of action (hours) and is adminis-tered bid. Astemizole has a slow onset (days) and a long half-life. Its use precludes skin testing for several weeks after cessation of the medication. In general, all antihis-tamines can make patients somnolent. Patients should be allerted of this possibility.

(2) **Sympathomimetic** medications with alpha-receptor ac-tivity can be given with or instead of an antihistamine. Pseudoephedrine is taken in 30- to 60-mg doses qid. This medication causes stimulation in some patients and somnolence in others. All patients must be advised of the potential side effects.

Sympathomimetics are contraindicated in patients with any form of arteriosclerotic cardiovascular disease. As is discussed under rhinitis medicamentosa (see **7.**), nasal drops or sprays containing sympathomimetic medica-tions should not be used over prolonged periods of time.

(3) **Steroids.** Aerosolized dexamethasone spray can be used for acute exacerbations. Patients must be cautioned not to overuse this medication, as adrenal suppression can result. Beclomethasone can be used intranasally with a decreased potential for adrenal suppression. Patients who are skin test–positive for specific allergens often benefit from a course of desensitization therapy.

For patients with edematous inferior turbinates occlud-ing the nasal airway, electrocautery of the turbinates or site steroid injection may also afford relief.

3. **Nasal polyps** represent localized areas of swelling within the nasal or sinus mucosa, usually arising in the ethmoid sinuses. The polyps can progressively enlarge, obstructing the nasal air-way. They can be associated with either allergic rhinitis or in-fectious rhinosinusitis. Treatment is necessary when there is (1) symptomatic nasal obstruction, (2) recurrent or chronic in-fection, or (3) a consideration of malignant change.

Medical therapy can be initiated with Beclomethasone spray. For allergic-type polyps, the usual dosage is 2 sprays bid or tid. A short course of systemic steroids can also be tried in acute situations, if no associated infection is present. Intranasal chromalyn spray is an adjunctive preparation. Antibiotics are necessary with associated infection.

Patients not responding to medical therapy frequently benefit from a **nasal polypectomy.** Choanal polyps appearing in the nasopharynx may originate in the maxillary sinus, making surgical autrostomy either by ESS or open (Caldwell-Luc) tech-nique a consideration.

4. **Cystic fibrosis.** Patients with cystic fibrosis have a thick, viscid mucus, their main symptoms being nasal obstruction

and rhinorrhea. Often, secondary nasal and sinus infections occur. On examination, tenacious mucus and polyps are observed in 10–20% of the cases.

Therapy is directed toward reducing secondary infection and establishing a nasal airway. Nasal cultures should be taken and the patient appropriately treated. A bedside humidifier and nasal irrigations with normal saline can prove beneficial. Polypectomy may be needed repeatedly to maintain a patent nasal airway. Maintaining a patent airway is not a simple task, often requiring extensive resections in the form of endoscopic intranasal ethmoidal surgery.

5. **Atrophic rhinitis (ozena)** is associated with an offensive nasal odor, epistaxis, anosmia, nasal obstruction, and purulent nasal crusting. On examination, there is nasal crusting, atrophy of the turbinates, and secondary enlargement of the nasal cavity. The etiology of the primary condition is unknown, but it can be a sequela of excess fibrosis following nasal surgery. Histologically, there is fibrosis of the submucosa, without inflammatory infiltration.

   Medical therapy consists of nasal irrigations with isotonic saline and correction of underlying medical problems when feasible. For those not responding to medical therapy, there are two surgical procedures currently used. One procedure is an endonasal microplasty in which the internal nasal dimensions are markedly decreased. The other is staged complete closure of the nostrils. Neither procedure is common.

6. **Vasomotor rhinitis** presents with symptoms of nasal obstruction or rhinorrhea or both. On physical examination, these patients may not have swollen, edematous turbinates or excessive nasal mucus. An allergy evaluation is negative. Some benefit may be obtained from aerosolized steroids. Symptomatic relief at times is obtained from antihistamines and decongestants (see **2.c.**).

   Patients with edematous turbinates not responding to medical therapy often benefit from electrocautery of the inferior turbinate or from submucosal injection of long-acting corticosteroids, e.g., prednisolone tebutate (Hydeltra-TBA). Intranasal cryosurgery to the postganglionic parasympathetics in the medial aspect of the pterygomaxillary fossa provides relief for many patients.

7. **Rhinitis medicamentosa** develops after prolonged use of topical vasoconstrictors. Symptomatically, the effective duration of the medication decreases, and rebound develops. Subsequently, marked erythema with edema of the nasal mucosa evolves.

   The patient's understanding of the condition is the cornerstone of management. Vasoconstrictor usage is curtailed with the assistance of aerosolized intranasal beclomethasone or injections of prednisolone tebutate. Normal saline spray intranasally may give some symptomatic relief during the period of withdrawal.

Systemic decongestants, such as pseudoephedrine, are also of some value. A brief course of oral steroids (less than 1 week—methylprednisolone) may rapidly improve symptoms of withdrawal while topical therapy begins to take effect.

8. **Intranasal neoplasms** can cause nasal obstruction as a primary symptom, in addition to epistaxis, external nasal swelling, and sinusitis secondary to obstruction of the sinus ostia. Symptoms are usually unilateral. Pain is frequently present with malignancy.

   Intranasal neoplasms include inverted papilloma, hemangiopericytoma, melanoma, esthesioneuroblastoma, squamous cell carcinoma, plasmacytoma, lymphoma, and rhabdomyosarcoma.

D. **Nasopharyngeal obstruction**

1. **Adenoid hypertrophy.** Enlarged adenoids often obstruct the posterior nasal choanae in childhood. Snoring, mouth breathing, slow eating, nasal discharge, drooling, and adenoid facies are all potential sequelae. A narrow, high-arched palate with associated malocclusion may occur. The degree of facial alteration can be measured on cephalometric radiographs. Rarely, a child will develop cor pulmonale from upper airway obstruction secondary to adenoid or tonsillar hypertrophy or both. This condition is an absolute indication for adenoidectomy and tonsillectomy.

   Other indications for adenoidectomy due to upper airway obstruction are not clearly defined, and the decision to perform surgery must be individualized. The relationship of adenoid hypertrophy to otitis media is still being investigated. Recent data suggest some efficacy in removing the adenoids in selected cases.

2. **Choanal polyps.** Choanal polyps originate in the maxillary sinus and extend through the sinus ostia to the nasal cavity and posteriorly into the nasopharynx. These polyps can cause nasopharyngeal obstruction. The treatment is surgical; a maxillary antrostomy is necessary to ensure complete removal. Endoscopic techniques are becoming more commonplace in the management of the condition.

3. **Angiofibromas** of the nasopharynx are rare lesions, occurring primarily in adolescent males.

   a. **Signs and symptoms.** Epistaxis and nasal obstruction are the primary symptoms. Less frequent are serous otitis, anosmia, hyponasal speech, and sinusitis. With skull base involvement, the second, third, fourth, and sixth cranial nerves can be affected.

   b. **Physical.** Mucus secondary to obstruction may preclude visualization on anterior rhinoscopy. Nasopharyngeal examination frequently demonstrates a purplish, lobulated mass.

   c. **Studies**

      (1) **Lateral skull films** in most instances demonstrate a soft tissue mass.

(2) Extension is seen on **computed tomography (CT)** scans of the region. Bone destruction is evident in approximately 50% of cases.

(3) Arteriography is essential to delineate the major contributing vessels.

d. Pathology. The ratio of vascular to connective tissue varies signficantly from tumor to tumor.

e. Treatment

(1) Surgery

(a) Blood loss is markedly reduced by preoperative **embolization.**

(b) Estrogen therapy has been reported to decrease vascularity. It is not indicated if embolization is used.

(c) Cryosurgery was used prior to embolization. It now has merit for accessible recurrences.

(d) Surgery is the treatment of choice. Biopsy is not indicated, as bleeding can be profuse. Wide exposure is essential to minimize recurrence.

(2) Radiotherapy. Most feel radiotherapy should be reserved for lesions not amenable to resection; however, long-term control of primary lesions has been reported.

f. Prognosis. A 50% incidence of recurrence was not uncommon in the past. Better imaging, decreasing blood loss, and more aggressive surgery should decrease the recurrence rate.

4. Squamous cell carcinoma. Squamous cell carcinoma of the nasopharynx may present with cervical lymphadenopathy but more frequently will present with nasal obstruction, frank epistaxis, or bloody nasal discharge. This entity must be ruled out whenever an adult presents with a unilateral serous otitis. Squamous cell carcinoma is less frequent in children.

5. Stenosis of the nasopharynx. Nasopharyngeal stenosis can be congenital or acquired. Congenital stenosis may be incomplete choanal atresia (see Chap. 1) or a hypoplastic nasopharynx. The latter is usually associated with generalized skull deformities.

Acquired stenosis may be posttraumatic, iatrogenic, or secondary to granulomatous infection such as tuberculosis, syphilis, or diphtheria. Acquired stenosis usually has a gradual onset and can be asymptomatic until the obstruction is nearly complete. Nasal obstruction, discharge, and secondary bacterial rhinitis herald the diagnosis. On anterior rhinoscopy there may be contraction of the posterior intranasal space. The diagnosis can be established by indirect mirror examination, transnasal fiberoptic study (giving a dynamic functional assessment), cinefluoroscopy with contrast media and CT scan. Many surgical procedures have been described for restoring patency; however, adequate functional dimensions are frequently difficult to achieve.

IV. Nasal discharge

A. **Purulent rhinitis** rarely occurs as a primary problem. It is associated with acute problems such as sinusitis, nasopharyngitis, nasopharyngeal obstruction, intranasal foreign body, or as a secondary bacterial infection associated with a viral URI. Resolution depends on treatment or recovery from the primary disorder. Chronic disease states (e.g., cystic fibrosis) are noted for frequent exacerbations and usually are slow to respond to medical measures. (See sec. **II.E.4.**)

B. **Acute sinusitis** presents with pain, malaise, nasal obstruction, and purulent rhinorrhea. Often the onset follows a viral URI or an exacerbation of allergic rhinitis. Patients with nasal polyposis, septal deviation, allergic rhinitis, sinus ostial obstruction, or cystic fibrosis are more commonly affected. *Streptococcus pneumoniae* and non-typable *Haemophilus influenzae* remain the most common pathogens isolated. Anaerobic bacteria are found in up to 10% of cases. *Staphylococcus aureus* is rare, and *Moraxella catarrhalis* is more common in children; however, *S. pneumoniae* and *H. influenzae* predominate. Carefully performed cultures yield a viral etiology in up to 20% of cases of acute adult sinusitis.

1. **Acute frontal sinusitis** presents with a unilateral or bilateral frontal headache. Concomitant nasal obstruction and discharge are not constant features. The sinus is tender to palpation and percussion. A Caldwell view of the skull demonstrates either an air-fluid level or opacification of the affected frontal sinus.

   a. The **primary treatment** of frontal sinusitis includes the administration of oral antibiotics. Although *S. aureus* is an uncommon sinus pathogen, should this organism be etiologic, the frontal sinus is the most likely to be affected. Amoxicillin-clavulinate 500 mg q8h is a good initial drug. A vasoconstrictor mucolytic preparation such as pseudoephedrine and guaifenisin provides symptomatic relief in conjunction with steam inhalation, warm compresses, and humidification. A short-duration of a topical nasal spray (oxymetazoline hydrochloride—2 sprays tid for 3 days) encourages ostial patency.

   Adults allergic to the penicillin group should be started on trimethoprim-sulfamethoxazole (160/800 mg) PO bid. Those with significant arteriosclerotic cardiovascular disease are best not given pseudoephedrine.

   b. **Complications.** Complications of acute frontal sinusitis include osteomyelitis, meningitis, epidural abscess, subdural abscess, and brain abscess. When frontal sinusitis is associated with severe pain, with or without swelling, frontal bossing, and edema of the upper lids, hospitalization and intravenous antibiotics are necessary. In this situation, purulent material in the middle meatus should be cultured and a Gram stain made. The reliability of intranasal cultures in frontal sinus infection has not been established; however, when choosing an antibiotic, any predominant organism on Gram stain and culture should be covered. Blood cultures should also be obtained.

Hospitalized patients should be started on ceftriaxone. If a patient is allergic to penicillin, a careful history of the reaction must be obtained. Patients who have had only a rash can be placed on cephalosporins; however, patients with a history of significant urticaria, anaphylaxis, or upper airway or laryngeal edema must not be given a cephalosporin because of the possibility of cross sensitivity. Alternatively, these patients should be placed on clindamycin.

If a positive response, evidenced by decreasing pain, temperature, and percussion tenderness, is not noted within 36–48 hours, trephination of the affected sinus should be performed.

c. **Chronic frontal sinusitis** is a low-grade infection. It presents with headache, intermittent rhinorrhea, and sinus tenderness. Antibiotic management should be predicated on nasal culture whenever possible. An increasing number of anaerobes are being identified with chronic sinus disease. Often, the infection resolves only after a surgical procedure is performed to establish drainage and eradicate the chronically infected mucosae.

When a mucopyocele is present, surgery is necessary. Exploration can be accomplished by an osteoplastic frontal procedure with obliteration of the sinus, by a frontoethmoidectomy with reconstruction of the nasofrontal duct or, in selected cases, by ESS.

2. **Ethmoiditis** usually presents with a persistent dull medial orbital sensation of pressure. There may be an associated diffuse headache, lacrimation, or lid edema. Lateral displacement of the globe suggests that the process has extended through the lamina papyracea. Sinusitis in children frequently involves the ethmoid sinuses, given that these sinuses are partially developed at birth.

On examination, pus can be seen emanating from the middle or superior meatus. Radiographs show opacification of the affected sinus. Primary therapy is similar to that outlined for acute frontal sinusitis (see **1.a.**). However, amoxicillin is the initial antibiotic to consider.

a. **Complications of ethmoiditis** include orbital cellulitis, orbital abscess, and intracranial extension.

(1) **Orbital cellulitis** is suspect when purulent rhinorrhea antedates the rapid onset of periorbital erythema, conjunctival engorgement, and associated pain and toxicity, including an elevated temperature. When present or sus-

pect, cultures must be taken and IV antibiotic therapy initiated as part of a hospital management regimen. Chloramphenicol is often used in combination with ampicillin, in appropriate dosage, as the initial form of medical management until culture specific antibiotics can be started. Ceftriaxone is an excellent alternative.

Both oral and topical **decongestants** should be used in a cooperative adult patient. The nose is packed with cotton pledgets, saturated with a 4% cocaine solution, providing a measure of pain relief in addition to vasoconstriction. Ophthalmologic consultation should be considered immediately, to assess the presence or absence of spontaneous venous pulsations. Visual acuity must be assessed and frequently monitored for signs of deterioration.

(2) Orbital abscess presents much the same clinical picture as orbital cellulitis, but exophthalmos and orbital fixation are more common.

(3) Surgical management. Evidence of deteriorating vision or a failure of a favorable response to IV antibiotic therapy within 48 hours mandates surgical drainage. The documentation of an abscess with CT scan mandates drainage acutely via an external ethmoidectomy approach.

b. Chronic ethmoiditis occurs alone, in association with nasal polyps, or with isolated allergic diathesis. If there is no response to antibiotic therapy, ethmoidectomy is required. Endoscopic sinus surgery has become the procedure of choice because of the precise nature of this technique, which encourages normal tissue preservation. A trial of antibiotic therapy following appropriate cultures is warranted prior to surgical intervention.

3. Maxillary sinusitis

a. Signs and symptoms. The maxillary antra are the most frequently infected sinuses in the adult. Infection often presents with dental pain, pressure over the maxilla, nasal obstruction, and purulent rhinorrhea. The affected sinus is tender to palpation, and purulent discharge may emanate from the middle meatus. The infection can occur as a sequela of a periapical infection of an upper tooth. Affected teeth are usually tender to percussion.

b. Diagnosis. In most instances the diagnosis can be made on the clinical information available, and therapy is instituted. X rays in this setting need not be ordered before initiating therapy. Three weeks after the onset of treatment, a follow-up film will provide a base line for future use and a test of the completeness of resolution. In questionable cases, x rays should be ordered when the symptoms first present. A Waters' projection is the most informative plain view, often demonstrating a thickened lining, an air-fluid level, or total opacification.

c. **Therapy**

(1) **Acute.** Assuming patient compliance, proper medical management almost always effects resolution of the uncomplicated acute process.

(a) **Antibiotics.** The proper choice of antibiotics reflects a knowledge of the most common organisms, as noted above (**IV.B.**). Amoxallin or TMP-SMZ are two excellent choices. A minimum of 14 days of treatment is essential, and frequently 21 days are necessary. Close patient observation is mandatory to ensure complete resolution.

(b) **Rest.** For the first 48 hours rest is important.

(c) **Vasoconstrictors.** Early drainage speeds resolution. A topical nasal vasoconstrictor spray used tid for a maximum of 5 days should be prescribed. Vasoconstrictor preparations may be beneficial, and their use appears to be warranted for patients readily tolerating them.

(d) **Heat.** Moist heat also seems beneficial when applied over the infected sinus.

(2) **Ancillary measures**

(a) **Culture.** A nasal culture does not necessarily reflect the organisms present in the sinus. It is reserved for cases not responding to initial therapy and should be combined with culture data from the involved antra. Aspiration of the sinus contents provides material for staining and culture.

(b) **Antral puncture.** Often, gentle irrigation with saline can speed resolution in selected cases. Aspiration and irrigation are procedures best performed by an experienced physician. Although exceedingly rare in competent hands, injury to the globe, air embolus, bleeding, and osteomyelitis are potential complications of antral lavage.

d. **Chronic maxillary sinusitis** develops after prior acute episodes of infection with subsequent irreversible mucosal change, or OMC obstruction. Chronic rhinorrhea, halitosis, and occasionally mild pharyngitis, secondary to the persistent posterior nasal discharge, are the most consistent diagnostic features. Cultures of the infected sinus frequently grow anaerobes, and antibiotic therapy must cover these organisms. With chronic disease the antibiotic response is limited, and judicious surgery is often necessary.

4. **Sphenoiditis** rarely occurs as an isolated sinus infection. Acute sphenoiditis can present with severe retroorbital pain, and fre-

quently the pain is also referred to the vertex and basiocciput. The diagnosis is confirmed radiographically when clouding or opacification of the sinus is evidenced on lateral and submental vertex skull films.

Therapy. All patients with obstructive sphenoid sinusitis should be hospitalized and placed on antibiotics as for complications of frontal sinusitis (see **1.b.**). Any purulent drainage in the sphenoethmoid recess should be Gram stained and cultured. Blood cultures should be obtained, and 4% cocaine-impregnated strips should be placed in the nose for 10 minutes q8h until drainage is achieved. Oral decongestants such as pseudoephedrine are indicated (60 mg q6–8h). A bedside humidifier should be considered. If there is no response to the medical regimen within 36 hours, a sphenoidotomy is performed. Impending complications mandate drainage.

5. **Sinus ostial closure** can occur from secondary scarring induced by infection or iatrogenically from repeated cannulation of the ostium. Stenosis decreases effective drainage as well as aeration, predisposing the sinus to infection. Surgical intervention should be directed whenever possible toward establishing drainage. Frontal ablation is reserved for the most refractory cases or those with major associated complications.

6. **Barosinusitis** refers to paranasal sinus symptomatology due to a pressure differential between the sinus cavity and the environment. This condition most frequently occurs during flying, especially on descent. Altered function is often fostered by inflammation, redundant tissue, or an anatomic aberration obstructing the normal sinus ostium.

   Symptoms range from a sensation of fullness over the affected sinus to local excruciating pain. The ideal therapy is to return the patient to the initial altitude, slowly repeating the descent. Oral decongestant preparations and topical vasoconstrictors are indicated. Only with associated infection are antibiotics warranted.

7. **Immunosuppression** in patients with AIDS or receiving chemotherapy may predispose to infections from a number of uncommon bacterial or fungal pathogens. Sinus aspiration must be performed early in the course of the disease so that appropriate therapy is instituted. Surgical drainage may be required as initial treatment, because antimicrobial agents previously discussed may be ineffective. Evidence is emerging that MRI is useful in identifying mycotic infections of the paranasal sinuses.

C. **CSF rhinorrhea** may occur spontaneously or after an episode of trauma. Frontoethmoid fractures can be complicated by a CSF leak. Watery or blood-tinged nasal discharge should be analyzed for glucose. A level of 40–100 dl is diagnostic for a CSF leak. Dipstick and tablet-type analysis of glucose levels are not reliable.

Unless the rhinorrhea is profuse, the initial management is conservative. Hospitalization and the consideration of IV antibiotics are warranted. A semisitting position is beneficial, and the patient is instructed to abstain from nasal blowing and straining. Most traumatic CSF leaks resolve without intervention.

1. **Complications.** Undiagnosed CSF rhinorrhea can lead to recurrent meningitis.

2. The **site** of the **leak** must be located. Topical vasoconstriction in the office setting and subsequent endoscopic evaluation can disclose the site of leakage. For cases in which a diagnosis cannot be made by this method, fluorescein and radioactive indium are adjunctive diagnostic measures.

   Technique. Three cotton pledgets are placed in each nasal chamber—one in the sphenoethmoid recess, a second in the cribriform region, and a third in the middle meatus. Each pledget is appropriately labeled prior to placement. A spinal tap is performed, with the removal of 10 ml of CSF. Next, 0.5 ml of 5% fluorescein is mixed with 10 ml of CSF, and the mixture is slowly injected intrathecally. *It is important to use fluorescein approved for intravenous injection and not topical fluorescein.* In addition, 500 μCi of indium is injected intrathecally. Between 2 and 4 hours postinjection the patient is scanned. Frequently, the site of the leak can be identified on this scan. The cotton pledgets are removed and each examined under a Wood's lamp for fluorescence. Subsequently, the pledgets are evaluated for their radioactivity. An increased pledget count is considered a positive test result, and the location of the pledget is compared to the scan. Preoperative identification of the leak helps to define the appropriate corrective surgical procedure.

V. **Olfaction.** The olfactory cells of the first cranial (olfactory) nerve pass into the superior nasal fossa through the cribriform plate. Synapsing, second-order neurons enter the rhinencephalon where the olfactory stimulus is processed. All patients complaining of olfactory dysfunction should have a complete otorhinolaryngologic and neurologic examination. In patients complaining of dysosmia (alteration in smell), it is important to rule out sources such as bronchiectasis, caries, or sinusitis.

The initial evaluation can be performed using coffee, chocolate, lemon oil, tobacco, ammonia, menthol, and acetone. The last three are strong trigeminal stimulants. Malingering should be suspected whenever a patient cannot "smell" these. Commercial tests for olfaction are also available and may be more reliable.

CT scans are appropriate if a symptom or sign other than anosmia can be found.

A. **Etiology.** Olfactory aberrations can be related to nasal obstruction, congenital dysfunction, trauma, infection, neoplasms, or environmental pollutants. Hyposmia is seen as part of the aging process. As many as 80% of individuals over the age of 60 years will note some decrease in the sense of smell awareness. Investigations have linked the early onset of anosmia with the subsequent development of Alzheimer's disease.

1. **Nasal airway obstruction** due to any of the factors previously discussed can influence olfactory function. Opinions differ as to whether septal deviation can affect the sense of smell. Relief of anosmia, secondary either to nasal polyposis or to allergic rhinitis, has been reported with steroids.

2. **Complete congenital anosmia** is rare and has been reported as an isolated familial disorder. It occurs in Kallmann's syndrome (agenesis of the olfactory lobes and secondary hypogonadism due to lack of gonadotropins). Many patients have a specific anosmia for a limited number of odors; however, this is usually asymptomatic.

3. **Trauma.** Anosmia can occur after head trauma. Most commonly, it is related to occipital or frontal blows. Unilateral anosmia can be present in conjunction with CSF rhinorrhea following head trauma.

4. **Infection.** Viral upper respiratory tract infections can alter the sense of smell directly by affecting the olfactory cell or secondarily by effecting nasal airway obstruction. Anosmia is especially frequent following influenza. Postinfluenza patients may continue to have anosmia, and others have transient parosmia as olfaction returns.

5. **Neoplasia.** Neoplasms known to cause altered olfaction include meningiomas of the dura of the cribriform plate, tumors of the third ventricle, frontal lobe glioma, sphenoidal ridge meningioma, temporal lobe tumors, and suprasellar meningioma.

6. **Pollutants.** Industrial exposure to benzene, ethyl acetate, formaldehyde, menthol, paint solvents, oil of peppermint, butyl acetate, carbon disulfide, and trichloroethylene has been reported to cause anosmia or hyposmia.

7. **Olfactory disturbances** can occur with psychiatric disorders such as schizophrenia, hysteria, confusional states, and depression.

B. **Therapy** is directed toward removing the causative agent or toward correcting the underlying disturbance. Therapy for postviral or idiopathic smell disorders is limited. The use of zinc sulfate has been occasionally successful. Vitamin A as a therapy is currently being investigated.

VI. **Facial pain** has multiple etiologies, including tumors, neuralgia, inflammation of the paranasal sinuses, or vascular occlusion. All patients with facial pain must have a complete otolaryngologic and neurologic evaluation.

A. **Sinus pain.** Maxillary sinus pain usually presents with a sensation of pressure over the sinus. As the pain intensifies, it involves all areas abutting the sinus walls, including the ipsilateral orbit. Ethmoid sinusitis produces orbital pain and pain between the eyes, which can extend to the temporal region. Frontal sinus pain is usually localized over the affected sinus. Sphenoid sinusitis causes severe pain behind the eyes, which can radiate to the parietal or occipital regions (see sec. **IV.B.4.**).

B. Neuralgia is typified by paroxysms of lancinating pain of a few seconds' to a few minutes' duration. The paroxysm is usually initiated by any stimulus to a trigger point or region.

1. **Trigeminal neuralgia (tic douloureux).** The brief, lancinating, paroxysmol pain of trigeminal neuralgia is confined to the branches of the fifth cranial nerve. The maxillary division is most frequently affected, followed in frequency by the mandibular. On sensory testing the nerve is found to be intact. Facial trigger points are frequently found, with symptoms brought on by chewing, yawning, swallowing, shaving, etc. Most patients are over the age of 40 years, with women affected more often than men. Rarely, further investigation of trigeminal neuralgia with associated hypesthesia in the distribution of the facial nerve, other cranial neuropathies, and with onset before age 40 years may disclose multiple sclerosis or a posterior fossa tumor.

   Therapy. Oral carbamazepine and phenytoin have each been used with limited success. The usual adult dose of phenytoin is 100 mg tid. Phenytoin can have detrimental effects on the endocrine, nervous, integumentary, gastrointestinal, cardiac, and hemopoietic sytems. It frequently causes gingival hyperplasia.

   Carbamazepine should be prescribed only by a physician who will be following the patient closely. The initial adult dose is 200 mg PO qid. Among the more significant side effects are aplastic anemia, agranulocytosis, jaundice. Stevens-Johnson syndrome, congestive heart failure, and cardiovascular collapse. Baclofen may be used alone or in conjunction with phenytoin or carbamazepine. The initial dosage is 5–10 mg tid, with gradual increase to 20 mg qid as needed.

2. **Glossopharyngeal neuralgia** begins with severe pain, starting in the lower pharynx, tonsil, or base of the tongue. It can radiate to the ipsilateral ear, mandible, and teeth. The pain is unilateral and so intense that patients will not speak during an episode. The trigger point is often in the base of the tongue or tonsillar region. In some individuals, the pain is initiated by deglutition. The diagnosis is made if local anesthesia to the trigger point provides temporary relief of the pain. Once recognized, nerve section can provide relief.

3. **Sphenopalatine neuralgia** presents with lower facial pain radiating to the orbit, temple, forehead, and upper cervical region. It is accompanied by ipsilateral lacrimation, conjunctivitis, rhinorrhea, and nasal congestion. If local anesthesia to the sphenopalatine ganglion provides symptomatic relief, the diagnosis is confirmed. Local anesthesia can be accomplished by topical placement of a cocaine-soaked cotton pledget in the posterior nasal chamber.

4. **Atypical facial neuralgia** is a unilateral aching pain of hours' or days' duration that is not limited to a specific nerve distribution. It often spreads over the cervical root distribution and can involve the nose, eye, cheek, ear, neck, and shoulder. Attacks

have been precipitated by fatigue, tooth extractions, tension, and anxiety. Associated autonomic symptoms can include pallor, diaphoresis, lacrimation, and rhinitis. This pain is refractory to section of the trigeminal nerve, local anesthesia to the sphenopalatine ganglion, and resection of the superior cervical sympathetic ganglion. The etiology of atypical facial neuralgia is unknown, and multiple causation is likely. Patients presenting with these symptoms should be evaluated to rule out local pathology as well as any depressive symptoms. Treatment includes phenytoin and carbamazepine.

C. Carotidynia is pain that comes from the carotid artery and radiates to the ipsilateral eye, ear, and malar region. The episodes are periodic, and there are no associated visual disturbances. On examination, the common carotid is tender to palpation. The pain usually resolves within 2 weeks. Symptomatic relief is often provided by aspirin, or nonsteroidal anti-inflammatory agents. Occasionally, ergotamine can diminish the pain.

D. Migraine headaches may start in childhood, adolescence, or early adulthood. An aura precedes the pain, and the prodromes include scintillating scotomas, flashing lights, hemianopsia, paresthesias, and hemiparesis. The pain is localized to one part of the head, usually unilateral, and can vary in intensity from mild discomfort to severe throbbing pain. There is often associated photophobia, nausea, emesis, altered taste, or smell. Migraine headaches can last from a few hours to 3 days. Females are more frequently affected. Basilar artery migraine can produce occipital head pain and is often accompanied by episodes of vertigo that recur with the headache.

1. Therapy

a. For an **acute attack,** a combination of ergotamine tartrate and caffeine often provides relief. This medication can be prescribed as a tablet or suppository. Initial adult PO dosage is 2 mg ergotamine tartrate and 200 mg of caffeine taken during the onset of the attack. If necessary, an additional 1 mg ergotamine and 100 mg caffeine can be taken PO one-half hour after the initial dose for further relief of symptoms. This medication is contraindicated with arteriosclerotic cardiovascular disease, hypertension, impaired hepatic function, impaired renal function, or pregnancy.

b. Prophylaxis. A 50% reduction in symptoms should be considered successful management. Prophylaxis should not be continued beyond 1 year. Multiple medications have shown efficacy for prevention, but methysergide and propanalol are time-tested and remain appropriate.

(1) Methysergide has been used for long-term prophylaxis of migraine; it is not effective for acute attacks. The standard dosage is 2 mg, 2 to 4 times daily. Methysergide should be prescribed only by a physician who will be following the patient closely, since it has serious adverse effects including retroperitoneal fibrosis and fibrosis of cardiac valves. Contraindications include pregnancy, any form of arteriosclerotic cardiovascular disease, pulmonary disease, impaired hepatic or renal function, valvular heart disease, serious infection, and phlebitis or cellulitis of the lower limbs.

(2) Propranolol can be used for prevention of the migraine attack. The initial dose is 20 mg PO qid. This dose can be gradually increased to 40–60 mg qid. The patient's blood pressure and pulse must be monitored while adjusting the propranolol dose. It is contraindicated in patients with bronchial asthma, congestive heart failure, and sinus bradycardia. Abrupt withdrawal of propranolol in patients with angina pectoris has resulted in myocardial infarction.

E. Cluster headache (Horton's cephalgia)

1. Signs and symptoms. Cluster headache is idiopathic, excruciating, knifelike pain that involves the ipsilateral temple, forehead, face, head, and neck but spares the lips and tongue. There is no preceding aura; it lasts from 10 minutes to several hours. The attacks can recur several times within 24 hours; they often repeat daily for several weeks, followed by a prolonged symptom-free interval. Males are affected 4–6 times as often as females. The first attack usually occurs between the ages of 20 and 35.

2. Therapy

a. Acute. Ergotamine tartrate and caffeine can be used for relief of the pain. The total maximum weekly dose, however, is 10 mg of ergotamine. Therefore, patients should take only 1–2 mg of ergotamine initially. Some patients require injection of ergotamine tartrate, since they do not benefit from the oral medication. These patients require 0.25 mg IV qid. The contraindications for this medication have been discussed (see **1.a.**).

b. Prophylaxis. Methysergide calcium channel blocking agents are both effective (see **1.b.**). Prophylactic lithium has been given when the attacks begin, with doses necessary to obtain a blood level of 0.6–1.2 mEq/l should be used. Methysergide is contraindicated in pregnancy, renal disease, cardiovascular disease, and in patients on diuretics. There are several serious reactions, including an encephalopathic syndrome, hypothyroidism, seizures, peripheral circulatory collapse, arrhythmias, stupor, and coma. Serum levels must be monitored and should be drawn 8–12 hours after the oral dose is taken.

F. Tension headaches commonly start in the occipital region and spread in a band distribution around the head. Patients often describe a viselike sensation over the entire head. These headaches can be intermittent or can persist throughout a 24-hour period with varying intensity. Muscle relaxants are occasionally of value, along with an analgesic.

G. Glaucoma can present with an acute, unilateral, deep penetrating pain or with a chronic, dull pain. All patients presenting with a headache should be evaluated to rule out glaucoma.

H. Temporal arteritis is an illness of patients over 50 years of age and is characterized by a severe inflammatory reaction around the vessels and with multinucleated giant cells in the media. It is similar to periarteritis nodosa.

1. **Signs and symptoms** include pain in the distribution of the temporal artery, along with systemic symptoms of lethargy, low-grade fever, and weight loss. Visual loss can occur when the central retinal artery is involved.

2. **Diagnosis** is made with an elevated erythrocyte sedimentation rate (ESR) of 60–120 mm/hour. Biopsy of the artery confirms the diagnosis; however, angiography may be needed in some cases.

3. **Management** is with corticosteroids at high doses (prednisone 45 mg/day) particularly if vision is affected. Steroids frequently can be discontinued after 6 months, because temporal arteritis is a self-limiting disease.

I. Other causes of facial pain include temporomandibular joint syndrome and muscular spasm.

Selected Readings

Axelsson, A. The correlation between bacteriological findings in the nose and maxillary sinus in acute maxillary sinusitis. *Laryngoscope* 83:2003, 1973.

Blickerstaff, G. R. Cluster Headaches. In P. J. Vinken and G. W. Bruyn (eds.), *Handbook of Clinical Neurology: Headaches and Cranial Neuralgias* (vol. 5). New York: Wiley, 1968. Pp. 111–118.

Blitzer, A., Lawson, W., and Friedman, W. H. *Surgery of the Paranasal Sinuses* (2nd ed.). Philadelphia: Saunders, 1991.

Chapnik, J. S., and Bach, M. C. Bacteria and fungal infections of the maxillary sinus. *Otolaryngol. Clin. North Am.* 9:43, 1976.

Dalessio, D. J. Atypical Facial Neuralgia(s). In *Wolff's Headache and Other Head Pain* (3rd ed.). New York: Oxford University Press, 1972. Pp. 452–462.

Doty, R. L. A review of olfactory dysfunctions in man. *Am. J. Otolaryngol.* 1:57, 1979.

Duvall, A. J., and Banovetz, J. D. Nasoethmoidal fractures. *Otolaryngol. Clin. North Am.* 9:507, 1976.

Duvall, A. J., and Banovetz, J. D. Maxillary fractures. *Otolaryngol. Clin. North Am.* 9:489, 1976.

Fischer, T. J., Entis, G. N., Winant, J. G. Jr., and Bernstein, I. L. Basic Principles of Therapy for Allergic Disease. In G. J. Lawlor Jr. and T. J. Fischer (eds.), *Manual of Allergy and Immunology, Diagnosis and Therapy*. Boston: Little, Brown, 1988. Pp. 46–95.

Frederick, J., and Braude, A. I. Anaerobic infection of the paranasal sinuses. *N. Engl. J. Med.* 290:135, 1974.

Fried, M. P., Kelly, J. H., and Strome, M. Pseudomonas rhinosinusitis. *Laryngoscope* 94:192, 1984.

Graham, J. R. Migraine: Clinical Aspects. In P. J. Vinken and G. W. Bruyn (eds.), *Handbook of Clinical Neurology: Headaches and Cranial Neuralgias* (vol. 5). New York: Wiley, 1968. Pp. 45–48.

Hier, D. B. Headache. In Samuels, M. A. (ed.), *Manual of Neurology, Diagnosis and Therapy* (4th ed.). Boston: Little, Brown, 1991. Pp. 17–31.

Hill, D. P., and Jafek, B. W. Initial otolaryngologic assessment of patients with taste and smell disorders. *Ear Nose Throat J.* 68:362, 1989.

Karma, P., Jokiph, L., and Sipila, P. Bacteria in chronic maxillary sinusitis. *Arch. Otolaryngol.* 105:386, 1979.

Kennedy, D. W., Zinreich, S. J., Rosenbaum, A. E., and Johns, M. E. Functional endoscopic sinus surgery, theory and diagnostic evaluation. *Arch. Otolaryngol.* 111:576, 1985.

Knight, A., and Kolin, A. Long-term efficacy and safety of beclomethasone dipropionate aerosol in perennial rhinitis. *Ann. Allergy* 50:81, 1983.

Kortekangas, A. E. Antibiotics in the treatment of maxillary sinusitis. *Acta Otolaryngol. [Suppl.]* (Stockh.) 188:379, 1964

Lystad, A., Berdal, P., and Lauritz, L. I. The bacterial flora of sinusitis with an in vitro study of the bacterial resistance of antibiotics. *Acta Otolaryngol. [Suppl.]* (Stockh.) 188:390, 1964.

McGrail, J. D. Management of maxillary fractures. *Otolaryngol. Clin. North Am.* 9:223, 1972.

Montgomery, W. W. Facial Fractures. In W. W. Montgomery (ed.), *Surgery of the Upper Respiratory System* (vol. I) (2nd ed.). Philadelphia: Lea & Febiger, 1979. Pp. 280–285.

Montgomery, W. W. Repair of Dural Defects. In W. W. Montgomery (ed.), *Surgery of the Upper Respiratory System* (vol. I) (2nd ed.). Philadelphia: Lea & Febiger, 1979. Pp. 175–208.

Montgomery, W. W. Surgery of the Frontal Sinus. In W. W. Montgomery (ed.), *Surgery of the Upper Respiratory System* (vol. I) (2nd ed.). Philadelphia: Lea & Febiger, 1979. Pp. 165–173.

Pollak, K., and Payne, E. E. Fractures of the frontal sinus. *Otolaryngol. Clin. North Am.* 9:517, 1976.

Poser, C. M. Facial pain: Diagnostic dilemma, therapeutic challenge. *Geriatrics* 30:110, 1975.

Rachelefsky, G. S., Katz, R. M., and Siegal, S. C. Chronic sinusitis in children with respiratory allergy: Role of antimicrobials. *J. Allergy Clin. Immunol.* 69:382, 1982.

Reed, S. E. The aetiology and epidemiology of common colds and the possibilities of prevention. *Clin. Otolaryngol.* 6:379, 1981.

Ritchie, J. M., and Cohen, P. J. Local Anesthetics. In L. S. Goodman and A. Gilman (eds.), *The Pharmacological Basis for Therapeutics* (5th ed.). New York: Macmillan, 1975. Pp. 379–394.

Ritter, F. N. Ethmoidal and Sphenoidal Sinus Disease. In G. M. English (ed.), *Otolaryngology* (vol. 2). Hagerstown, Md.: Harper & Row, 1990.

Schramm, V. L., Jr., Curtin, H. D., and Kennerdell, J. S. Evaluation of orbital cellulitis and results of treatment. *Laryngoscope* 92:732, 1982.

Scott, A. E. Clinical characteristics of taste and smell disorders. *Ear Nose Throat J.* 68:297, 1989.

Stammberger, H. *Functional Endoscopic Sinus Surgery.* Philadelphia: B. C. Decker, 1991.

Toohill, R. J., et al. Rhinitis medicamentosa. *Laryngoscope* 91:1614, 1981.

Weld, E. R. Rhinitis and Acute and Chronic Sinusitis. In C. D. Bluestone and S. E. Stool (eds.), *Pediatric Otolaryngology* (2nd ed.). Philadelphia: Saunders, 1990. Pp. 729–744.

Zinreich, S. J., Kennedy, D. W., Rosenbaum, A. E., et al. Paranasal sinuses: CT in assessing requirements for endoscopic surgery. *Radiology* 163:769, 1987.

Appendix: Antihistamine Usage

Class	Generic examples	Trade name	Oral dosage Pediatric	Oral dosage Adult	Characteristics
Ethylenediamines	Pyrilamine maleate	Triaminic preparations	Infant 16 mg qid /2 lbs	75–200 mg/24 hr in divided doses	Low sedative and anticholinergic effects; gastrointestinal complaints common (reduced by giving drug with meals)
Ethanolamines	Clemastine fumarate	Tavist preparations	6–12 yr, 1–2 tsp bid	1.34 mg bid–2.68 mg (max. 8.04 mg/24 hr)	Drowsiness most frequent complaint but no marked sedation; anticholinergic effects weak and gastrointestinal complaints uncommon
	Diphenhydramine hydrochloride	Benadryl	6–12 yr, 5 mg/kg/24 hr, in 4 divided doses	25–100 mg q6–8h	Sedative effects high; anticholinergic effects moderate; gastrointestinal complaints uncommon
Alkylamines	Brompheniramine maleate	Dimetane Dimetapp	0.5 mg/kg/24 hr in 4–6 divided dosages (max. 6 mg/24 hr for ages 2–6 yr; 12 mg/24 hr for ages 6–12 yr)	4 mg q4–6h (max. 24 mg/24 hr), or 8–12 mg q8–12h using time-released form	Low sedative, anticholinergic, and gastrointestinal effects; approximately 75% of over-the-counter preparations contain an alkylamine antihistamine
	Chlorpheniramine maleate	Chlor-Trimeton Novahistine Ornade Numerous over-the-counter preparations	0.35 mg/kg/24 hr in 4 divided doses. Over 7 yr, 8 mg q12h (time-released)	2–4 mg q6–8h, as time-released form, 8–12 mg q12h	As above

Class	Generic name	Trade name	Pediatric dosage	Adult dosage	Comments
Piperazines	Hydroxyzine hydrochloride	Atarax	2–5 mg/kg/24 hr in 3 divided doses	25–100 mg q6–8h	Drowsiness and dry mouth common; used to treat pruritus
	Meclizine hydrochloride	Antivert	Not recommended <12 yr	25–100 mg/24 hr in 3–4 divided doses	As above; used primarily for motion sickness and vertigo
Phenothiazines	Promethazine hydrochloride	Phenergan	0.5 mg/kg/dose q6–8h	25 mg at bedtime or 12.5 mg qid	Marked sedative effect; used primarily as sedative and antiemetic
Piperidines	Azatadine maleate	Trinaline	Dosage not established <12 yr	1–2 mg bid	Drowsiness most common side effect; chemically similar to cyproheptadine
	Cyproheptadine hydrochloride	Periactin	2–6 yr, 2 mg q8–12h (max. 12 mg/24 hr)	4–20 mg/day in divided doses (max. 0.5 mg/kg/24 hr)	Drowsiness most common side effect; weight gain common; useful for pruritus and especially for cold urticaria; do not use in newborn or premature infants
Nonsedating anti-histamines	Terfenadine	Seldane	Not recommended <12 yr	60 mg bid	Well accepted; rapid onset nonsedating; negligible side effects
	Astemizole	Hismanal	Not recommended <12 yr	10 mg qid	Well accepted; half life 1 day; diminishes response to skin testing for up to two weeks

Source: Adapted from G. L. Lawlor, Jr., and T. J. Fischer, *Manual of Allergy and Immunology.* Boston: Little, Brown, 1981.

4

Oral Cavity, Pharynx, and Esophagus

Oro-Naso-Hypopharynx

I. **Anatomy.** The pharynx is a musculomembranous tube posterior to the oral cavity that extends from the base of the skull to the larynx. Posteriorly, the pharynx is connected to the cervical vertebral column by loose areolar tissue; laterally, it is bordered by the constrictor muscles; superiorly, it is limited by the occipital bone and sphenoid sinus; inferiorly, it joins the esophagus at the cricopharyngeus muscle level; and anteriorly, it is incomplete, with an opening communicating with the nasal cavities, the oral cavity, and the larynx. The pharynx is divided into the nasopharynx, the oropharynx, and the hypopharynx (laryngopharynx) (Fig. 4-1).

   A. The **nasopharynx** is situated above the soft palate and communicates anteriorly with the nasal cavities via the choanae. The roof and posterior wall contain the adenoids, or pharyngeal tonsils, lymphatic tissue that often attains considerable size, especially in children. The paired eustachian tube orifices are situated on the lateral walls of the nasopharynx, behind the posterior ends of the inferior turbinates.

   B. The **oropharynx**, visible directly by depressing the tongue, extends from the soft palate to the hyoid bone, opening anteriorly into the oral cavity and containing on its lateral wall the palatine, or faucial, tonsils.

   C. The **hypopharynx** is inferior to the base of the tongue and extends from the hyoid bone to the lower border of the cricoid cartilage. It contains the triangular-shaped entrance to the larynx, the base of which is the epiglottis and the sides, the aryepiglottic folds. The oropharynx and hypopharynx are actually a muscular cone. Swallowing is made possible by the specialized constrictor muscles, and the attached accessory muscles protect the airway when gag and cough reflexes are initiated by unwanted material threatening the airway.

II. **Physical examination**. Most conditions of the pharynx are readily diagnosed from the history and physical examination.

   A. **Systematic examination** of the oral cavity and oropharynx is imperative so that no abnormalities are overlooked. Dentures should be removed. Attention should be directed to the lips, buccal mucosa,

137

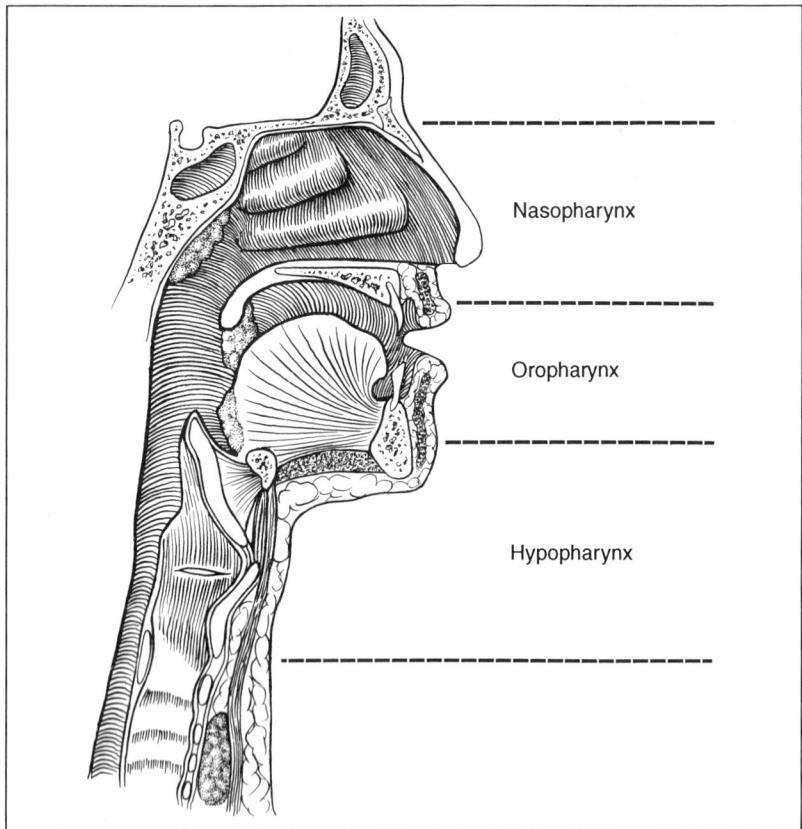

Fig. 4-1. Anatomy of lateral upper airway. Anatomic divisions of oro-, naso-, and hypopharynx.

teeth, gingiva, floor of mouth, tongue, hard and soft palates, and posterior pharyngeal wall. Effects of both local and systemic disease can be noted.

Palpation of lesions in the oral cavity and base of tongue is imperative in suspected neoplastic disease. The oropharynx can best be visualized with a tongue depressor. The palatine tonsils lie between the anterior and posterior tonsilar pillars, and are accessible to direct inspection and palpation. The tonsils are normally the same color as the surrounding oral mucosa and often contain visible crypts, in which exfoliated epithelium and debris can accumulate. Lymphoid nodules on the posterior pharyngeal wall appear as discrete submucosal masses. The lateral pharyngeal bands, also lymphoid-containing tissue, are located behind the posterior tonsilar pillar and descend from the nasopharynx toward the lingual tonsils at the base of the tongue. The adenoids, palatine, and lingual tonsils, along with the lateral pharyngeal bands, compose Waldeyer's ring.

B. Nasopharyngeal examination requires either proper use of the indirect mirror or direct visualization with rigid or flexible fiberoptic telescopes. An indirect, defogged No. 0 or No. 00 mirror is placed to one side of the uvula, nearly touching the posterior pharyngeal wall. A light beam from a head mirror or headlight is reflected from the nasopharyngeal mirror into the nasopharynx. The patient is instructed to breathe through the nose so that the palate will relax. The posterior ends of the nasal turbinates, the eustachian tube orifices with adjacent torus tubarius and fossa of Rosenmüller, the posterior end of the vomer, adenoid tissue, and the entire choanal circumference can be visualized. Direct nasopharyngoscopy is best performed after shrinking and anesthetizing the nasal mucous membranes. The scope is passed through one nasal chamber along its floor, into the nasopharynx, and manipulated so as to view the above structures.

C. Hypopharyngeal examination is performed with either a mirror or flexible fiberoptic telescope. The tongue is retracted anteriorly by grasping it with a gauze pad. A defogged No. 4 or No. 5 mirror is placed with the back touching the midline soft palate. A light is directed onto the mirror to visualize the base of tongue, valleculae, pharyngeal walls, piriform sinuses, and larynx.

III. Infectious pharyngitis. Sore throat is the outstanding symptom of acute pharyngitis, no matter what the etiology.

A. Acute bacterial pharyngotonsillitis

1. Signs and symptoms

a. Bacterial tonsillitis or pharyngitis, usually caused by group A beta-hemolytic streptococci, presents with the sudden onset of sore throat, malaise, fever, anorexia, and odynophagia. Temperature may rise to 102.2–104°F over the first 24–48 hours, often to 104–105°F in children. Dehydration may result from the odynophagia and fever. Myalgias, arthralgias, headache, and vomiting may occur. Cough and rhinorrhea make a viral etiology more likely.

b. On **physical examination,** the patient appears ill with pharyngeal erythema (sometimes deeply red-purple), patchy yellow-white exudate, and hypertrophy of all local lymphoid tissue. Edema of the soft palate, as well as tender cervical adenopathy, may be evident. There may be a patchy yellow-white exudate, which easily can be wiped away. The presence of exudate does not establish a specific etiology and may be seen in infections due to *S. pyogenes, S. pneumoniae, H. influenzae, H. parainfluenzae* (children), and *Corynebacterium diptheriae,* as well as some viruses (adenovirus and mononucleosis).

2. Diagnosis is made by throat culture (on 5% sheep blood agar), which will usually grow group A beta-hemolytic streptococci in this clinical picture. Culture accuracy varies with the aggressiveness of the technique. Sampling both sides of the pharynx yields a higher percentage of positive growth. A single, representative throat culture has approximately 95% of the accuracy of serial cultures. New rapid tests for group A streptococci can provide information in hours. However, false-negatives occur, and follow-up traditional cultures should be performed when the clinical picture suggests streptococci. A leukocytosis and negative mononucleosis spot test aid in making the diagnosis.

3. Therapy

   a. Treatment consists of bed rest, hydration, warm saline pharyngeal irrigations hourly while awake until pain subsides, antipyretics, and an antibiotic.

   b. Penicillin is the drug of choice unless allergy precludes it. Two regimens should be considered:

   (1) Oral penicillin V, 250 mg PO tid or qid for 10 days; 500,000 units/kg/day PO tid or qid for 10 days in children.

   (2) IM benthazine penicillin, a single dose, 600,000 units for children less than 6 years of age; 900,000 units between 6 and 9 years old; and 1.2 million units for those over 9 years old. Higher initial levels can be achieved with the addition of IM procaine (IM Bicillin R, 1.2 million units) or oral penicillin along with benzathine penicillin.

   Benzathine, 900,000 units, plus procaine penicillin G, 300,000 units, may be better tolerated than plain benzathine penicillin G in the pediatric patient. In cases of penicillin allergy, erythromycin estolate, in a dose of 10–20 mg/kg/day for 10 days, is effective therapy. For erythromycin intolerance, clindamycin should be considered.

   c. An occasional patient needs hospitalization for IV hydration because of dehydration secondary to severe odynophagia.

   d. Recurrent acute or chronic tonsillitis may require tonsillectomy. The indications are seven episodes in 1 year, five episodes per year for 2 years, or three episodes per year for 3 years.

   e. For symptomatic bacteriologic failure, rifampin 20 mg/kg, not exceeding 600 mg/day, administered as a single daily dose for the last 4 days of a new primary regimen (cephalosporin), is frequently effective.

B. Diphtheria is a rare disease today, but it must be considered in any pharyngeal infection, especially in those demonstrating a membranous exudate. Required immunization has decreased the incidence during the past 40 years, but nonimmunized patients are common and endemic. Occasional epidemics (e.g., San Antonio, 1970) are still seen. Immediate and specific treatment is necessary to prevent the serious complications of paralysis or myocarditis.

1. **Signs and symptoms**

    a. Onset is more insidious than streptococcal pharyngitis, with several days of sore throat, low-grade fever, and increasing swelling of the anterior cervical nodes. Associated symptoms are headache, malaise, nausea, and increasing toxemia.

    b. The patient presents with a characteristic, adherent dirty gray membrane over the tonsils, extending over the pillars and sometimes onto the soft palate; when removed with a culture swab, the underlying area bleeds. The mucosa of the nose, larynx, and hypopharynx may also be involved. Ulcerations are not common. Complications can include airway obstruction and cardiac toxicity.

2. **Diagnosis.** Direct cultures should always be obtained for smear (Gram) and culture (on Klebs-Löffler and tellurite agar media). Patients treated with penicillin or erythromycin before being seen may have less marked symptoms and eradicated organisms, but antibiotics are totally ineffective against circulating toxin.

3. **Therapy**

    a. Prompt treatment with specific diphtheria antitoxin should be initiated if the smears are questionable and if strong clinical suspicion prevails. After appropriate skin sensitivity testing, 20,000–50,000 units of antitoxin are given IM or IV (100–200 ml saline diluted over 30 minutes). This should be given within the first 48 hours of the disease onset.

    b. Isolation until three consecutive daily nose and throat cultures are negative, strict bed rest, and antibiotics are ordered while carefully observing the patient's airway for signs of obstruction. Tracheotomy may be necessary.

    c. Antibiotic therapy for the pediatric patient should be procaine penicillin, 25,000–50,000 units/kg/day IM q12h, or erythromycin, 50 mg/kg/day PO for 7–10 days. In the adult, procaine penicillin, 1.2 million units IM, or erythromycin, 250–500 mg PO qid, is used.

C. **Infectious mononucleosis** is an acute disease, occurring most commonly among adolescents and young adults; it is caused by the Epstein-Barr virus (EBV). It is characterized by fever, pharyngitis, lymphadenopathy, lymphocytosis with atypical cells, a positive heterophile antibody titer, and persistent EBV-antibody responses. CMC and Toxoplasma gondii infections can mimic mononucleosis, presenting with atypical circulating lymphocytes and peripheral lymphocytosis.

1. **Signs and symptoms**

    a. Sore throat is the most common symptom. Over 80% of patients demonstrate sore throat, fever, and anterior and posterior cervical lymphadenopathy.

    b. Other symptoms are malaise, persistent fever, and headache. These symptoms can be present in spite of previous treatment with antibiotics, further aiding the diagnosis.

    c. Physical examination reveals a febrile (101–103°F) patient (although children often have no fever), with marked hyperplasia, inflammation, and edema of the pharyngeal lymphoid tissue. In 50% of cases, a gray-white membrane covers the tonsils for 7–10 days. There is anterior and posterior cervical adenopathy. Palatal petechiae are seen in about one-third of patients, splenomegaly occurs in about one-half, and a transient faint maculopapular rash is present on the trunk and extremities of about 10% of patients. Fifty percent of patients develop hepatomegaly, and 70–75% develop splenomegaly. There is anterior and posterior cervical adenopathy.

2. Diagnosis. Laboratory findings include a leukocytosis of 10,000–20,000 with 40–60% lymphocytes and monocytes, including 10–20% atypical forms. A positive Monospot test and high or rising heterophil antibody titers support the clinical diagnosis. Eighty percent of patients have abnormal liver function tests. EBV seroconversion makes the diagnosis.

3. Therapy

    a. Treatment of infectious mononucleosis includes penicillin for secondary bacterial infection if throat cultures are indicative of such; symptomatic measures for fever, pharyngitis, and headache (analgesics, warm saline irrigations); and, in patients with severe pharyngotonsillitis with edema, steroids.

    b. Prednisone, 40–80 mg the first day and decreasing this dosage daily over 7–10 days, is very effective in reducing inflammation.

4. Complications of mononucleosis include splenic rupture (often from vigorous palpation), hepatitis, myocarditis, ascending paralysis, hemolytic anemia, and airway obstruction.

D. Vincent's angina (gangrenous pharyngitis). Vincent's angina is usually found in older patients with poor oral hygiene and general lowered resistance to infection. Tissue destruction seems to be caused by the synergistic interaction between several endogenous mouth organisms under anaerobic conditions. The lesions contain large numbers of fusiform bacilli (*Borrelia vincenti*), spirochetes, and other normal mouth flora.

1. Signs and symptoms

    a. Symptoms of sore throat, dysphagia, salivation, fetid breath, bad taste in the mouth, and tender gingiva are typical.

    b. Physical findings include low-grade fever, submandibular lymphadenopathy, ulcerative lesions on the pharyngeal mucous membranes, with a dirty, gray-yellow membrane covering the tonsils and occasionally the tonsillar pillars and soft palate. As opposed to the diphtheritic membrane, this membrane peels off easily. The gingiva and interdental papillae are ulcerated, bleed easily, and are also covered with a membrane.

2. **Diagnosis** by laboratory depends on demonstrating typical organisms in cultures and on biopsy sections of the necrotic lesions.

3. **Therapy.** Treatment is with penicillin (250 mg PO qid) or tetracycline (1.0 gm PO qid), along with frequent gargles with oxidizing agents (half-strength hydrogen peroxide or sodium perborate, 1 tsp : 1 glass of warm water) or sodium perborate pastes applied several times a day.

E. **Candidiasis (moniliasis).** *Candida albicans* is a yeast found in 15–25% of normal mucous membrane surfaces. The normally saprophytic organism becomes pathogenic in states of impaired tissue resistance (debilitated, diabetic, immunocompromised patients) or in those patients on prolonged antibiotic regimens or receiving radiation therapy. A mild form is seen in normal infants and is commonly known as "thrush."

1. **Signs and symptoms**

   a. Sore mouth and throat and odynophagia can occur.

   b. **Examination** reveals a red, edematous mucous membrane with a soft, white mucoid exudate present on the tonsils, buccal, and gingival mucosa. These patches are easily scraped off and reveal a reddened, slightly ulcerated surface beneath. Cervical adenopathy and fever are usually absent.

2. **Diagnosis** is confirmed by a potassium hydroxide preparation of the scrapings from the lesion or by culture on Sabouraud's agar.

3. **Therapy.** Nystatin oral suspension (200,000 units/ml), 2–3 ml swished in the mouth and then swallowed q4h until inflammation is controlled, is an appropriate treatment regimen. If candida esophagitis is present, systemic treatment with oral ketoconazole can be given.

F. **Syphilis**

1. **Signs and symptoms.** Syphilis, caused by *Treponema pallidum,* may produce pharyngeal lesions that are relatively asymptomatic in any of the three states of the disease.

   a. **Primary stage.** The primary chancre is seen as a firm, indurated, painless lesion with superficial ulceration, usually on the lip, tongue, tonsil, or soft palate. Regional adenopathy accompanies the primary chancre. The nodes are firm and painless and may persist long after the chancre heals (in 4–6 weeks).

   b. **Secondary stage.** Superficial mucosal ulcerations, called mucous patches, are characteristic of secondary stage syphilis. These lesions vary and appear as painless silver-gray erosions surrounded by a red periphery, white papules or macules, or as a large, deep, ulcerated unilateral tonsillitis. Posterior cervical lymphadenopathy, a macular rash, and other mucocutaneous lesions may accompany the oropharyngeal findings.

      c. Tertiary stage. These lesions, called gumma, may affect the maxilla, mandible, or oral cavity. The tongue lesions can mimic carcinoma.

  2. Diagnosis

      a. Except for gummatous lesions, darkfield examination is positive. Care must be taken to differentiate *Treponema microdentium,* which is part of the normal oral flora, from *Treponema pallidum.*

      b. The serologic tests for syphilis are positive, with the fluorescent treponemal antibody absorption test (FTA-ABS) being the confirmatory test of choice. All patients being tested for syphilis should be HIV tested.

      c. The mucous membrane lesions must be differentiated from follicular tonsillitis, diphtheria, Vincent's angina, pemphigus, herpes simplex, minor trauma, and infectious mononucleosis. Infectious mononucleosis poses a special problem in that false-positive serologic tests for syphilis can occur.

  3. Therapy. Treatment entails benzathine penicillin G, 2.4 million units IM biweekly to total 4.8 million units. Doxycycline 100 mg bid for 2 weeks or tetracycline 500 mg qid for 2 weeks should be used in penicillin-allergic patients. Erythromycin must be used with caution, because increasing resistance is being noted.

G. Gonococcal pharyngitis. Gonorrhea is the most prevalent of all the venereal diseases and may be transmitted both heterosexually and homosexually. Pharyngitis is seen following oral–genital transmission of organisms, often in male homosexuals.

  1. Signs and symptoms

      a. Symptoms are sore throat and perhaps mild temperature elevation.

      b. Examination of the oropharynx may reveal erythema and edema, with or without exudate of the uvula, soft palate, and tonsillar pillars.

  2. Diagnosis. Culture of the areas on Thayer-Martin medium reveals typical gram-negative, oxidase-positive colonies, and smear of the mucous membranes demonstrates gram-negative intracellular cocci.

  3. Therapy. Treatment is with ceftriaxone 250 mg IM in a single dose. Ofloxacin 500 mg PO as a single dose may be appropriate. Tetracycline resistance is widespread in the United States, and tetracycline therefore is no longer considered adequate.

H. Tuberculosis. The pharyngeal mucosa is not a common site of involvement in extrapulmonary tuberculosis but must be considered in a patient with active cavitary pulmonary tuberculosis and indolent, punched-out ulcers of the gingivae and pharyngeal mucosa.

  1. Signs and symptoms. Hoarseness, dysphagia, and extreme odynophagia suggest laryngeal tuberculosis in this setting.

2. **Diagnosis.** Confirmational biopsy, smear, and culture identification of the tubercle bacilli are necessary prior to treatment.

3. **Treatment** is with isoniazid and rifampin for 6 months, with pyrazinamide added during the first 2 months. In patients exposed to drug-resistant organisms, treatment is with isoniazid, rifampin, and ethambutol, with pyrazinamide added during the first 2 months.

I. **Viral pharyngitis.** Most cases of mild pharyngitis are due to viruses and are manifested by mild pharyngeal erythema associated with cough, rhinorrhea, myalgias, headache, and fever. Also favoring a viral origin are a normal white blood count, hoarseness, and absence of lymphadenopathy, which is present usually in bacterial pharyngitis or mononucleosis. Exudative pharyngitis may be caused by adenoviruses, EBV, as well as other viruses, so the presence of exudate does not rule out viral etiology. Two characteristic, viral-caused diseases are listed below.

1. **Herpangina** is a benign, infectious disease of childhood, less common in young adults, caused by various cocksackie and ECHO viruses. It occurs in epidemic form, usually during the fall and summer months.

   a. **Signs and symptoms.** Characteristic symptoms include sudden onset of high fever (104°F), severe sore throat, odynophagia, nausea and vomiting, and malaise with absence of rhinorrhea and other respiratory tract symptoms. The tonsillar pillars, tonsils, and soft palate demonstrate marked erythema, injection, and numerous 1- to 2-mm vesicles, which soon rupture and enlarge into 3- to 4-mm, punched-out, shallow ulcers with gray craters surrounded by deep red areolas. These ulcers heal in 4–5 days with regression of local symptoms, and total recovery is within 7–10 days.

   b. The **diagnosis** is usually made clinically. Clinically these lesions are for the most part difficult to differentiate from herpes simplex virus (HSV). The site can help, with HSV involving the gingiva more frequently. Throat cultures and acute and convalescent antibody titers confirm the diagnosis.

   c. **Therapy.** Treatment consists of local and symptomatic measures. Topical anesthetics may be used if the patient has difficulty eating or drinking. Saline gargles and irrigations, a soft diet, and antipyretics are also helpful.

2. **Herpes** (primary herpetic gingivostomatitis). Either the type 1 or type 2 herpes simplex virus can cause primary infection of the oral cavity and pharynx. Transmission is via close personal contact. Children between ages 2 and 5 years are usually affected.

   a. **Signs and symptoms.** Symptoms include a prodrome of fever, headache, malaise, nausea and vomiting, irritability, oral fetor, and tender submaxillary lymphadenopathy. Physical examination reveals erythema and edema of the gingival and anterior oropharyngeal mucous membranes, with multiple vesicles present. These vesicles quickly rupture and form ulcers that heal in 1–2 weeks. An important diagnostic sign is the generalized acute marginal gingivitis. Systemic symptoms cease within 3–5 days. As opposed to herpangina, the vesicles are usually confined to the anterior portion of the mouth, and the disease does not occur in epidemic form.

   b. Diagnosis. Impression smears (Giemsa stain) of the clear liquid from an opened vesicle reveals syncytial giant cells with intranuclear inclusions. Viral culture and immunofluorescence can confirm the diagnosis.

   c. Therapy. Symptomatic therapy as outlined for herpangina (see **1.c.**) is usually the only treatment necessary. Antibiotics and steroids are of no help in primary herpes infections. Acyclovir is given only to immunosuppressed patients with chronic oropharyngeal herpes.

J. Lingual tonsillitis. Although commonly occurring with tonsillitis, lingual tonsillitis can be an isolated infection. It is characterized by a mild temperature elevation, odynophagia, and a burning or painful sensation localized deep in the throat. The patient is tender over the hyoid bone and may have altered phonation, the typical "hot potato" voice. Mirror examination demonstrates pooled secretions, red and edematous lingual tonsils with patchy exudate, and a normal epiglottis. Treatment is essentially the same as that for acute bacterial pharyngitis (see **A.**).

K. Nasopharyngitis. The adenoid tissue is usually simultaneously inflamed in a bacterial or viral pharyngitis, especially in children. Symptoms include those of acute pharyngitis along with nasal obstruction or pain, rhinorrhea, and burning behind the nose and above the palate with respiration or swallowing. Indirect nasopharyngoscopy reveals a yellowish exudate in the shallow clefts of the red and edematous adenoid folds. Treatment is dependent on culture results and is identical to those listed for specific pharyngeal infections.

L. Acquired immunodeficiency syndrome (AIDS) is caused by infection with the human immunodeficiency virus (HIV). It manifests as the presence of one or more opportunistic diseases associated with immunodeficiency.

Disease transmission is usually through sexual contact, parenteral exposure to blood or blood products, and perinatally from mother to child.

Currently, high-risk groups are homosexual men, intravenous drug users, children born to HIV-infected mothers, and blood transfusion recipients of unscreened blood products. Sexual contact with HIV-infected persons has increased the rate of infection in the heterosexual population.

   1. Signs and symptoms. Otolaryngologic manifestations of AIDS include Kaposi's sarcoma (skin, external ear canal, nose, nasopharynx, oropharynx, and larynx), candidiasis (oropharyngeal, esophageal), parotid enlargement (sometimes cystic), cervical lymphadenopathy, herpetic ulcers (nasal vestibule and upper lip), and sensorineural hearing loss.

2. Diagnosis is made by serologic tests, which require patient consent.

3. Therapy

a. Azidothymidine (AZT) prolongs patient survival but has a significant incidence of serious side effects.

b. Treatment for specific infections (such as antifungal therapy for candidiasis) is employed whenever possible.

c. Preventative measures such as condom use for sexually active people, clean needles for intravenous drug users, screening of blood products, and universal precautions for health care workers are all essential.

IV. Noninfectious etiology

Pharyngeal trauma (e.g., heat, foreign body), irritant inhalation or ingestion (ammonia, lye, acid), and dryness (e.g., mouth breathing) are among some of the causes to be considered in a patient presenting with pharyngeal lesions, pain, or both. These causes are not detailed here.

A. Pemphigus is a progressive disease of unknown etiology. Skin and mucous membranes are characterized by scattered bullae, which can involve other organs and lead to death unless treated with immunosuppressive agents or steroids.

1. Signs and symptoms

a. More than half of the patients first present with oropharyngeal lesions. Patients complain primarily of throat pain, odynophagia, or tongue pain. The vesicles and bullae are painless at first, but with rupture and secondary infection, the pain is severe.

b. On physical examination, the fibrinous exudate covering tender, superficially eroded areas of the oral cavity and oropharynx is characteristic. Often the lesions remain limited to this area for several weeks before spreading to other skin and mucous membrane sites.

2. Diagnosis is made by a high index of suspicion prompting a subsequent biopsy, which reveals acantholysis of the suprabasal cell region and immunofluorescent antibodies to a specific intracellular antigen at the site of acantholysis.

3. Therapy. Management involves vigorous and early systemic corticosteroid therapy (prednisone, 120–240 gm), along with adjuvant immunosuppressive drugs (methotrexate, azathioprine). Hospitalization, isolation (if the skin is denuded, as in a burn patient), and topical and systemic antibiotics for secondary infection may be necessary. Viscous lidocaine, milk of magnesia, diphenhydramine (Benadryl), dyclonine (Dyclone 0.5%), and saline mouth washes may be helpful for local pain and oropharyngeal cleansing.

B. Pemphigoid includes bullous pemphigoid and benign mucous membrane pemphigoid (BMMP).

1. **Signs and symptoms.** These diseases are usually much more benign than pemphigus. BMMP often presents with oral cavity lesions, most commonly affecting the buccal mucosa, gingiva, and palate. The lesion begins as a blister, which then ruptures, leaving a denuded area. The gingiva may be diffusely friable and hemorrhagic.

2. **Diagnosis** is made by immunofluoresence study of the biopsied lesion. IgG antibodies react with the basement membrane, as opposed to in pemphigus, where the antibodies react at the site of acantholysis.

3. **Therapy.** Systemic steroids are used in these diseases, which respond much better than does pemphigus.

C. Erythema multiforme is an acute, self-limited disease of the skin and mucous membranes in response to various etiologies, including drugs (e.g., penicillin, sulfa) and infection (e.g., herpes, mycoplasma). Over half the cases are idiopathic.

1. **Signs and symptoms.** Oral vesicles and bullae quickly rupture to become erosions that are friable and bleed. Ulcerations covered with a white pseudomembrane are characteristic. Cutaneous manifestations, often involving the palms and soles, consist of the sudden onset of erythematous patches or plaques that erupt symmetrically. They may then develop into characteristic "target lesions." These oral lesions are extremely painful. The lips are frequently covered with a dark, hemorrhagic crust. This symptom complex may be initiated by drug reactions, herpes infections, or by an internal malignancy.

2. **Diagnosis** is made clinically.

3. **Therapy.** Treatment is supportive with hydration and topical anesthetic mouth rinses (dyclonine, diphenhydramine, plus milk of magnesia). Systemic steroids are sometimes used.

D. Recurrent aphthous stomatitis

1. **Signs and symptoms.** This disorder is characterized by recurring buccal and labial painful mucosal ulcers in an otherwise healthy patient. These patients usually have between two and six lesions with each episode and may experience several exacerbations per year. The etiology is unclear, but factors such as heredity, hormones, nutrition, stress, and local trauma have been suggested to play a role. An altered immune response remains a postulated etiology. Patients should be queried as to inflammatory bowel disease and diabetes.

2. **Diagnosis.** Physical examination reveals round, symmetric, shallow painful lesions on the buccal and labial mucosa. The hard palate and attached gingiva are spared. Major aphthous ul-

cers can be as large as 2–3 cm. Healing without scarring within 2 weeks is the rule for smaller lesions. It may take months for larger lesions to heal and scarring is common.

3. **Therapy.** Treatment with topical corticosteroid preparations, e.g., tramcinolone acetonide (Kenalog in Orabase, qid), may be palliative. In severe cases, tetracycline mouth rinses (250-mg capsule dissolved in 50 ml of water qid) may be used, but with the risk of oral candidiasis and allergic reactions. For large ulcers, prednisone may be necessary 40 mg daily until healing is complete.

E. **Agranulocytosis.** Agranulocytosis is believed to occur as a rare reaction to a wide variety of drugs (e.g., phenytoin [Dilantin], phenylbutazone, chloramphenicol, chlorpromazine, and meprobamate).

1. **Signs and symptoms**

   a. These patients are acutely ill with fever, sore throat, malaise, and prostration.

   b. Physical examination reveals an ulcerative, sometimes gangrenous mucositis of the oropharynx, demonstrated by lesions that range from small superficial ulcers to a membranous gingivitis and pharyngitis.

2. **Diagnosis.** The total leukocyte count is often 1000–2000 cells/ μl, and neutrophils are absent from the bone marrow. The differential must include leukemia, Vincent's angina, mononucleosis, diphtheria, or acute tonsillitis on initial examination.

3. **Therapy.** Immediate discontinuance of the offending drug— supportive measures and antibiotics to control secondary infections sustain the patient until bone marrow recovery occurs.

F. **Leukemia.** As opposed to agranulocytosis, leukemia is characterized by neoplastic proliferation of one of the blood-forming cells, which then replaces the normal hematopoietic cells in the bone marrow.

Signs and symptoms. Symptoms are usually abrupt and consist of fever, prostration, infection, or bleeding, but may be insidious with progressive weakness, low-grade fever, bleeding tendencies, and recurrent infections. Often the patient presents to the otolaryngologist with fever, sore throat, and gingival bleeding. Findings can include swollen, purplish gingivae, tonsillar enlargement with exudate or necrotic ulcers, and pharyngeal mucous membrane ulcerations. These necrotic lesions must be differentiated from diphtheria, tuberculosis, Vincent's angina, pemphigus, and other bacterial or viral entities.

V. **Deep neck space abscess**

A. **Peritonsillar abscess (quinsy)** is a purulent collection between the tonsillar capsule and the fascia of the superior constrictor muscle (i.e., the peritonsillar space). Organisms involved are streptococci (anaerobic species) and occasionally staphylococci. It is believed that infection deep in the tonsillar crypts penetrates the capsule (usually in the supratonsillar fossa) to spread into the peritonsillar space. The process may be localized to a collection of minor salivary glands (Weber's glands) in the superior pole of the tonsil. The abscess may occur early or late in the course of an acute tonsillitis and is often seen during or after appropriate antibiotic treatment of the initial tonsillitis. The abscess is usually unilateral and is rare in children.

1. Signs and symptoms

   a. Symptoms. The patient often gives a history of a sore throat that initially improved but subsequently worsened, progressing to a unilateral painful throat. This can occur with or without antibiotic treatment. The temperature may be elevated and the patient demonstrates a thickened or "hot potato" voice. Odynophagia, drooling, and trismus (due to irritation of the internal pterygoid muscle) are common.

   b. Physical examination reveals unilateral edema and erythema of the soft palate and anterior tonsillar pillar with medial displacement of the tonsil. Examination is often difficult due to trismus. Spontaneous drainage, if present, usually occurs in the superior portion of the anterior pillar area.

2. Diagnosis. Differentiation between cellulitis and abscess can be made with needle aspiration of the area lateral to the superior pole or at any point of obvious fluctuation. A large-bore (16- or 18-gauge) spinal needle, after topical or local anesthesia, should be used. The aspirate is sent for Gram stain and anerobic and aerobic culture and sensitivity.

3. Therapy

   a. Needle aspiration is the treatment of choice. If there is a concern regarding potential reaccumulation, incision and drainage under local anesthesia is done immediately after aspiration.

   b. Aspiration is followed by outpatient treatment with oral antibiotics (penicillin 500 mg PO qid, modified by the results of the culture and sensitivity). Hourly irrigations with warm saline, liquid oral analgesics, and hydration are all important.

   c. Hospitalization for IV antibiotics and hydration is indicated for significant trismus, dehydration, inability to swallow, and significant obstruction.

   d. Immediate bilateral tonsillectomy is advocated for the pediatric patient in whom patient anesthesia would be required for incision and drainage.

   e. There is debate as to whether "interval tonsillectomy," performed 6–8 weeks after initial treatment for the peritonsillar abscess is indicated. In the absence of a prior history of recurrent tonsillitis, there is only a 10% chance of recurrent peritonsillar abscess.

B. **Retropharyngeal abscess** (see Chap. 1, **IV.B.**) is usually a disease of children less than 3 years of age. This relatively uncommon abscess is due to necrosis and suppuration of the lymph nodes in the retropharyngeal space, which lies between the buccopharyngeal fascia and the prevertebral fascia. The nodes, which drain the nasal passages, eustachian tube, sinuses, and pharynx, usually regress by age 3 or 4 years. This abscess may follow penetrating pharyngeal injuries, neglected middle ear infections, suppurative parotitis, or during active tuberculosis (Pott's disease).

1. **Signs and symptoms**

    a. **Symptoms.** The child lies with the head extended and tilted toward the uninvolved side, refuses food, and demonstrates nuchal rigidity. If old enough, the patient complains of odynophagia or dysphagia but does not have trismus. If the swelling becomes massive, obstructive symptoms of snoring, muffled cry, or dyspnea may be present. Later in the course, respiratory embarrassment occurs.

    b. **Physical examination.** There is cervical adenitis and a soft unilateral red bulging of the posterior pharyngeal wall, visible directly or by mirror examination.

2. **Diagnosis.** Fluctuance to palpation is often present, but caution must be exercised so as not to precipitate rupture with possible aspiration of pus, causing asphyxia or pulmonary infection. The temperature and white count are elevated. An inspiratory hyperextended lateral neck film shows an anterior bulging of the posterior pharyngeal wall. Fluoroscopy is beneficial and reveals decreased mobility of the posterior pharynx. CT can help define the extent of an abscess. A chest film is indicated, because a retropharyngeal abscess is a likely source of mediastinitis.

3. **Therapy**

    a. If seen early, before suppuration occurs, most cases of retropharyngeal adenitis are successfully treated with parenteral antibiotics that cover anaerobes, staphylococci, streptococci. *H. influenzae,* and other oral flora. A third-generation cephalosporin (ceftriaxone) should be considered initially.

    b. Abscess formation necessitates incision and drainage in the operating room with the patient in the extreme Trendelenburg position (head down) to avoid aspiration of the pus from a ruptured abscess.

C. **Pharyngomaxillary space (parapharyngeal) abscess.** This space is pyramid shaped, with its base located at the base of the skull and its apex at the hyoid bone. Its lateral boundary is the fascia covering the internal pterygoid muscle, mandible, and deep surface of the parotid gland. Fascia covering the superior constrictor muscle serves as the medial boundary. The styloid process and its muscular attachments divide the space into anterior (the tonsillar fossa medially and internal pterygoid laterally) and posterior spaces (containing the carotid sheath and the ninth through twelfth cranial nerves). Pharyngeal infection is the most common source, but direct extension from infection in other cervical spaces (submaxillary, retropharyngeal, peritonsillar, masticator, parotid) is commonly seen. Bezold's abscess results from infection breaking through the mastoid tip cells medial to the digastric muscle and dissecting inferiorly into the pharyngomaxillary space.

1. **Signs and symptoms**

   a. Fever, odynophagia, sore throat, ipsilateral otalgia, and neck rigidity are common.

   b. Marked trismus is due to internal pterygoid muscle inflammation. There is lateral neck swelling, especially posterior to the angle of the mandible. The posterior tonsillar pillar is deviated medially.

   c. Cranial neuropathies, as well as septic thrombosis of the internal jugular vein or carotid artery rupture, can lead to disastrous complications.

2. **Diagnosis.** The x-ray findings of posterior pharyngeal swelling assist in the diagnosis; however, a computed tomography (CT) or MRI scan may give information as to the extent of the abscess.

3. **Therapy.** Treatment includes parenteral antibiotics to cover anaerobes, streptococci, and staphylococci (especially if there is a history of trauma, iatrogenic or otherwise). The choice of antibiotics includes penicillin G, clindamycin, or cefoxitin, pending culture and sensitivity results. Surgical drainage may be indicated. High doses of penicillin or cephalosporin should be started and maintained until culture and sensitivity results are available. Nafcillin or oxacillin should be used if *Staphylococcus* is suspected.

D. **Submandibular space abscess (Ludwig's angina)** (see Chap. 1, **IV.A.**). The submandibular space consists of the sublingual space (between the floor of the mouth and mylohyoid muscle) and the submaxillary space (below the mylohyoid). Most abscesses ($> 80\%$) are due to dental infections, but they can also be caused by trauma, lingual tonsillitis, or salivary gland disease. The submaxillary space is involved by abscesses of the first, second, or third molars breaking through the mandibular cortex below the mylohyoid line, while the sublingual space is infected with abscesses of the premolars or first molars, whose roots are above the mylohyoid insertion. Often a history of dental work within the past week is elicited.

Ludwig's original description in 1836 is still valid and describes the angina as (1) a rapidly spreading gangrenous cellulitis or phlegmon, which causes the brawny hardness of the tissues; (2) originating near the submandibular gland, but never involving only one space; (3) arising from direct extension rather than by lymphatics; and (4) producing gangrene and serosanguineous, putrid infiltration but little or no frank pus.

1. **Signs and symptoms**

   a. The patient experiences odynophagia, drooling, trismus, and cannot speak or swallow due to tongue involvement. Dyspnea, agitation, and aspiration occur as the swelling increases. Very high fevers are characteristic.

   b. Floor-of-mouth edema forces the tongue upward and posteriorly with sublingual infection, whereas submandibular induration, tenderness, and swelling are evident with submaxillary space involvement. Ludwig's angina is present when both spaces are affected. As with the other neck space infections, a leukocytosis with left shift is present.

2. **Therapy.** Treatment is with surgical decompression, high-dose parenteral antibiotics (see parapharyngeal abscess), control of the airway either by tracheotomy or by nasotracheal intubation, and removal of suspected teeth if panorex evaluation identifies a source. Early control of the airway is of utmost importance, whether or not surgery is performed.

VI. Allergic edema

A. Quincke's edema, presumed to have an allergic etiology, involves acute uvular and soft palatal edema.

1. **Signs and symptoms.** The patient presents with the sudden onset of a muffled voice and fullness of the throat. Clinical examination reveals a watery palatal and uvular edema, often with the uvula resting on the tongue. One should question the patient for a history of trauma, caustic substance ingestion, known allergies, and be alert for developing laryngeal edema.

2. **Therapy.** Treatment with IM or SQ epinephrine (1:1000 units, 0.3–0.5 ml) and steroids—hydrocortisone sodium-succinate (100–200 mg IV) or dexamethasone (Decadron, 10 mg IV)—is indicated if edema is massive. Antihistamines, such as diphenhydramine (25–50 mg IV), have also been used, although their effects are not as immediate as epinephrine. Steroids are used q6–8h for resistant cases.

B. Angioedema (see Chap. 1, **VI.**). Angioedema is characterized by transient, localized, painless swelling of the subcutaneous tissue or submucosa of various parts of the body, including the skin and mucosa of the oral cavity, pharynx, larynx, and gastrointestinal tract. Episodes may be triggered by exposure to specific allergens, physical stimuli, or emotional stress. Two forms occur: a well-publicized but rare hereditary angioedema (occurring in fewer than 0.5% of cases of chronic urticaria or 2% of all cases of angioedema) and a more common nonhereditary allergic form. Pharyngeal and laryngeal involvement is more common in the hereditary form, where mortality ranges from 5–50% due to glottic edema. Hereditary angioedema is an autosomal dominant genetic disease in which there is a deficiency of the inhibitor of the first component of complement (C1 esterase).

1. **Signs and symptoms** involve nonpitting swelling without the sharply defined, raised border characteristic of urticaria of the face, extremities, genitalia, lips, tongue, or pharynx. Pain or itching is absent. The edema may cause respiratory obstruction.

2. **Diagnosis.** Angioedema is suspected in the patient with a history of previous episodes, a positive family history (in the hereditary form), the typical clinical presentation, and the absence of signs of infection. Laboratory confirmation of low or absent levels of C1 esterase inhibitor or low levels of C4 or C2 secures the diagnosis.

3. **Therapy.** Treatment is prevention, with avoidance of provocative factors. For an acute attack, epinephrine, 0.5 ml of 1:1000 solution IM, and steroids should be administered, with prompt airway control by intubation or tracheotomy if laryngeal involvement is progressing. Distinction between hereditary and nonhereditary forms is important, as long-term use of such drugs as epsilon aminocaproic acid has been used in the familial disorder. Purified C1 esterase inhibitor, if available, reverses the acute episode. Danazol, a synthetic androgen, or stanazolol, an anabolic steroid, appear to be effective for long-term therapy, bringing the C1 esterase inhibitor into normal range.

VII. Tissue hypertrophy

A. Adenotonsillar hypertrophy. The adenoid is a mass of lymphoid tissue located on the posterosuperior wall of the nasopharynx, which forms part of Waldeyer's ring. This lymphoid tissue undergoes physiologic hypertrophy and hyperplasia in response to upper respiratory infections, usually greatest between 2 and 5 years of age. Infection of the adenoids rarely occurs alone and usually involves an adenotonsillar inflammation with hypertrophy and enlargement as a response. Repeated infections lead to hyperplasia with microscopic demonstration of active germinal centers, inflammatory infiltrates, and scanty fibrosis in surgical specimens.

1. **Signs and symptoms**

   a. Symptoms are usually obstructive and include mouth breathing, restless sleep, nasal obstruction with snoring, purulent rhinitis, and hyponasal speech.

   b. Nasal airway obstruction may cause altered midface development, with a narrow and arched palate, demonstrable in serial cephalometric radiographs.

   c. Eustachian tube obstruction with subsequent serous otitis media, hearing loss, and perhaps recurrent acute otitis media, may occur. Adenoid hypertrophy alone rarely appears to be the sole factor causing otitis media.

2. **Diagnosis.** Direct examination of the oral cavity shows enlarged tonsils. Lateral radiographs of the nasopharynx reveal narrowing or obliteration of the airway by enlarged adenoid tissue. Obstructive apnea can be demonstrated on a sleep study (see next section).

3. Therapy. Adenotonsillectomy is required and may occasionally be done emergently to relieve airway obstruction. Noninfectious indications for an adenotonsillectomy include cor pulmonale, sleep apnea, severe upper airway obstruction, and malocclusion secondary to chronic mouth breathing.

B. Obstructive sleep apnea. Sleep apnea is defined as cessation of airflow at the nares and mouth for at least 10 seconds. Central apnea is the absence of both airflow and respiratory effort; obstructive apnea is the absence of airflow in the presence of respiratory effort; and mixed apnea is a combination of both central and obstructive apneas. Sleep apnea is defined by 5 episodes of apneas and hypopneas per hour of sleep or 30 episodes over 7 hours.

Obstructive sleep apnea syndrome (OSAS) is caused by collapse and obstruction of the upper airway at the level of the oropharynx and/or hypopharynx; often the exact site(s) of obstruction is difficult to pinpoint. Contributing factors may include obesity, adenotonsillar hypertrophy, redundant oropharyngeal soft tissue, macroglossia, micrognathia, pharyngeal neoplasms, and certain medications.

1. Signs and symptoms. There is usually a history of loud snoring and restless sleeping; there may be enuresis and impotence. Daytime symptoms include hypersomnolence, early morning headaches, and difficulty concentrating.

Physical examination should include a Müller maneuver, where the flexible nasopharygoscope is used to visualize the degree of collapse at first the level of the soft palate, and then the base of tongue, while the patient is inspiring against a closed mouth and nose.

2. Diagnosis

a. A polysomnogram is used to measure the frequency and type of apneic spells, oxygen saturation, stages of sleep, and cardiac arrythmias.

b. Other tests include cephalometric x rays, CT scan, and/or fluoroscopy to measure the pharyngeal airway; pulmonary function tests, sleep latency tests, and continuous performance measures are also useful.

3. Therapy

a. Medication, such as protriptyline, may be helpful, but side effects limit its usefulness.

b. Weight-control measures are clearly beneficial for some patients.

c. Stimulants such as coffee and colas, as well as alcohol, should be avoided at bedtime.

d. Nasal CPAP (continuous positive airway pressure) is known to be effective for OSAS, but some patients will not tolerate the use of a mask.

e. Uvulopalatopharyngoplasty (UPPP) widens the oropharyngeal airway by excising portions of the soft palate, uvula, tonsils, and posterolateral pharyngeal walls. This alleviates snoring in most patients, but the number of patients where sleep apnea is cured depends in part on the experience of the operating surgeon, and whether the surgery is pre- or post-tonsillectomy. Fifty to ninety percent of patients experience symptomatic improvement. Negative prognostic factors include retro- or micrognathic mandible, a narrow mandibular arch, macroglossia, hypopharyngeal collapse, and weight greater than 125% of ideal body weight.

f. Nasal airway surgery, such as septal reconstruction, turbinate reduction, and polypectomy, can be done at the same time as the UPPP in patients with known nasal obstruction.

g. Mandibular advancement, geniotubercle and anterior hyoid advancement, and hyoid expansion are other surgical options that are not yet as well studied as UPPP.

h. Tracheotomy is indicated for patients with cor pulmonale, serious cardiac nocturnal arrythmias, and chronic alveolar hypoventilation.

VIII. Congenital obstruction

A. Pierre-Robin syndrome. This congenital complex of U-shaped cleft palate, micrognathia, glossoptosis, and associated eye, ear, skeletal, and cardiac defects (esotropia, cataracts, deafness, spina bifida occulta) is present in about 1 of every 30,000 live births. An arrest in development, probably with multiple etiologies, is the basic defect. Neonatal airway obstruction and feeding problems due to the hypoplastic mandible and relative glossoptosis can be remedied by placing the infant in the prone position or by suturing the tongue to the mandibular labial sulcus until the mandible reaches more normal proportions. The use of the McGovern nipple (a baby nipple with a large open tip) to provide an oral airway is of value until more definitive repair is undertaken. The prognosis is good if the patient survives infancy.

B. Thornwald's bursa or nasopharyngeal cyst represents a midline persistence of an embryonic communication between the notochord and the roof of the pharynx.

1. Signs and symptoms

a. Occlusion of the ostia by inflammation causes cyst formation. Subsequent infection may cause headache, persistent postnasal discharge, unpleasant taste sensation, nasopharyngeal crusting, and nasal or eustachian tube obstruction.

b. Examination reveals a cystic, perhaps fluctuant, lesion of the posterior wall of the nasopharynx.

2. Therapy. Treatment requires use of antibiotics and drainage, if necessary, with definitive marsupialization and excision of epithelial lining at a later date.

C. Choanal atresia (see Chap. 1, **VII.A.**) Failure of the buccopharyngeal membrane to become patent during the seventh and eighth weeks of embryonic life results in choanal atresia. It may be unilateral (right side is affected more than the left) or bilateral, bony (90%) or membranous, complete or incomplete. A familial tendency is recognized.

1. Signs and symptoms

   a. Symptoms of bilateral nasal obstruction should be noted immediately after birth. Cyclic dyspnea and cyanosis, which disappears with crying and mouth breathing, is classic. Oropharyngeal breathing is an acquired habit, not learned for weeks, and neonates may die unless an oral airway is provided. Affected infants tightly purse their lips, struggle for air, have sternal retractions, and become cyanotic. Unilateral atresia is not ordinarily life-threatening.

   b. Less immediate signs are feeding difficulties (cyanosis while sucking), aspiration, viscid nasal discharge, or constant mouth breathing.

   c. Unilateral obstruction obviously has less marked symptoms and may not be discovered for years. There is chronic unilateral rhinorrhea and a hyponasal voice. The suggestion of chronic unilateral maxillary sinusitis may lead to the proper diagnosis.

2. Diagnosis should be made in the delivery room by passing a soft catheter through each nares into the nasopharynx to assess choanal patency. Radiologic confirmation can be performed with Lipiodol or other radiopaque substance placed in the nares. A CT scan delineates this skull base anomaly and is the diagnostic procedure of choice.

3. Therapy. Immediate treatment is establishing an oropharyngeal airway. Intubation or tracheotomy is usually not necessary. The McGovern nipple technique (see **A.**) or variations of it have proved successful over the years. The infant may eventually learn to coordinate breathing and feeding, but modern anesthesia and surgical techniques are now available for definitive surgical repair in the neonatal period, so surgery is no longer delayed. A transnasal or transpalatal approach is used.

IX. Cysts and neoplasms

A. Nasopharyngeal. Nasal obstruction, rhinorrhea (especially unilateral), epistaxis, hyponasal voice, cranial nerve palsy, hearing loss secondary to serous otitis media, facial pain, or a neck mass should alert the physician to the possibility of a nasopharyngeal mass.

1. Benign masses of the nasopharynx

   a. Nasopharyngeal angiofibroma (juvenile angiofibroma). This uncommon, highly vascular neoplasm predominantly affects adolescent males and arises from tissue in the vault of the nasopharynx. The etiology and pathogenesis are poorly understood, but an endocrine-related phenomenon is suspected. The tumor is locally destructive and commonly erodes the base of the skull. Intracranial extension can occur.

(1) Signs and symptoms are often not representative of the size of the lesion. Nasal obstruction (90%), epistaxis (80%), palatal or cheek fullness, and exophthalmus may be present.

(2) Physical examination reveals a grayish or red mass in the nasopharynx.

(3) Diagnosis can consistently be made with radiologic techniques; thus, biopsy is not recommended, as significant hemorrhage can result. Plain films demonstrate "bowing" of the posterior wall of the maxillary sinus, and the carotid arteriographic appearance is diagnostic of a vascular tumor. CT scan with enhancement demonstrates a vascular mass lesion. Erosion of the orbital wall, zygomatic arch, and base of skull may also be noted.

(4) Treatment is surgical removal, preceded by embolization of arterial feeders. Irradiation as a primary treatment is rarely indicated.

b. Choanal polyps. These large, soft, gelatinous masses originate from the mucosa of the maxillary sinus and extend through the sinus ostia into the nasal cavity; they then prolapse through the choana into the nasopharynx. Traditional treatment is by excision through a Caldwell-Luc approach to the maxillary antrum and polyp base. Endoscopic removal is sometimes possible by a combined intranasal and anterior wall antrotomy approach.

c. Other benign neoplasms and **pseudotumors** of the nasopharynx are teratomas (usually seen shortly after birth as obstructive upper airway masses), mixed tumors, adenomas, chondromas, and cysts.

2. Malignant neoplasms of the nasopharynx

Nasopharyngeal malignancies represent approximately 2% of all malignancies in Caucasians and up to 15% in the Southern Chinese population. The male-female ratio is approximately 3:1. No familial tendency has been established, and most patients in the United States are 50–70 years old. High titers of antibody to the EBV appear in about 70% of patients.

Eighty-five percent of these malignant neoplasms are epidermoid carcinomas (this includes lymphoepitheliomas or nonkeratinizing epidermoid cancers). Of the remainder, half are lymphomas, with adenocarcinomas, plasmacytomas, melanomas, or sarcomas occasionally seen. Fifty percent of cases present with metastatic cervical nodes as the chief complaint.

a. Signs and symptoms. Nasal symptoms include purulent or bloody rhinorrhea, posterior epistaxis, or nasal obstruction.

Obstruction of the eustachian tube by edema or tumor results in a conductive hearing loss secondary to serous otitis media. An adult with unilateral serous otitis media must be suspected of having a nasopharyngeal cancer. Ophthalmic symptoms may be related to neurologic compromise, with tumor involvement of the fifth and sixth cranial nerves being the most frequent. Ophthalmoplegia, pain, diplopia, or a decreased corneal reflex may occur. Metastasis to the jugular foramen nodes (jugular foramen syndrome) may involve the ninth through twelfth cranial nerves and the sympathetic trunk (causing unilateral Horner syndrome). Due to the rich lymphatic supply and late symptomatology, 60–80% of patients will already have cervical metastasis on admission to the hospital.

b. Examination with direct or indirect nasopharyngoscopy, careful neurologic evaluation, radiologic evaluation of the skull base, with eventual transnasal or transoral biopsy, establishes the diagnosis.

c. The **primary treatment** is radiation therapy directed to the nasopharynx and both sides of the neck. Repeated radiation may be used for the 30–60% of patients with recurrent disease. Interval neck dissection should be considered in cases with persistent cervical nodes after the completion of radiation. Carefully selected recurrences may be removed via an infratemporal skull base approach. The prognosis is guarded with a 5-year overall survival rate of about 30–35% for all stages of disease.

B. Oro- and hypopharyngeal. Depending on the anatomic location, these masses present with sore throat, a sensation of a lump in the throat, dysphagia, voice changes, odynophagia, otalgia, and possible trismus.

1. Benign lesions

a. Mucous retention cysts arising from minor salivary glands occur in the valleculae and aryepiglottic folds, and may cause respiratory distress in the newborn; however, they are usually seen as incidental findings on indirect laryngeal examination and most often require no therapy.

b. Squamous papillomas are small, pink, mulberrylike masses on the soft palate, uvula, or tonsillar fossae. They are viral in origin and do not portend malignancy. Surgical excision of persistent papillomas is advised. These may be associated with respiratory papillomatosis.

c. Parapharyngeal tumors present as lateral oropharyngeal or palatal masses with few symptoms. Most are benign (pleomorphic adenomas, neurilemmomas, lymphangiomas, teratomas, or leiomyomas) and are approached surgically through an upper lateral neck incision. Large tumors in the region may require an intraoral as well as external approach with a mandibular osteotomy, or parotidectomy.

d. Aberrant thyroid tissue located in the base of the tongue in the region of the foramen cecum or between the epiglottis and circumvallate papillae may result from failure of the thyroid anlage to descend into its normal position in the neck. Females are predominantly affected and may complain of a foreign body sensation, dysarthria, or dysphagia, especially during periods of increased endocrine activity.

A biopsy will differentiate thyroid tissue from other tumors such as amyloid, angiomas, fibromas, papillomas, gummas, lingual tonsil carcinomas, lymphomas, or sarcomas. A thyroid scan must be performed, as this aberrant tissue may be the patient's only thyroid tissue, and in many cases it is hypofunctional. Rarely is therapy necessary although thyroid supression may be necessary in symptomatic patients.

2. Malignant neoplasms of the oropharynx. Smaller tumors of the tonsil, pharyngeal walls, or base of the tongue are often asymptomatic, and growth is usually advanced by the time the patient seeks medical care.

a. Signs and symptoms. Vague sore throat, foreign body sensation, local irritation with rough or hot food, odynophagia, referred otalgia, and a neck lump are common presenting complaints. Most patients are males, 50–80 years old, and have a history of chronic alcohol or tobacco use. More than 50% will have clinically positive cervical nodes when first examined. About 90% of tonsil cancers are epidermoid carcinomas, with about 10% being lymphomas. Ninety-five percent of base of tongue cancers are epidermoid in type.

b. Physical examination reveals a firm exophytic or ulcerated lesion. Direct visualization and palpation of both the primary tumor and the neck at the time of biopsy are important for proper staging and therapy.

c. Combined therapy with radiation, surgery, and/or chemotherapy can be planned. Endoscopic evaluation of the entire upper aerodigestive tract should be performed because of the high (up to 15%) incidence of multiple separate tumors.

3. Malignant tumors of the hypopharynx include cancers of the pyriform fossa, posterior hypopharyngeal wall, and postcricoid region. Ninety-five percent of pyriform sinus and posterior pharyngeal wall cancers are epidermoid carcinomas. Most are poorly differentiated infiltrating tumors. These neoplasms spread by direct as well as lymphatic extension. More than half of the patients present with palpable cervical nodes, and local disease is often extensive by the time symptoms of dysphagia, voice alteration, otalgia, aspiration, stridor, throat pain, or weight loss prompts the patient to seek medical assistance.

Indirect laryngoscopy demonstrates a large sessile or exophytic superficially ulcerative mass. MRI and CT scans and barium swallows are helpful in delineating the extent of disease, but tumor mapping at the time of direct laryngoscopy and biopsy are of utmost importance in treatment planning. Combined treatment with surgery, irradiation, and chemotherapy is then coordinated.

Postcricoid carcinoma usually presents with dysphagia, intermittent cough secondary to aspiration, a lump-in-the-throat sensation, local pain, excess salivation, and weight loss. Indirect laryngoscopy may reveal only interarytenoid edema and pooling of secretions. Radiologic studies confirm the presence of a mass, and direct endoscopy determines the geography of the disease. The inferior boundary must be defined for the proper application of surgery and/or radiation therapy.

4. **Dysphagia (oropharyngeal).** Dysphagia is defined as difficulty swallowing. It is distinguished from odynophagia, which is pain on swallowing.

The swallow is divided into the oral, pharyngeal, and esophageal phases. The oral phase starts when the tongue begins its anterior to posterior motion, which strips the bolus along the hard palate. The oral phase ends when the bolus passes the anterior tonsillar pillars, which begins the pharyngeal phase. The pharyngeal phase ends when the bolus passes through the pharyngoesophageal segment (PES). The esophageal phase then begins; it ends when the bolus passes through the lower esophageal sphincter (LES).

a. **Signs and symptoms.** The patient who has difficulty propelling the bolus through the oropharynx may describe the bolus getting stuck in the throat, often requiring regurgitation to dislodge the bolus. Nasal regurgitation implies palatal dysfunction. Coughing, sometimes associated with aspiration, may lead to pneumonia. Other associated symptoms include a change in voice, weight loss, or diet change. Odynophagia may indicate the presence of either neoplasia or infection.

b. Physical examination includes assessment of palatal elevation, tongue strength and mobility, vocal cord mobility, pooling of secretions, presence of masses in the neck, naso-, oro-, or hypopharynx.

c. **Diagnosis**

(1) Oropharyngeal swallowing videofluoroscopy studies the oropharyngeal phases of the swallow by giving the patient small amounts of liquid, paste, and solid barium. Various parameters are studied, including the presence and mechanisms of aspiration. Therapeutic maneuvers such as variations in bolus texture and head position are attempted to facilitate a normal swallow. A swallowing videofluoroscopy should be done for any patients with dysphagia, especially if aspiration is suspected.

(2) A standard barium swallow uses a large bolus of liquid barium. It is helpful for visualizing any structural lesions, esophageal motility, or gastroesophageal reflux. Patients with solid food dysphagia, odynophagia, history

of reflux, or persistent dysphagia with a normal swallowing videofluoroscopy should have a standard barium swallow.

(3) Other diagnostic procedures include manometry, swallowing ultrasound, and EMGs.

d. There are numerous diseases that are associated with dysphagia. These include neurologic (CVA, cerebral palsy, multiple sclerosis, and Parkinson's), musculoskeletal (polymyositis, oculopharyngeal muscular dystrophy), idiopathic (cricopharyngeal achalasia), and structural (neoplasms, oropharyngeal or laryngeal resections). Two diseases will be discussed:

(1) Hypopharyngeal diverticulum (Zenker's diverticulum). Patients with Zenker's diverticulum are usually males over 40 years of age and complain of longstanding dysphagia, food sticking in the throat, and noisy deglutition. They often must swallow water with their food and give a history of regurgitation of undigested food when supine. Aspiration pneumonia may result. The diverticula is thought to be caused by incoordination of the upper esophageal sphincter, with a congenital or acquired weakness in the muscular hypopharyngeal wall between the inferior constrictor muscle and the cricopharyngeus muscle. A sack forms from the posterior hypopharyngeal mucosa, entering the prevertebral space and protruding to the left as it enlarges. Physical examination may reveal a soft, compressible, nontender mass deep to or behind the left sternocleidomastoid muscle. Barium swallow with cineradiography should be diagnostic.

Treatment is a diverticulectomy or diverticulopexy combined with cricopharyngeal myotomy through an external approach. Endoscopic cautery or laser division of the common wall between the diverticulum and the pharyngeal lumen is reserved for poor surgical candidates.

(2) Cricopharyngeal achalasia. The PES, sometimes called the upper esophageal sphincter (UES), is contracted at rest and relaxes during a swallow period. PES dysfunction may result in a failure, incomplete, or delayed relaxation of the sphincter. This causes dysphagia, mostly for solids, which have difficulty passing through the PES. Pure cricopharyngeal achalasia is rare; it is most often seen in conjunction with diffuse pharyngeal phase dysfunction.

e. Treatment

(1) The underlying disease should be treated if possible.

(2) A cricopharyngeal myotomy (cutting the muscles of the PES) is indicated in patients with predominantly PES dysfunction. Oculopharyngeal dystrophy patients may also benefit from a myotomy. Any patient who undergoes a Zenker's diverticulectomy should have a concomitant myotomy.

(3) Swallowing therapy, performed by a trained swallowing therapist, may be quite helpful. This includes teaching the patient various maneuvers which, on video, have demonstrably improved the patient's swallowing dysfunction.

(4) If oral intake results in significant aspiration or inadequate caloric intake, non-oral feeding such as a gastrostomy or jejunosotomy tube may be necessary.

Esophagus

I. Congenital

A. Cysts. Esophageal cysts are embryologic remnants of uncertain origin, lined by the types of epithelium from which they arise (stratified squamous and ciliated columnar epithelia), with or without a muscle coat. **Duplication of the esophagus** is less common but may have a similar embryologic derivation. Both anomalies rarely connect with the esophagus and may be associated with vertebral anomalies such as spina bifida and Klippel-Feil deformity, as well as intraspinal malformations.

1. Signs and symptoms. These anomalies are usually asymptomatic in adults and are discovered as incidental findings on chest or spine roentgenograms. If symptoms occur, they can include dysphagia, pain, bleeding, choking, and retrosternal discomfort.

2. Diagnosis. Plain films of the esophagus may demonstrate a posterior mediastinal mass. Contrast films of a cyst demonstrate a smoothly rounded extramucosal mass, usually in the middle or lower third of the esophagus. CT scans delineate a cystic mass.

3. Treatment of the symptomatic lesions is transthoracic enucleation, without opening the esophageal lumen.

B. Atresia. Esophageal atresia and tracheoesophageal fistula are believed to result from incomplete formation of the tracheoesophageal septum during the fourth week of gestation. The anomalies are commonly associated with defects of the gastrointestinal, genitourinary, and neurologic systems. Five categories of malformation have been described:

Type C accounts for 85–90% of these anomalies. The distal end of the upper esophagus ends blindly, and the superior end of the lower esophagus attaches into the posterior tracheal wall.

Type A. There is no communication between the upper and lower esophageal segments and no communication with the trachea.

Type B. The distal end of the upper esophageal segment communi-cates with the trachea, while the proximal end of the lower esophageal segment is blind.

Type D. Both the upper and the lower esophageal segments com-municate with the trachea.

Type E, otherwise known as the **H-fistula.** The esophagus is unin-terrupted but communicates with the trachea.

1. **Signs and symptoms.** Infants in whom the upper esophageal segment ends blindly are unable to swallow even their own se-cretions, with resultant regurgitation, choking, and aspiration. Infants in whom the upper esophageal segment fistulizes to the trachea frequently experience life-threatening pulmonary com-plications, particularly if the anomalies are not noted immedi-ately after birth and the infants are fed. H-fistulae may be relatively asymptomatic if the fistula tract is small and may go undetected for many years. Symptoms include recurrent pneu-monitis, failure to thrive, and coughing, especially when swal-lowing liquids.

2. **Diagnosis.** In all but the H-fistula, a catheter passed through the nose will not enter the stomach. Anteroposterior (AP) and lateral chest and abdominal films with a catheter in position are often sufficient to make the diagnosis. In the type A and B anomalies, no abdominal gas is visible, whereas gas is present in types C, D, and E. If the diagnosis is still in doubt, instilla-tion of a small amount of sodium diatrizoate (Hypaque) under fluoroscopic control may be helpful, though at the risk of addi-tional soiling of the tracheobronchial tree.

3. **Treatment** is surgical repair of the fistula and atresia as soon as the infant is medically stabilized. Repair usually consists of a one-stage esophageal anastomosis and closure of the fistula. If a primary anastomosis is not feasible, the procedure may be per-formed in two or more stages.

C. **Stenosis and webs.** Congenital stenoses and congenital webs are discussed together, since the terms **webs, bands, strictures, stenoses,** and **rings** have all been used to refer to similar anom-alies. These entities are rare, usually identified in the midesoph-agus, and may be associated with tracheoesophageal fistula.

1. **Signs and symptoms.** The degree of dysphagia is a function of the amount of esophageal obstruction. Infants with significant narrowing may be unable to handle their own secretions. With a minimum of narrowing, however, they may have no difficulty swallowing until solid food is added to their diet, at which time intermittent regurgitation of undigested food may develop with or without aspiration.

2. **Diagnosis.** Contrast studies of the esophagus constitute the most reliable means of demonstrating such anomalies. As webs frequently project from the anterior wall of the esophagus, it is important to obtain oblique or lateral views as well as AP views.

3. **Treatment.** Symptomatic webs and stenoses usually respond to dilatation. If the narrowing is secondary to the presence of a cartilaginous ring (a tracheobronchial tree remnant), surgical resection with esophageal reanastomosis may be necessary.

II. Motility disorders

A. **Achalasia** denotes the combination of impaired relaxation of the gastroesophageal sphincter with abnormal esophageal motility. Its etiology is unknown, but it has been associated with a decreased number of ganglion cells in Auerbach's plexus and with a decreased number of cells in the dorsal motor nucleus of the vagus nerve. Chagas's disease, caused by Trypanosoma cruzi, produces changes similar to those seen in achalasia but is also associated with dilatation of the colon, ureters, and other viscera.

1. **Signs and symptoms.** Patients experience the gradual onset of dysphagia, with the sensation of food sticking in the lower esophagus, or discomfort referred to the area of the suprasternal notch. These symptoms may be precipitated by the intake of cold food or liquid. The patient may find that by making repetitive swallowing efforts or by washing the food down with fluids the discomfort is temporarily relieved. Regurgitation of undigested food, either delayed or immediate, may occur. In advanced achalasia, repeated aspiration of esophageal contents may lead to pneumonitis, lung abscess, and bronchiectasis. Bleeding and pain are uncommon.

2. **Diagnosis.** Early in the course of achalasia, the distal esophagus may appear tapered on barium swallow, with disorganized contractions. Later, the esophagus dilates and may assume a sigmoid shape. An air-fluid level may be identified, and passage of contrast material into the stomach is slow. Manometry demonstrates a lack of esophageal peristalsis and impaired relaxation of the gastroesophageal sphincter on deglutition, with normal or elevated resting pressures. Esophagoscopy is not necessary to make the diagnosis of achalasia but should be performed in patients whose symptoms are of short duration to rule out a distal esophageal malignancy.

3. **Treatment**

   a. **Dilatation.** Mechanical dilatation of the gastroesophageal sphincter with bougies provides only transient improvement. However, balloon dilators positioned within the gastroesophageal sphincter and expanded with air or fluid offer 60–70% of patients long-term improvement after only one or two dilatations.

   b. **Surgery.** Surgical therapy consists primarily of modifications of the Heller procedure, in which a transthoracic esophagomyotomy is performed, incising the circular fibers of the gastroesophageal sphincter and leaving the esophageal mucosa intact. These procedures provide long-term improvement in approximately 80% of patients. They may be considered as alternatives to balloon dilatation or employed if dilatation fails.

B. Diffuse esophageal spasm (DES) is a disorder in which the smooth muscle contractions are simultaneous and repetitive.

1. **Signs and symptoms.** Pain referred to the neck, jaw, arms, or shoulders is the usual symptom. Dysphagia and regurgitation may also be seen.

2. **Diagnosis.** Contrast cineradiography may reveal diffuse irregular esophageal spasm, diffuse constant narrowing, or pseudodiverticulosis. Hiatal hernias are often seen. Manometry of the lower esophageal sphincter may demonstrate increased tone but complete relaxation on swallowing.

3. **Treatment**

   a. **Medical.** Medications including sedatives, tranquilizers, anticholinergics, antispasmodics, and H_2 blockers each have a modicum of success. Oral or sublingual nifedipine (10–20 mg before meals) may provide relief of associated chest pain and has efficacy for the subgroup with less pressure elevation.

   b. **Dilatation.** A few patients will benefit from bouginage.

   c. **Surgery.** Surgical therapy consisting of an extended esophagomyotomy and repair of hiatal hernia, if present, may be helpful for severely symptomatic patients.

C. Gastroesophageal reflux (GER) is the result of an incompetent gastroesophageal sphincter. It is commonly associated with a sliding (but not paraesophageal) hiatal hernia; however, not all patients with sliding hiatal hernias have reflux and not all patients with reflux have sliding hiatal hernias. Esophageal damage, the result of the erosive activity of regurgitated gastric contents, may range from diffuse erythema to deep ulceration and transmural fibrosis. Complications include bleeding, stricture formation, shortening of the esophagus, perforation, replacement of the lower esophageal squamous epithelium by columnar epithelium (Barrett's esophagus), and motility disturbances. Patients with Barrett's esophagus have a 10–15% incidence of esophageal carcinoma.

1. **Signs and symptoms.** The most common symptom is "heartburn," burning substernal or epigastric distress. Dysphagia is common and is manifested as food "sticking" during the first few swallows of a meal, perhaps secondary to spastic contraction of the lower esophagus or to spasm of the upper esophageal sphincter. Coughing secondary to regurgitation and aspiration noted with recumbency may also occur.

2. **Diagnosis.** The most sensitive studies for reflux are the acid perfusion, pH monitoring, and acid-clearing tests. Contrast cineradiography is not as accurate for this entity, although reflux of contrast material into the lower esophagus may be observed. Esophagoscopy is used to examine the esophageal mucosa for the pathologic sequelae of reflux.

3. **Treatment**

   a. **Reflux precautions** include elevation of the head of the bed, weight reduction, bland diet, the wearing of loose-fitting abdominal garments, and refraining from heavy lifting, alcohol, coffee, and tobacco. H_2 blockers have made symptom relief possible for most patients.

b. Medications include antacids, cimetadine, ranitadine, and omeprazole.

c. Surgery. Symptoms that are refractory to medical therapy often respond to a fundopliction, which restores the competence of the gastroesophageal sphincter. Strictures usually respond to dilatation with subsequent fundoplication, although severe strictures may require resection with interposition of small bowel or colon.

III. Acquired

A. Foreign bodies. Dysphagia secondary to pharyngeal or esophageal obstruction from foreign bodies is usually observed in children less than 10 years old, in the mentally retarded, and in adults over 50 years of age who obstruct with meat or bones. The narrowest part of the gastrointestinal tract is the upper esophageal sphincter and one-half to two-thirds of foreign bodies are found at this level, primarily in children. Mid- or lower esophageal obstruction is more common in adults.

1. Signs and symptoms. Foreign body obstruction produces dysphagia and occasionally pain of sudden onset. Associated coughing or choking is seen if the foreign body is impacted at or just below the laryngeal inlet. The degree of dysphagia correlates with the amount of obstruction.

2. Diagnosis. Plain AP and lateral roentgenograms of the chest and neck may demonstrate the foreign body if it is radiopaque. The mediastinum and prevertebral space should be examined for the presence of air, which would indicate an esophageal perforation. Only in questionable cases, with normal plain films and without significant obstruction, is the use of contrast material indicated. Contrast studies may be performed with barium or with a small piece of cotton coated with barium.

3. Treatment

a. Emergency. Difficult respiration, aspiration, or the suspicion of a perforation warrant emergency esophagoscopy.

b. Medical. Sedation with narcotics, barbiturates, or diazepam may produce sufficient esophageal relaxation in milder cases to permit passage of the foreign body. The use of papain to digest foreign bodies consisting of meat is not recommended, as necrotic esophageal epithelium may also be digested.

c. If the foreign body does not pass or is unlikely to do so because of its size or shape, removal using a rigid esophagoscope is recommended.

B. Diverticula. Nearly all esophageal diverticula are acquired and seen in adults. Pulsion diverticula are the result of prolonged or excessive intraesophageal pressure that produces mucosal herniation through weak points in the esophageal musculature. The pharyngoesophageal and gastroesophageal sphincter areas are common sites. These diverticula are usually not covered by muscle. Traction diverticula are most often the result of inflammatory mediastinal lymph nodes and differ also from pulsion diverticula by having a muscular coat.

1. **Parabronchial (midesophageal) diverticula** are rarely symptomatic. Affected individuals infrequently experience dysphagia, odynophagia, or suffer the complication of fistulization to the respiratory tract.

2. **Epiphrenic diverticula of the lower esophagus** are less common than pharyngoesophageal diverticula and are usually secondary to functional or mechanical obstruction of the gastroesophageal sphincter.

    a. **Signs and symptoms.** Although epiphrenic diverticula are usually asymptomatic, symptoms may include dysphagia, food retention, and regurgitation. Since these diverticula are often associated with other lower esophageal disorders such as achalasia, diaphragmatic hernia, esophagitis, and stricture, symptoms of these other disorders may predominate.

    b. **Diagnosis.** Epiphrenic diverticula are most accurately diagnosed with contrast radiography. Other diagnostic tests may be performed if other lower esophageal disorders are found or suspected.

    c. **Treatment.** The only available therapy is surgical and is reserved for severely symptomatic patients. Transthoracic diverticulectomy is performed with a gastroesophageal myotomy.

IV. Tumors

A. Benign

1. **Intramural tumors.** The most common benign esophageal tumor is the leiomyoma, which is usually seen in the middle or lower third of the esophagus.

    a. **Signs and symptoms.** Leiomyomas are usually asymptomatic until they reach a diameter of approximately 5 cm. Dysphagia, fullness, and retrosternal pressure are then noted.

    b. **Diagnosis.** A barium swallow demonstrates a smoothly rounded filling defect that appears to be half in and half out of the esophagus. Less often, the leiomyomas may be large and circumferential. On esophagoscopy, they are generally seen to be covered with normal esophageal epithelium, although ulceration may also be seen.

    c. **Treatment.** A thoracotomy is performed and the tumor enucleated, leaving the esophageal epithelium intact.

2. **Pedunculated intralumenal tumors.** Pathologically, such tumors are fibromas, myxomas, and lipomas, and they are usually found in the cervical esophagus.

   a. **Signs and symptoms.** Symptoms include dysphagia, aspiration, and regurgitation. Because these tumors are pedunculated, they may prolapse into the hypopharynx and even the
   larynx, producing dyspnea and choking.

   b. **Diagnosis.** Carefully performed contrast studies and esophagoscopy are necessary to detect these tumors. They may
   easily be overlooked because they are often not bulky and
   may be covered with normal esophageal epithelium.

   c. **Treatment.** Therapy consists of surgical removal, either endoscopically or through a lateral neck incision.

3. **Other benign tumors** include sessile mucosal and submucosal
   lesions, such as papillomas. Hemangiomas usually present
   with bleeding, which may be life-threatening, and therefore
   should be removed.

B. **Malignant.** Dysphagia and odynophagia may result from malignant tumors located in the base of the tongue, hypopharynx
   (including the pyriform sinuses and postcricoid area), and esophagus. Ninety percent are squamous cell carcinomas, and the remainder, located near the gastroesophageal sphincter, are largely
   adenocarcinomas. Leiomyosarcomas, melanomas, and verrucous
   carcinomas have also been reported. Factors implicated in the etiology of these tumors include tobacco, alcohol, nitrosamines, lye
   burns, achalasia, reflux esophagitis, and Plummer-Vinson syndrome. They are usually seen in the sixth and seventh decades of
   life.

1. **Signs and symptoms.** The most common symptom is progressive dysphagia. Other symptoms include weight loss, vague retrosternal pressure, and hematemesis.

2. **Diagnosis** is usually made by a combination of contrast radiography and esophagoscopy with biopsy of the mass or cytologic
   washings if no mass is apparent.

3. **Treatment.** Surgery, and to date, chemotherapy, have not favor-
   ably altered survival. Radiotherapy is used either alone or in
   combination. The overall 5-year survival is a dismal 15–25%,
   except for squamous cell carcinoma of the lower esophagus,
   which carries a somewhat more favorable prognosis. Carcinoma
   of the body of the esophagus may be radiated or resected, and a
   gastric pull-up or colonic interposition procedure performed.
   Lower tumors may require esophagogastrectomy. Similar procedures may be performed for the purpose of palliation. Other
   palliative procedures include dilatation, gastrostomy, jejunos-
   tomy, and insertion of a bypass tube. The Nd-YAG laser has
   been used endoscopically to establish a serviceable lumen.

Selected Readings

Batsakis, J. G. *Tumors of the Head and Neck* (2nd ed.). Baltimore: Williams &
Wilkins, 1979.

Biller, H. F., Sessions, D. G., and Ogura, J. M. Angiofibroma: A treatment approach. *Laryngoscope* 84:695, 1974.

Fairbanks, D. N. F. *Pocket Guide to Antimicrobial Therapy in Otolaryngology—Head and Neck Surgery* (5th ed.). Alexandria, Va.: American Academy of Otolaryngology—Head and Neck Surgery, 1989.

Fairbanks, D. N. F., Fujita, S., Ikematsui, T., and Simmons, F. B., eds. *Snoring and Obstructive Sleep Apnea.* New York: Raven, 1987.

Ferguson, C. F., and Kendig, E. L. Pediatric Otolaryngology. In C. F. Ferguson and E. L. Kendig (eds.), *Disorders of the Respiratory Tract in Children* (vol. III). Philadelphia: Saunders, 1972.

Fineman, S. M. Urticaria and Angioedema. In G. J. Lawlor, Jr. and T. J. Fischer (eds.), *Manual of Allergy and Immunology: Diagnosis and Therapy* (2nd ed.). Boston: Little, Brown, 1988. Pp. 214–224.

Fiumara, N. J., Wise, H. M., Jr., and Mamy, M. Gonorrheal pharyngitis. *N. Engl. J. Med.* 276:1248, 1967.

Goode, R. L. Sleep Disorders. In C. W. Cummings, J. M. Fredrickson, L. A. Harker, C. J. Krause, and D. E. Schuller (eds.), *Otolaryngology—Head and Neck Surgery—Update I.* St. Louis: Mosby, 1989.

Goodman, R. M., and Gorlin, R. J. *Atlas of the Face in Genetic Disorders* (2nd ed.). St. Louis: Mosby, 1977.

Holinger, L. D. Foreign Bodies of the Larynx, Trachea, and Bronchi. In C. Bluestone and S. Stool (eds.), *Pediatric Otolaryngology* (vol. II, 2nd ed.). Philadelphia: Saunders, 1990.

Kenna, M. A. Sore Throat in Childhood: Diagnosis and Management. In C. Bluestone and S. Stool (eds.), *Pediatric Otolaryngology* (vol. II, 2nd ed.). Philadelphia: Saunders, 1990.

Levy, A. M. Hypertrophied adenoids causing pulmonary hypertension and severe congestive heart failure. *N. Engl. J. Med.* 227:606, 1967.

Lucente, F. E., Dull, H. B., and Pincus, R. L. Acquired Immunodeficiency Syndrome in Otolaryngology. In C. W. Cummings, J. M. Frederickson, L. A. Harker, C. J. Krause, and D. E. Schuler (eds.), *Otolaryngology—Head and Neck Surgery—Update I.* Saint Louis: Mosby, 1989.

Mandell, G. L., Douglas, R. G., Bennett, J. E. (eds.). *Principles and Practice of Infectious Disease.* New York: Churchill Livingstone, 1990.

Marks, J. E., et al, Floor of mouth cancer: Patient selection and treatment results. *Laryngoscope* 93:475, 1983.

McGovern, F. M. Bilateral choanal atresia in the newborn: A new method of medical management. *Laryngoscope* 71:480, 1961.

Paparella, M. M., Shumrick, D. A., Gluckman, J. L., and Meyerhoff, W. L., eds. *Otolaryngology, Vol. III—Head and Neck* (3rd ed.). Philadelphia: Saunders, 1991.

Paradise, J. L., Bluestone, C. D., Bachman, R. Z., et al. Efficacy of tonsillectomy for recurrent throat infection in severely affected children: Results of parallel randomized and nonrandomized clinical trials. *N. Engl. J. Med.* 310: 674, 1984.

Pletcher, J. D., et al. Preoperative embolization of juvenile angiofibromas of the nasopharynx. *Ann. Otol. Rhinol. Laryngol.* 84:740, 1975.

Powell, K. R., and Hall, C. B. Infections of the Upper Respiratory Tract. In R. E. Reese and R. F. Betts (eds.), *A Practical Approach to Infectious Diseases* (3rd ed.). Boston: Little, Brown, 1991.

Sessions, R. B., et al. Juvenile nasopharyngeal angiofibroma: Radiographic aspects. *Laryngoscope* 86:2, 1976.

Shapiro, J., and Goyal, R. K. Disorders of the Upper Esophageal Sphincter. In M. P. Fried (ed.), *The Larynx: A Multidiscipliniary Approach*. Boston: Little, Brown, 1988. Pp. 293–318.

Singleton, M. A. Peritonsilar Abscess. In Gates (ed.), *Current Therapy in Otolaryngology—Head and Neck Surgery—3*. Philadelphia: Decker, 1987.

Suberman, S., and Healy, G. B. Sleep apnea syndrome associated with upper airway obstruction. *Laryngoscope* 89:878, 1979.

Thawley, S. E., ed. Symposium on sleep apnea disorders. *Med. Clin. North Am.* 69: 1985.

Wall, M. C. Management of chronic urticaria: A review. *Immunol. Allergy Prac.* 1:117, 1979.

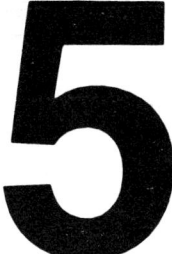

Larynx

I. Anatomic considerations

The **skeletal larynx** is derived from the branchial arch system. The hyoid bone is derived from the second and third arches, and the thyroid cartilage and epiglottis are derived from the fourth arch. The cricoid arises from the sixth branchial arch.

The **skeletal support** of the **larynx** is derived from the hyoid bone and the thyroid cartilage. The cricoid cartilage is the only truly circumferential portion of the entire airway and supports the arytenoid cartilages, which articulate on the posterior cricoid lamina (Fig. 5-1). The trachea begins below the level of the cricoid cartilage and consists of 16–20 U-shaped cartilaginous rings, which eventually bifurcate at the carina into two mainstem bronchi. These bronchi further arborize in the pulmonary tree.

The superior margin of the larynx is the tip of the epiglottis; the inferior border is the undersurface of the cricoid cartilage. The two vocal folds (true vocal cords) form the glottis. The region above the glottis to the tip of the epiglottis is defined as the supraglottic larynx, while the area below the vocal folds is designated as subglottic. The superior and inferior thyroid arteries supply blood to the larynx via the laryngeal vessels. Innervation of the larynx is primarily from the superior and inferior laryngeal nerves. The superior laryngeal nerve is largely sensory and is motor only to the cricothyroid muscle. The inferior laryngeal nerve is derived from the recurrent laryngeal branch of the vagus. Although the inferior laryngeal nerve is sensory below the vocal cords, it supplies the predominant motor innervation to the laryngeal musculature (Fig. 5-2).

II. Evaluation

The external framework of the larynx can be palpated; however, the intrinsic form and function require more sophisticated methods for assessment. The hyoid bone can be noted in the midline, with the prominence of the thyroid notch below. Moving inferiorly, the cricoid cartilage is often palpable, with the tracheal rings below this. Various techniques for examination of the intrinsic larynx are discussed in the next section.

A. Physical examination

1. **Mirror.** Because the location of the larynx renders it difficult to visualize, the following techniques are used. The head mirror and laryngeal mirror afford indirect visualization. The patient is seated upright, leaning forward slightly. The examiner,

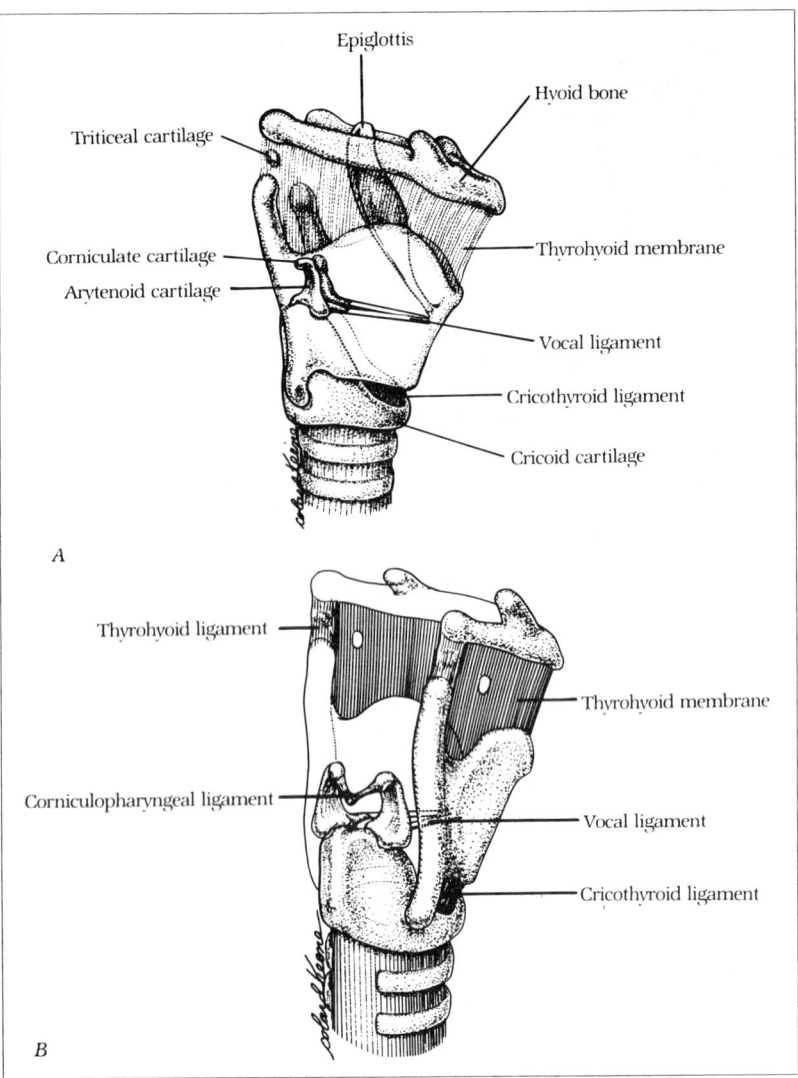

Fig. 5-1. Intrinsic laryngeal ligaments viewed laterally (A) and obliquely from posterior (B). (From M. P. Fried, *The Larynx: A Multidisciplinary Approach.* Boston: Little, Brown, 1988.)

seated just to the side of the patient, uses a light source that parallels his or her visual axis. This light source can be either a head mirror that uses reflected light from a separate source or a headlamp. The tongue is protruded and held firmly in a gauze pad by the examiner. Quiet breathing and relaxation are encouraged. The examiner's opposite hand is used to introduce the laryngeal mirror, which just abuts the soft palate.

Provided that the tongue base and posterior pharyngeal wall are not stimulated by the advancing mirror, a gag reflex will

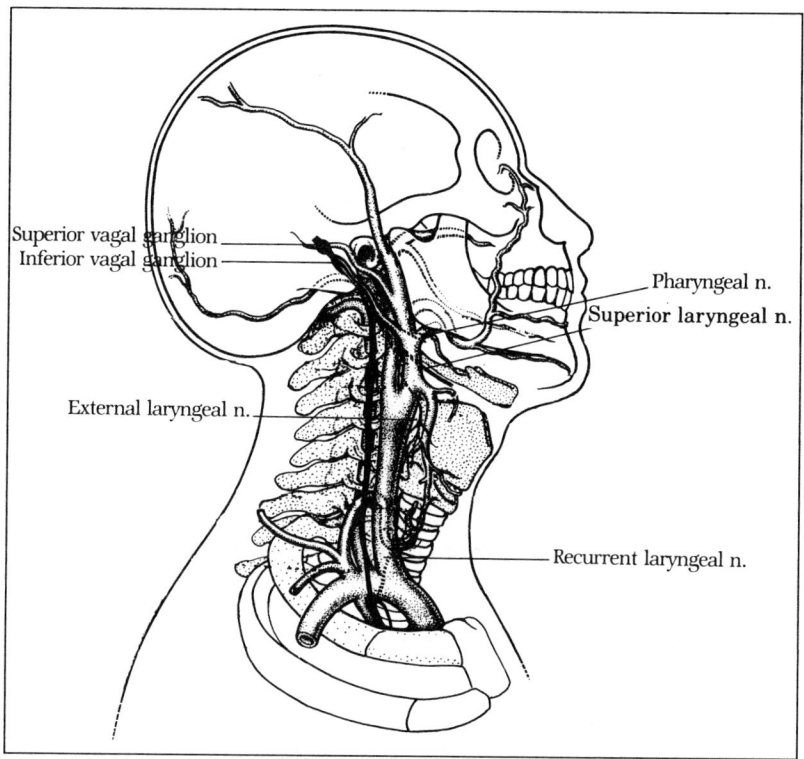

Superior vagal ganglion
Inferior vagal ganglion
Pharyngeal n.
Superior laryngeal n.
External laryngeal n.
Recurrent laryngeal n.

Fig. 5-2. The laryngeal innervation on the right side. (From M. P. Fried, *The Larynx: A Multidisciplinary Approach.* Boston: Little, Brown, 1988.)

not be elicited in most patients. Some individuals with a hyper-active gag reflex may be difficult to examine, even under the best of circumstances. A topical anesthetic spray (e.g., benzocaine) can facilitate the examination. Phonating the vowel "e" elevates the epiglottis and exposes the laryngeal inlet, vocal folds, and upper trachea.

2. **A rigid fiberoptic laryngoscope,** with a distal light source, is inserted through the oral cavity to visualize the laryngeal structures below. New models are smaller in size with improved optics and offer teaching side arms. Miniaturized video cameras allow for excellent visualization for the patient and observer as well as documentation. Videolaryngeal stroboscopy can be added to rigid fiberoptic laryngoscopy in order to evaluate vocal cord motion. This technique uses a flashing stroboscopic light source that appears to slow the motion of the vocal folds. It permits assessment of the laryngeal mucosal wave, symmetry of cord motion, and the presence of pathological conditions such as small cysts, polyps, or nodules that otherwise would be difficult to see. A permanent record is also available for later comparison, after treatment has been instituted.

3. **A flexible fiberoptic laryngoscope** uses a fiberoptic principle to visualize the structures of the pharynx, larynx, and subglottis. It is placed through the nares after topical anesthesia is applied intranasally (e.g., 4% cocaine solution or, alternatively, a 50:50 solution of 4% lidocaine and 1% ephedrine). Because the tip is flexible, excellent visualization may be obtained of the hypopharynx and larynx while the patient is swallowing or speaking. Attachments are available for photographic documentation.

4. **A rigid endoscope** can be used to visualize the larynx and tracheal bronchial tree directly. This procedure is most often performed under general anesthesia and is especially useful when obtaining biopsies and when removing foreign bodies. A **rigid laryngoscope** is used in conjunction with an operating microscope for precise tissue sampling and surgical procedures. A **rigid bronchoscope** is invaluable for aspirating thick tracheobronchial secretions in relieving distal airway obstruction. Smaller distal bronchial passages are visualized with the aid of a telescopic attachment.

5. **Flexible bronchoscopy** is often performed under local anesthesia. Tissue samples can be obtained using a brush or biopsy forceps. These instruments enable the examiner to have access to segmental bronchi. It is superior to the rigid endoscope in assessing the site of hemoptysis and in evaluating small distal lesions.

6. **Voice analysis** should be performed on patients with persistent vocal symptoms or on those considered for surgical correction of voice pathology. Newer, computerized instrumentation can evaluate air flow and vibratory characteristics such as breathiness, intensity, pitch, and perturbations. See the appendix to this chapter.

B. **History.** There are no specific features of the history for laryngeal disease that are diagnostic. The two most common complaints are hoarseness and difficulty breathing. The onset of each complaint should be noted, as well as its duration and change in severity. Stridor is frequently associated with respiratory difficulty (dyspnea). Inquiry should be made as to the presence of pain, whether it is associated with speaking or swallowing, and its location. Hemoptysis is rarely present. The presence of antecedent trauma or surgical procedures, as well as the possibility of a foreign body, should be noted. Systemic symptoms may be absent in the presence of localized laryngeal disease.

C. **Ancillary diagnostic techniques**

1. **Radiographs**

a. **Anteroposterior (AP) neck x ray.** Although of limited value because of the superimposition of the cervical spine on the laryngeal architecture, the AP view is useful when evaluating air-fluid levels (i.e., laryngoceles), subcutaneous emphysema, calcific nodules, as well as distortion of the upper airway. A copper grid filtration can be used to enhance the image. When specifically looking for the air column, an over-penetrated film may provide the necessary contrast.

b. **Lateral neck view.** A lateral neck radiograph is particularly useful in evaluating the epiglottis, the retropharynx, and the general configuration of the airway. Often, the nasopharynx is included in this projection. In both this view and the frontal AP projection, radiopaque foreign bodies can be visualized.

c. **Fluoroscopy.** Fluoroscopy affords visualization of the functions of respiration and phonation, with or without the use of contrast or cineradiographic films. It may demonstrate vocal cord dysfunction or other neuromuscular disorders of the upper aerodigestive tract. Fluoroscopy is invaluable in assessing the presence of a foreign body in the distal airway when comparison of movement of the lung fields is mandatory.

d. **Barium swallow.** A barium swallow is particularly useful as a contrast radiographic technique when radiolucent foreign bodies are suspected. The study also delineates neoplasia within the hypopharynx and cervical esophagus. Esophageal diverticula, tracheoesophageal fistulas, potential causes of dysphagia, and neuromuscular disorders can be evaluated. Often there is some degree of aspiration of barium with upper airway dysfunction, beneficially coating the intralaryngeal structures. This technique has additional value in assessing upper airway anomalies in the infant and should be performed prior to direct examination of the larynx.

e. **Contrast laryngography.** A laryngogram is obtained by coating the laryngeal structures with a contrast medium, often an oily radiopaque substance, e.g., propyliodone (Dionosil). This procedure is performed after atropine is given to dry the mucous membranes and after a topical anesthetic is applied. By having the patient carry out various maneuvers such as quiet breathing, expiratory phonation of a high-pitched "e," a modified Valsalva maneuver, and inspiratory phonation, the larynx and hypopharynx can often be clearly visualized. Specific details as to structures within the pyriform sinuses, laryngeal ventricle, and subglottis are demonstrated. The quality of the film often depends on patient cooperation. Shortcomings include the need for premedication as well as topical anesthesia before adequate radiographs can be obtained. Contrast laryngography may be hazardous in the presence of airway compromise. Currently, this study is infrequently performed.

f. **Computed tomography.** Computed tomography (CT) has become increasingly valuable in assessing lesions of the head and neck. It is specifically useful in diagnosing soft-tissue densities when other radiographic techniques fail. CT can delineate destruction of bony and cartilaginous structures, as well as distortions of the airway. CT is a precise method of assessing the airway radiographically. In conjunction with contrast enhancement of vascular structures, it affords a panoramic visualization of the entire neck. CT has supplanted the use of polytomography and contrast laryngography in evaluation of the larynx.

g. **Magnetic resonance imaging (MRI).** Although an excellent modality to evaluate the soft tissue, lymphatics, and vascular structures of the neck, current MRI methods do not offer any benefit in imaging the laryngeal framework. Motion can induce artifact, and small lesions may not be visualized. Rapid improvement in imaging times and three-dimensional reconstruction by new computer software programs, however, may add detail and information not otherwise obtainable.

2. **Cultures.** If laryngeal or tracheal infection is suspected, appropriate cultures should be obtained. Most often, aerobic bacteria are detected; however, in immunocompromised patients, such as those receiving chemotherapy, having AIDS or neoplastic disorders, or who are transplant recipients, special care should be taken in obtaining cultures for fungi and anaerobic bacteria. Often, only the predominant organism can be obtained from a surface smear, yet it enables the appropriate antibiotic therapy. Occasionally, a biopsy is needed to define the causative organism, especially with mycoses.

III. Stridor

It must be remembered that **stridor** is a **symptom** and is not indicative of any particular disorder. It signifies airway turbulence and often narrowing of the airway. High-pitched inspiratory stridor usually indicates a problem at the laryngeal level. Low-pitched stridor may signify a pharyngeal location. Wheezing stridor points toward bronchiolar constriction. A high-pitched inspiratory stridor plus a low-pitched expiratory phase usually indicates obstruction below the level of the larynx.

A. Congenital

1. **Laryngomalacia.** An immature and flaccid larynx is the most common cause of childhood stridor.

   a. **Signs and symptoms.** The stridor often begins at birth and is inspiratory as well as variable in severity. It is due in part to a flaccid supraglottic structure that collapses into the airway with inspiration. It is aggravated in the supine position and improved when prone. Vocal quality is unimpaired.

   b. **Physical examination.** Intermittent inspiratory stridor is noted, but in general the child appears healthy without significant respiratory distress.

   c. **Diagnosis.** Fiberoptic or direct laryngoscopy confirms the diagnosis of laryngomalacia. It is important to control respirations and motion of the glottic stenosis. Intubation may limit visualization at the time of laryngoscopy; consequently, inspection of the entire larynx must be accomplished at some point without the endotracheal tube in place.

d. Therapy. The symptoms usually regress spontaneously by 12–18 months of age, and management with intubation or tracheotomy is rarely necessary. For a marginal airway, laser lysis of the tethered aryepiglottic folds has been beneficial.

2. Stenosis. Subglottic laryngeal stenosis may be congenital or acquired. It is difficult to make the diagnosis of congenital subglottic stenosis if there has been a history of intubation. Episodic and recurrent croup should suggest subglottic stenosis.

   a. Important pathologic correlations

   (1) There are three forms of **subglottic stenosis:**

   (a) A normal-shaped cricoid that is small for the patient's age and weight

   (b) A normal-sized cricoid but with submucosal fibrosis

   (c) An abnormally shaped cricoid

   (2) Associated anomalies may occur in the presence of congenital subglottic stenosis. Twenty percent of these patients may also have laryngomalacia.

   (3) Acquired subglottic stenosis is most commonly due to endotracheal intubation. Some of the predisposing factors are:

   Physical trauma during intubation
   Large endotracheal tube size
   Lack of humidification
   Piston action of a ventilator, allowing motion of the endotracheal tube
   Infection around the endotracheal tube
   Underlying systemic disease (diabetes, immunosuppressed hosts)
   Prolonged duration of intubation
   Overinflation of the endotracheal tube cuff in older patients

   b. Etiology. The pathogenesis of acquired subglottic laryngeal stenosis begins with the inciting event, which may be external trauma or internal trauma from intubation. Trauma leads to edema in the subglottic space that is limited by a fully circumferential cricoid cartilage. Ulceration or encrustation leads to infection, granulation tissue, and cicatrix with associated stenosis.

   c. Signs and symptoms. Stridor is almost invariably present in subglottic stenosis. Respiratory difficulty may be intermittent and frequently is associated with upper respiratory tract infection or progressive contracture. Dyspnea may be present.

d. Diagnosis is suggested by a history of recurrent episodes of stridor and croup, as well as intubation or laryngeal trauma. In the adult, CT scanning gives valuable preoperative information. The diagnosis is confirmed by direct inspection of the subglottis. Care must be taken during manipulation of these airways, since a minimum amount of edema may compromise a marginal airway, necessitating a tracheotomy.

e. Therapy. Early periodic dilatation in mild noncartilaginous stenosis is of value. Endoscopic laser resection of the stenotic segment is often applicable in more advanced cases. Judicious cryosurgery can also be beneficial. Occasionally, for severe stenosis, an open surgical procedure with insertion of autogenous tissue (i.e., hyoid bone, thyroid cartilage, or free rib) may be necessary. Hyoid grafts can be pedicled on the sternohyoid muscle, increasing vascularity and potential healing. On rare occasions, both the anterior and the posterior laminas of the cricoid cartilage may need to be transected to reconstruct a serviceable airway. In the infant with congenital subglottic stenosis, a surgical split of the cricoid cartilage may be therapeutic.

3. Vascular

a. Vascular rings. Most common vascular anomalies include either a double aortic arch or incomplete rings from aberrant development of the major vessels (aortic arch, subclavian arteries, pulmonary artery, persistent ductus arteriosus).

(1) Signs and symptoms. Anomalies of the great vessels produce respiratory difficulty from tracheal compression as well as dysphasia from esophageal compression. The stridor produced is frequently both inspiratory and expiratory, characteristics of tracheal involvement rather than laryngeal involvement. The vocal quality is not altered.

(2) Diagnosis

(a) X rays. Routine chest roentgenograms rarely demonstrate vascular anomalies. A barium swallow will show esophageal compression, and angiography will clearly delineate the lesion. MRI with contrast is the imaging modality of choice, yielding the most information concerning the airway and vascular anatomy.

(b) Endoscopy. Bronchoscopy and esophagoscopy are essential to demonstrate the magnitude of the functional compromise, thereby assisting in the decision as to whether corrective surgery is warranted.

(c) Therapy. Repair of vascular rings requires the expertise of a cardiothoracic or vascular surgeon.

b. Subglottic hemangioma. Fifty percent of subglottic hemangiomas are associated with cutaneous hemangiomas.

(1) Signs and symptoms. Although the hemangioma is present at birth, the patient may be asymptomatic. Hemangiomas often enlarge within the first year and may not present until 6 months or later. Stridor is the most common symptom of this disorder. Characteristically, subglottic hemangiomas enlarge with crying or straining, which makes the stridor more pronounced.

(2) Diagnosis

(a) Physical examination may reveal cutaneous lesions. Stridor, as noted above, may be present.

(b) Radiography. A lateral soft tissue x ray of the neck often demonstrates fullness in the subglottic area. MRI or CT scanning may clearly demonstrate the anomaly. Angiography is not required.

(c) Direct laryngoscopy affords visualization of the subglottic mass, which may not have a red or purple hue. The lesion is often soft and compressible.

(3) Therapy. Usually no therapy is necessary, because these lesions regress spontaneously. With severe obstructive symptoms, a tracheotomy must be considered. The use of endoscopic cryosurgery or laser excision may be considered beneficial for larger lesions.

4. Webs

a. Pathologic correlates. Laryngeal webs are thought to be due to failure of the larynx to reestablish its lumen at the tenth week of fetal life. Seventy-five percent are at the glottic level, the remaining being supraglottic and subglottic. The thickness of the web may vary from a thin, transparent membrane to full fusion of the vocal folds.

b. Signs and symptoms. The stridor is primarily inspiratory and is generally exacerbated by an upper respiratory tract infection. With significant narrowing, respiratory distress may be present at birth. Often there is an alteration in the vocal quality, secondary to decreased vocal cord movement.

c. Diagnosis. Radiographs frequently fail to delineate the lesion. The diagnosis is made on direct laryngoscopy.

d. Therapy. A tracheotomy may be necessary, depending on the extent of the web. Incision of the web, followed by repeated dilatations, may be required. A stent within the laryngeal lumen is occasionally needed after the web is resected. The laser or judicious cautery is helpful.

5. Cysts of the larynx are thought to be disturbances of fetal development.

a. Pathologic correlates. A laryngocele originates from the laryngeal saccule, which is the anterior portion of the ventricle and lies between the true and false vocal cords. It may extend into the larynx itself, most often into the false vocal cord, causing bulging of this structure. Occasionally, it traverses the thyrohyoid membrane and presents as a neck mass. Laryngoceles may be air or fluid filled and, although congenital, may not be diagnosed until adulthood. When infected, acute respiratory distress can occur with localized pain and neck tenderness.

b. Signs and symptoms. Children present with respiratory obstruction and inspiratory stridor, whereas adults often have hoarseness. Straining, coughing, and the Valsalva maneuver aggravate these symptoms.

c. Diagnosis. Radiographs are of value because they delineate cystic lesions that have an air-fluid level. MRI or CT scanning can localize the cyst. Direct laryngoscopy confirms the diagnosis.

d. Therapy. Surgery is required. Aspiration, marsupialization, and excision have proponents for the management of internal laryngoceles and supraglottic cysts. External laryngoceles require an external approach.

B. Acquired

1. Foreign body. The aspiration of a foreign body must always be suspected in cases of acute laryngeal stridor or respiratory distress, especially in infants.

a. Signs and symptoms. Obstruction at the level of the supraglottis or glottis usually produces the acute symptoms of inspiratory stridor and an alteration in vocal quality. Pain is infrequent. Foreign bodies lodged within the trachea similarly cause acute dyspnea and are true surgical emergencies. Objects lodged distally (bronchi) may present acutely with a short paroxysm of coughing and hoarseness, yet often are silent initially, ultimately presenting as atelectasis, chronic cough, or recurrrent pneumonitis.

b. Diagnosis

(1) The **history** is invaluable when specific inquiry is made as to the possibility of foreign body aspiration. A short paroxysm of coughing, followed by a localized peripheral auscultated wheeze, is classic. Occasionally, the initial episode may go unnoticed by the child's parents.

(2) **X rays** will detail a radiopaque foreign body. Atelectasis may be present distal to a foreign body; pulmonary infiltrates also may be present. Fluoroscopy will reveal paradoxical motion, since the obstructed pulmonary segment will not expand on inspiration. If a ball valve obstruction occurs, obstructive emphysema with increased lucency within a pulmonary segment may be present. In rare cases, a chest CT scan may be of value.

(3) **Therapy.** A Heimlich maneuver may be necessary for a totally obstructing laryngeal foreign body; however, it is preferable to remove a foreign body from the upper airway whenever possible by direct laryngoscopy and control of the airway. Forceful blind attempts at manual removal are ill-advised and may force a supraglottic or hypopharyngeal foreign body into the glottis, causing total respiratory obstruction. Moreover, if a foreign body presents in the tracheobronchial tree, turning the patient upside down may impact the foreign body in the subglottis, causing total obstruction. A controlled situation in the operating room is preferable.

2. **Acquired subglottic stenosis.** See sec. III.A.2.a.(3).

3. **Croup syndromes.** See Chap. 1, II.

4. **Pharyngeal abscess.** See Chap. 1, IV.C.

5. **Trauma.** See Chap. 1, V.

6. **Angioneurotic edema.** See Chap. 1, VI.

7. **Laryngitis.** See sec. IV.

8. **Neoplasia.** See sec. IV.

9. **Vocal cord paralysis.** See sec. IV.

10. **External compression of the larynx.** Although stridor is not found in isolation in these disorders, it may be a prominent symptom. Anterior compression usually arises from the thyroid gland and may be due to a goiter, thyroiditis, or carcinoma of the thyroid. When posterior compression occurs, it often arises from a carcinoma of the esophagus.

    a. **Signs and symptoms.** Associated physical findings are an obviously palpable mass or pain over the thyroid gland. Weight loss and dysphagia are common symptoms of carcinoma of the esophagus.

    b. **Diagnosis** is based on the history of a slow voice change and on the presence of a neck mass.

    c. **Radiographs.** Thyroid scanning assists in the delineation of a thyroid nodule. A barium swallow may show associated extrinsic or intrinsic compression as well as distortion. A neck CT scan will detail the airway and surrounding soft-tissue structures.

    d. **Therapy** is directed toward the underlying pathologic disorder.

11. **Tracheobronchial disease.** Carcinoma, tuberculosis, or adenomas may impinge on the airway, producing stridor that may be both inspiratory and expiratory.

IV. Hoarseness

Hoarseness reflects any abnormality of normal phonation. It has multiple causes that often require direct visualization of the larynx by one of the methods described. Although a breathy vocal quality may suggest a **vocal cords paralysis** and a coarse quality may suggest **nodularity,** there are no specific features of hoarseness that are definitively diagnostic.

A. Inflammatory

Acute laryngeal infections in adults may progress over several hours, but usually take several days from onset until the patient seeks medical care. This process is much more rapid in a child. Odynophagia and odynophonia are common. Chronic inflammations are more indolent, with symptoms extending over a period of weeks.

1. Acute

a. Viral and bacterial infections can cause an inflammatory response on the surface of the vocal cords (laryngitis).

(1) Pathologic correlates. Acute, simple laryngitis is almost invariably viral and is usually self-limited unless a complication develops. The viruses usually implicated are influenza, parainfluenza, rhinovirus, myxovirus, coxsackivirus, respiratory syncytial, paramyxovirus, and coronavirus of the RNA group. DNA viruses include adenovirus, herpes, Epstein-Barr, Varicella zoster, and variola. Complications include hemorrhagic nodules and acute membranous laryngitis, frequently secondary to colonization with *Streptococcus pneumoniae,* beta-hemolytic Streptococcus, or *Staphylococcus.* Diphtheria is now a rare cause of laryngitis.

(2) Signs and symptoms. Hoarseness usually occurs in the presence of the systemic symptoms of fatigue and occasionally fever. There may be associated hypopharyngeal pain, pain on phonation, or dysphagia. Such systemic symptoms may be associated with a generalized disorder.

(3) Diagnosis is confirmed via direct examination of the larynx. Erythema, either discrete or diffuse, is suggestive. Encrusted mucus is not unusual. Vocal cord motion is most often normal.

(4) Therapy. Antibiotics may be necessary for secondary bacterial infections and a cephalosporin is the treatment of choice for the adult. Voice rest and humidification are important adjuncts. If respiratory obstruction is present, hospitalization is essential and an antibiotic is administered parenterally. Removal of the obstructing crusts may be required.

b. Laryngeal abscess is rare and is usually secondary to irritation (endotracheal intubation) or direct trauma. The etiologic agent is usually *Staphylococcus, Pseudomonas,* or *Proteus.*

(1) Signs and symptoms. Severe throat pain is present, associated with odynophagia, fever, and signs of systemic toxicity. Cervical adenopathy may be present. Pain is precipitated by lateral motion of the larynx. Respiratory distress is to be expected.

(2) Diagnosis

(a) Radiographs demonstrate edema and distortion of the intralaryngeal structures, with occasional evidence of an air-fluid level within an abscess cavity.

(b) Fiberoptic laryngoscopy is required to assess the size of the glottic aperture for adequacy.

(3) Therapy. Broad-spectrum antibiotic therapy providing coverage for documented organisms is essential. A tracheotomy is frequently required. Open surgical drainage is necessary if a response to antibiotic therapy does not occur within 24–48 hours. Should chondritis with secondary necrosis ensue, judicious debridement may be required.

2. Chronic. Persistant irritation of the vocal cords leads to chronic hoarseness.

a. Etiology

(1) Most often, the irritation is due to chronic upper and lower respiratory tract infections or to the sequelae of the slowly resolving acute process. Aggravating factors, such as cigarette smoke in conjunction with excessive alcohol consumption, may be present. Other factors such as exposure to irritants at work (dust, fiber, asbestos) or at home (pet dander) must be considered.

(2) Granulomatous diseases

(a) Tuberculosis is caused by *Mycobacterium tuberculosis*. Although a common laryngeal infection in the past, it is currently rare and usually results from bronchogenic spread. Tissue culture and smears provide the definitive diagnosis, and standard therapy consists of a 3-month course of isoniazid, rifampin, and pyrazinamide, followed by a 9-month or longer course of isoniazid and rifampin.

(b) Syphilis is caused by *Treponema pallidum,* a spiral bacterium. Laryngeal involvement is seen in secondary and tertiary stages, with erythematous patches or gray lesions on the mucous membranes in the secondary stage. The tertiary stage is characterized by ulcers, granulomatous inflammation, and fibrosis. Stenosis can be a consequence of either stage. Penicillin is the treatment of choice.

(c) Rhinoscleroma is caused by *Klebsiella rhinoscleromatis,* a gram-negative rod also called the von Frish bacillus. It is endemic in Central America, South America, South and Central Europe, Egypt, the East

Indies, and Southwestern Asia. Diagnosis is made by culture, with standard treatment being Bactrim or tetracycline.

(d) Actinomycosis is a rare granulomatous disease caused by *Actinomyces israelii,* an anaerobic gram-positive bacteria. Diagnosis is culture-dependent, and penicillin is the treatment of choice.

(e) Fungal infections include histoplasmosis, blastomycosis, paracoccidioidomycosis, coccidiosis, candidiasis, and aspergillosis. These infections, although uncommon, are currently more frequently seen in immunocompromised hosts, such as patients with AIDS or those receiving chemotherapy. Culture is mandatory, and treatment is most often with amphotericin B.

(f) Sarcoidosis is an idiopathic, chronic, granulomatous multisystem disease that may involve the larynx. In the head and neck, the nose and paranasal sinuses are most frequently affected. Hoarseness, dysphagia and dyspnea, as well as progressive airway obstruction, can be found. Biopsy in conjunction with clinical findings is necessary to establish the diagnosis.

(g) Amyloidosis involves the larynx in either localized or systemic disease, a primary or idiopathic process, or as a result of other disorders, such as multiple myeloma. Hoarseness and obstruction are the most common laryngeal symptoms, with diagnosis based on histologic examination with documentation of amyloid deposits by special stains.

(h) Idiopathic granulomas include Wegener's granulomatosis, idiopathic midline granuloma, and polymorphic reticulosis. These disorders may form a continuum that leads to a true lymphoma. Differentiation among these lesions is important, because treatment for Wegener's granulomatosis is systemic (cyclophosphamide), as opposed to localized (radiation) for the other granulomas.

(i) Autoimmune processes, such as systemic lupus erythematosis or relapsing polychrondritis, may involve the larynx and cause hoarseness and pain, as well as airway compromise. Therapy is directed to the underlying disorder.

b. Diagnosis. Persistent hoarseness is the most common characteristic. Occasionally, the hoarseness fluctuates, being aggravated by voice abuse. Systemic symptoms of a granulomatous disease (see **a.(2)**) may also be present.

Laryngoscopy, most often indirect, reveals vocal cord edema and occasional erythema. Nodularity and thickening of the vocal cords may be noted, but this is usually diffuse, rather than unilateral or localized.

c. **Therapy.** Voice rest, limitation of irritant factors, and expectorants are current modes of treatment. In the early stages, a beclomethasone inhaler may assist in reversing the inflammation. Therapy should also be directed toward an underlying systemic disease, if present.

3. **Cricoarytenoid arthritis**

a. **Etiology.** Rheumatoid arthritis is the most common cause of cricoarytenoid arthritis. Other less common causes of arthritic change in the cricoarytenoid joint are gout, lupus erythematosus, tuberculosis, syphilis, and gonorrhea. Trauma may also result in arthritis to this joint.

b. **Diagnosis**

(1) **Hoarseness** is the most common symptom. It can occur after trauma from an external source or intubation. In cases of rheumatoid arthritis, however, the initial episode may be associated with exceptional throat pain, especially on swallowing or speaking. After the acute process subsides, the hoarseness may persist.

(2) **Indirect laryngoscopy** reveals a marked limitation or complete immobility of the vocal cord. In the acute stage, the mucosa overlying the arytenoid may be edematous and erythematous.

(3) **Direct laryngoscopy** with palpation of the arytenoid confirms the diagnosis. Decreased mobility on direct lateral pressure to the body of the arytenoid is present.

c. **Therapy.** Treatment is directed at the underlying disease whenever possible. If the airway is compromised due to poor motion of the involved vocal cord (cords), surgical intervention may be necessary with arytenoidectomy, arytenoidopexy, or even a tracheotomy. With the first two techniques, the airway is often improved at the expense of a weak, breathy voice and the possibility of intermittent tracheal aspiration. Techniques such as nerve-muscle pedicle grafts in the presence of a fixed joint are contraindicted.

B. **Vocal abuse**

1. **Etiology.** Nodules are usually caused by voice abuse and are the most frequent causes of persistent hoarseness, especially in children. These areas of fibrosis develop most characteristically at the junction of the anterior one-third and posterior two-thirds of the vocal cord and are often bilateral. Nodules of recent onset are discrete areas of inflammation and may be precipitated by viral laryngitis.

2. **Diagnosis.** A history of recent voice abuse is the most common preceding factor. Examination of the vocal folds reveals characteristic nodularity.

3. **Nodules** of recent origin are discrete areas of inflammation responding rapidly to voice rest, vocal therapy, or, occasionally, to

steroid spray (beclomethasone inhaler, two inhalations tid). More mature nodules are firm and fibrotic, usually requiring more prolonged therapy. Topical steroid spray is of less value in this situation.

4. Vocal polyps

  a. Etiology. Vocal polyps may be solitary or diffuse and are secondary to vocal abuse or irritation such as smoking. Solitary polyps may be traced to a single episode of voice strain or even to endotracheal intubation.

  b. Diagnosis

  (1) Physical examination most often reveals polyps to occur in the anterior portion of the vocal cords.

  (2) If polyps are noted overlying the vocal process of the arytenoids (posterior one-third of the vocal cords), an antecedent history of endotracheal intubation with or without reflux may often be present.

  c. Therapy. Voice rest, humidification, and a topical steroid spray are the initial forms of treatment. Laryngoscopic removal may be needed.

C. Hemorrhage

  1. Etiology. Hemorrhage of vocal cord vessels is uncommon but can occur secondary to anticoagulant therapy, bleeding diatheses, or trauma.

  2. Diagnosis. Visualization of the larynx and of possible sites of bleeding confirms the diagnosis. Although bleeding into the vocal cord substance may be localized, in patients on anticoagulants or with bleeding disorders, the bleeding and edema may be progressive. This progression is noted by diffuse ecchymosis of not only the glottic but also of the supraglottic structures.

  3. Therapy

  a. Therapy is usually directed toward correcting the underlying problem. Then the bleeding most often is self-limiting, and the alterations are reversible.

  b. With any airway compromise, hospitalization is mandatory. Intubation should precede any consideration of tracheotomy, the latter being a consideration after the hematologic condition is stabilized.

D. Intubation injury

  1. Pathophysiology. During endotracheal intubation, one or both arytenoids may become dislocated, or, rarely, the recurrent laryngeal nerves may be injured. If the vocal cords are traumatized, hemorrhage may occur or secondary granulomas may form over the vocal process. The incidence of such occurrences heightens with frequent attempts at intubation, local infection, motion of the endotracheal tube, or dehydration. Further injury can lead to the formation of a cicatrix or full stenosis.

2. **Diagnosis**

   a. **Pain** is not infrequent.

   b. Persistent **hoarseness** after extubation signifies an abnormality of the larynx.

   c. **Diagnosis** depends on direct visualization of the larynx with special emphasis on the posterior commissure and cordal mobility. Arytenoid dislocation is suggested by a foreshortened vocal cord with the arytenoid being tipped forward or laterally.

3. **Therapy**

   a. **Granulomas** may require removal if there is no response to topical steroids, but also raise the possibility of gastroesophageal reflux as a cause. Further investigation by barium swallow or 24-hour pH probe (with gastroenterology consultation) may be appropriate. Treatment in this circumstance is directed at the reflux, requiring altered diet, elevation of the head of the bed, antacids, and H_2 blockers.

   b. **Cicatrix formation** often requires endoscopic dilatation or lysing of the stenotic mucosa.

   c. **Cricoarytenoid dislocation** responds to replacement of the arytenoid surgically; however, endoscopic repositioning is usually only possible if the diagnosis is made within days of the injury.

   d. With **maturation** of **scar** tissue or persistent vocal cord paralysis, therapy is more problematic (see **III.A.2.e.** and **V.B.5.a.**).

E. **Allergy**

   1. **Etiology**

      a. **Irritative pollens** in atopic individuals occasionally produce hoarseness. Pollutants and smoking may cause irritation, mucosal hyperemia, and hoarseness.

      b. **Allergy** can also be responsible for altered capillary permeability and subsequent vocal cord edema (see Chap. 1, **VI.**). Laryngeal edema may follow drug ingestion, transfusion reactions, insect bites, food ingestion, or serum injection.

   2. **Diagnosis.** The acute condition is suspected when direct inspection of the larynx reveals diffuse edema not associated with mucosal alteration. Inhalants such as dust and smoke can be associated with hyperemia.

   3. **Therapy**

      a. Treatment of **angioneurotic edema** is outlined in Chap. 1, **VI.**

      b. **Allergic laryngeal edema** with associated obstructive symptoms requires epinephrine, 0.1–0.3 ml of 1 : 1000 solution SQ, steroids (dexamethasone, 4–10 mg, according to weight), diphenhydramine, 25–50 mg, and occasionally intubation or tracheotomy, if medical management fails.

   c. Less severe allergic responses require elimination or avoidance of identified irritating substances, humidification, and the occasional use of antihistamines (e.g., diphenhydramine). Topical steroid spray, beclomethasone, can also be beneficial.

F. Sicca syndrome

   1. Etiology

   a. The sicca syndrome is characterized by diminished flow from the salivary glands and can occur in conjunction with drying of the eyes, mucous membranes, and subsequent sialadenitis. It is often found in association with arthritis (Sjögren's syndrome). The sicca syndrome can progress to chronic laryngitis in which the laryngeal mucosa is persistently dry and subsequently undergoes atrophy.

   b. Other possible etiologies include external irradiation, chronic nonspecific laryngitis, mucoviscidosis, and medications such as antihistamines or gastrointestinal antispasmodics, phenothiazines, and tricyclics.

   2. Diagnosis

   a. History

   (1) A detailed history of pertinent medications must be sought, since their elimination may remedy the problem.

   (2) Dryness of the mouth or eyes with associated irritation may be present.

   (3) Arthritis, urethritis, and swelling of the parotid or submandibular glands must be noted.

   b. Physical examination. Hoarseness may be intermittent but is not associated with pain. Adenopathy is not present initially; however, salivary gland hypertrophy may be detected.

   (1) The oral mucosa is often dry, and viscid mucus can be expressed from the salivary ducts.

   (2) The vocal cords often are structurally unaltered, yet thick adherent mucous strands are almost always observed

   c. Biopsy of a minor salivary gland of the lower lip may assist in the diagnosis of Sjögren's syndrome.

   3. Therapy

   a. Elimination of offending medications is essential.

   b. Symptomatic treatment is often all that can be offered, paramount among which is humidification and hydration.

   c. Steroid therapy, whether topical or systemic, offers little in this disorder.

G. Endocrinopathy. Disorders of many of the endocrine glands may be associated with alterations in phonation. Therapy is directed toward the underlying imbalance. Although laryngeal alterations are not specific for each endocrinopathy, what follows is a general outline of the primary disorders.

1. **Pituitary**

   a. **Acromegaly,** such as that produced by pituitary adenomas, causes accelerated growth of the laryngeal structure, with hyperplasia of the laryngeal mucosa. This increased growth leads to a deep phonatory quality and hoarseness. The hoarseness is accentuated with involvement of the cricoarytenoid joint.

   b. In **primary pituitary hypofunction,** there is a lack of growth of the laryngeal architecture, with an immature high-pitched voice as seen in some dwarfs.

2. **Adrenal**

   a. **Adrenal hyperfunction** leads to virilization from hypersecretion of androgenic hormones. This condition also is associated with a lowered vocal pitch. Rarely, estrogenic hypersecretion may occur with feminization and elevation of the vocal pitch.

   b. **Adrenal hypofunction,** as found in Addison's disease, causes vocal weakness secondary to muscular asthenia, and the speech becomes listless and indistinct. Adrenal hypofunction may rarely lead to aphonia.

3. **Thyroid**

   a. **Hypothyroidism (myxedema)** can cause hoarseness and deepening of the voice due to hypertrophy of the vocalis muscle. Mucopolysaccharides may be deposited subepithelially, limiting vocal cord mobility. This deposition can lead to vocal cord enlargement and, on occasion, frank laryngeal polyposis.

   b. **Hyperthyroidism** has been associated with thyrotoxicosis, vocal fatigue, an increased respiratory rate, and a high-pitched voice.

   c. **Enlargement of the thyroid gland** may cause compression of the recurrent laryngeal nerve, thereby diminishing vocal cord mobility. Rarely, direct compression of the larynx by a massively enlarged thyroid can cause hoarseness.

4. **Gonadal**

   a. Hypogonadal syndromes are linked etiologically with persistence of a high-pitched juvenile voice in males.

   b. During pregnancy, hoarseness can occur, resolving after parturition.

   c. Virilizing tumors of the testicular Leydig cells may cause premature deepening of the voice.

H. Neoplasm

1. Benign

a. Papilloma. The squamous papilloma is the most common benign growth of the larynx and is the most common of all childhood neoplasms. Although these lesions usually occur in childhood, they can develop at any age.

(1) Etiology. Papillomas are suspected to be viral in origin. An association has been noted with upper respiratory papillomas and maternal condylomata acuminata of the genital tract. These growths can also be found in the oral cavity, independent of laryngeal involvement.

(2) Signs and symptoms. Hoarseness, beginning within the first few years of life, is the most common presenting symptom. Although usually observed at the level of the true and false vocal folds, papillomas can migrate subglottically and involve the entire tracheobronchial tree. Airway obstruction can occur.

(3) Diagnosis. A history of progressive hoarseness and, occasionally, respiratory distress are most common. The diagnosis is confirmed by endoscopic biopsy.

(4) Therapy

(a) The management is removal. Microsurgical instrumentation is essential, with the laser being most beneficial. Cryosurgery can be a useful adjunct. Often, repeated endoscopy and tumor removal are necessary before control is achieved.

(b) Antiviral vaccines have not been successful.

(c) Spontaneous regression may occur in late childhood.

(d) A tracheotomy should be avoided whenever possible as it has been associated with spread to the lower respiratory tract.

b. Cysts. See III.A.5.

(1) Other pathophysiology. In addition to laryngoceles, small mucous retention cysts can occur within the larynx, secondary to obstruction of mucous glands within the respiratory epithelium. These cysts are found at the level of the epiglottis, aryepiglottic fold, false vocal cords, or ventricle.

(2) Signs and symptoms. Except for infancy, rarely do laryngeal cysts produce symptoms of obstruction; however hoarseness or dysphonia may occur.

(3) Diagnosis is made by indirect examination videolaryngeal stroboscopy and confirmed at endoscopy.

(4) Therapy. Endoscopic excision or marsupialization is the treatment of choice. The laser is excellent for this.

c. Chondroma

(1) **Etiology.** These benign growths arise from hyaline carti-lage, which forms the skeletal support for the larynx. Chondromas occur most frequently on the posterior lam-ina of the cricoid cartilage.

(2) **Signs and symptoms.** Hoarseness, dyspnea, and dys-phagia are common.

(3) **Diagnosis.** Radiographs, including soft-tissue lateral films of the neck, MRI, and CT, show a dense mass con-tiguous with the cartilaginous structures of the larynx, especially the cricoid. This pathologic entity is confirmed by endoscopy and biopsy.

(4) **Therapy.** Complete extirpation is most often achieved through a laryngofissure and/or extended pharyngotomy. Surgery is the preferred treatment.

d. Hemangioma. See III.A.3.b.

e. Other benign neoplasms include neurofibromas that are found in association with von Recklinghausen's disease, li-pomas, chemodectomas, and adenomas arising from minor salivary glands.

2. Malignant

a. Epidemiology. Squamous cell carcinoma is the most fre-quent malignant neoplasm of the larynx, occurring in up to 95% of cases. The most consistent predisposing epidemio-logic factor associated with squamous cell carcinoma is cig-arette smoking. It has been shown that the correlation of incidence of laryngeal cancer is almost linear with the num-ber of cigarettes smoked per day. Heavy smokers have more than 3 times the risk of nonsmokers. Moreover, alcohol acts synergistically with tobacco in elevating cancer risks: the ef-fect of each is considerably greater as the levels of exposure to each factor increases. Numerous occupational risks have also been associated with cancer of the larynx, the most sig-nificant of which is asbestos exposure.

b. Staging. The American Joint Committee for Cancer Staging has detailed the following:

T_1. Tumor confined to one region within the larynx (e.g., vo-cal cord, laryngeal epiglottis, subglottis) with normal vo-cal fold mobility.

T_2. Tumor involving two adjacent regions (glottis and sub-glottis, glottis and supraglottis) with normal or impaired vocal fold mobility.

T_3. Endolaryngeal neoplasm with fixation of the vocal cord. T_3 supraglottic lesions may have tumor extension to in-volve the postcricoid area, medial wall of pyriform sinus, or preepiglottic space.

T_4. Massive tumor extending outside the confines of the larynx.

In conjunction with the above, nodal disease has also been classified:

N_0. No clinically positive nodes.
N_1. Single ipsilateral node that is less than 3 cm in diameter.
N_{2A}. Single ipsilateral node 3–6 cm.
N_{2B}. Multiple ipsilateral nodes, none greater than 6 cm.
N_{3A}. Clinically positive ipsilateral nodes, one over 6 cm in diameter.
N_{3B}. Clinically positive bilateral nodes (with each side staged separately).
N_{3C}. Clinically positive contralateral nodes.

Metastatic sites are classified as:

M_0. No distant metastatic deposits.
M_1. Distant metastatic deposits.

c. Signs and symptoms

(1) A suspicion of a malignancy should be heightened in a male aged 50–70 years with a history of heavy smoking and alcohol consumption.

(2) Characteristically, the most common symptoms are hoarseness, throat or neck discomfort, progressive dyspnea, hemoptysis, and weight loss.

(3) Tracheal carcinoma frequently presents with progressive dyspnea and hemoptysis; however, primary tracheal carcinomas are rare.

d. Diagnosis

(1) **Physical examination**

(a) Often no outward signs of laryngeal or tracheal carcinoma can be assessed. On occasion, palpation of the neck denotes a lack of lateral mobility of the cartilaginous laryngeal structural framework due to fixation to surrounding soft tissue, suggesting extension of tumor beyond the laryngeal confines.

(b) Cervical adenopathy must be noted as to size and location.

(c) Stridor or wheezing may be audible. Some patients may present initially with severe dyspnea and obvious signs of airway obstruction.

(2) **Radiographs.** Radiologic assessment is often of great value. Laryngeal CT scanning and MRI are invaluable in assessing the extent of laryngeal tumor involvement. These studies should be performed prior to biopsy so that subsequent edema does not alter the tumor configuration. Barium swallow can disclose esophageal involvement by a large tumor or a synchronous second primary. A chest x ray is mandatory, with CT scanning performed if a questionable lesion is found.

(3) Laryngoscopy

(a) Indirect laryngoscopy often suggests the location of the neoplastic process. This is the time to evaluate vocal cord mobility.

(b) A definitive **diagnosis** is made on direct visualization with operative laryngoscopy and biopsy. At the time of biopsy, it is wise to stage the tumor extent, i.e., tumor, node, or metastatic sites (TNM), and to diagram the lesion. Diagramming is essential so that, irrespective of the mode of therapy instituted, the original lesion can always be recalled.

Evaluation of the entire upper aerodigestive tract with bronchoscopy and esophagoscopy should be performed to rule out a second primary. Up to 20% of patients with one head and neck malignancy may have a second primary, either synchronously or metachronously. A thorough initial assessment is essential for proper treatment planning.

e. Therapy. The common therapeutic modalities for laryngeal carcinoma include chemotherapy, radiation therapy, and surgery. Each has its own role, but not infrequently two or three modalities are used in combination.

(1) For early carcinoma of the larynx (T_1), 90% 5-year survival rate can be anticipated with either **radiation therapy** or **partial laryngeal surgery.** With either modality, phonation and normal deglutition can be preserved. Each method has its proponents, yet radiation therapy is selected most often.

(2) For T_2–T_4 lesions or with associated nodal disease, combined therapy is becoming commonplace. Tumors confined to the supraglottic space can be resected with a **supraglottic laryngectomy** and still preserve vocal function. Large lesions, if treated surgically, require **total laryngectomy.** The latter does not relegate a patient to aphonia, given that the rehabilitative measures of esophageal speech and surgical reconstruction of a neoglottis may restore oral communication. Newer prostheses are available as well. Surgical treatment of neck disease includes neck dissection, either with or without preservation of the spinal accessory nerve, sternocleidomastoid muscle, and jugular vein, at the discretion of the operating surgeon and determined by the extent of the disease.

(3) Radiation therapy finds its greatest utility in lesions confined to the larynx and in neck disease staged N_0 (with a high suspicion of microscopic neoplastic nodal involvement) or N_1.

(4) Large lesions require **combined therapy.** Induction chemotherapy has been used with such agents as methotrexate, cisplatinum, and 5-fluorouracil to reduce tumor bulk, to eliminate possible microscopic distant metastasis, and to aid in controlling regional metastatic deposits. The role of induction chemotherapy has as yet not been established, although data are emerging that suggest that those patients who exhibit a complete response may go onto radiation therapy and possibly avoid total laryngectomy. Combined use of surgical resection and radiation therapy offers distinct advantages in larger lesions; the current trend is toward higher doses of postoperative radiation therapy. This combination (i.e., surgery followed by radiation) appears to diminish the incidence of surgical complications, without adding disproportionate morbidity.

(5) Conservation surgery of the larynx allows for tumor resection with preservation of vocal function by hemilaryngectomy, supraglottic laryngectomy, or other extended procedures. These procedures are based on the lymphatic anatomy of the larynx, which compartmentalizes various regions, preventing endolaryngeal tumor spread.

(6) Subglottic and tracheal tumors are usually diagnosed late in their course, as they remain silent for long periods. Hoarseness is not common. Survival for tumors in both of these regions is low, less than 36%. Metastatic disease is common, and radiation therapy combined with surgical resection offers the best possibility for cure.

f. Other neoplasms

(1) Verrucous carcinoma appears as a sessile filiform tumor that may first appear to be histologically benign. It has the same presenting signs and symptoms as epidermoid carcinoma. Although a verrucous carcinoma appears grossly benign, it is a variant of epidermoid carcinoma. Radiation therapy has been associated with progression of local and regional disease, and surgical excision is favored.

(2) Adenocarcinoma may occur in any region of the larynx, usually arising from a minor salivary gland. Surgery is the primary therapeutic consideration. With large tumors, postoperative radiation therapy may have merit.

(3) Rarely do tumors metastasize to the larynx; however, kidney, prostate, and breast have been implicated. Diagnosis is confirmed by endoscopy and biopsy, with the histology documenting the primary site. Control of the primary tumor dictates the laryngeal management. If the tumor obstructs the airway, a tracheotomy is essential.

I. Functional disorders. Occasionally, vocal disturbances have no detectable, physical aberration. These disturbances may be psychogenic in origin, while for some no specific etiologic basis can be ascertained. Often associated emotional problems, if allowed to proceed uncorrected, may lead to organic lesions such as vocal nodules or polyps.

1. **Dysphonia plica ventricularis (ventricular dysphonia)**

   a. **Etiology.** This disorder in phonation is produced by the false vocal cords being the sound source.

   b. **Signs and symptoms.** The voice is low-pitched, lacks projection, and is obviously hoarse. Dysphonia plica ventricularis often occurs as a hyperfunctional compensatory mechanism after an episode of laryngitis. On mirror examination, the false vocal cords (ventricular folds) can be seen to oppose before and override the true vocal cords. In longstanding cases of dysphonia plica ventricularis, the true vocal cords may not even be visualized.

   c. **Therapy.** Voice therapy is initiated in an effort to regain appropriate use of the vocal cords. Psychiatric consultation should be considered.

2. **Psychogenic aphonia**

   a. **Signs and symptoms.** Psychogenic aphonia represents a total loss of voice and may be associated with a traumatic emotional episode. It rarely occurs without other symptoms of emotional stress.

   b. **Diagnosis.** On mirror examination, no laryngeal pathology is noted. Rarely, the vocal cords may be seen to flutter, but they never approach the midline or produce sound.

   c. **Treatment.** Psychiatric consultation is essential. Although the symptoms may wax and wane, they reflect a significant emotional disturbance.

3. **Myasthenia laryngis**

   a. **Etiology**

      (1) Myasthenia laryngis, or phonasthenia, is a weakness of the voice that can be due to fatigue, emotional tension, anxiety, and distress. Affected patients are often those who need to use their voice at work or who develop symptoms in response to stressful situations. Occasionally, carcinophobia may give rise to this symptom.

      (2) It is imperative to rule out a neuromuscular disorder. Myasthenia gravis, amyotrophic lateral sclerosis, or primary muscle disease can produce a weak voice.

   b. **Signs and symptoms.** The vocal quality is often breathy and weak. The duration of the symptoms can vary but can become chronic.

   c. **Diagnosis.** Frequently, the laryngeal examination is normal. In some patients, however, such as the elderly, the vocal cords may appear thinner, having lost substance. With the latter, there is a true atrophy of the vocal cords leading to a loss of volume. Videolaryngeal stroboscopy can assist in diagnosis.

d. Therapy

(1) The patient must be reassured that no organic pathology exists. A consultation with a speech pathologist is beneficial.

(2) Humidification and minimization of excessive vocalization may prove to be helpful.

(3) If a systemic neuromuscular disorder is suspected, a neurologic consultation should be obtained.

4. Laryngeal spasm

a. Etiology. Hyperkinetic muscle activity like phonasthenia (see **3.a.**) can be emotional or neuromuscular in etiology. Spasmodic dysphonia, a variant of laryngeal spasm, has been attributed by some to a neurotropic virus, or to a central nervous system abnormality similar to other idiopathic dystonias such as torticollis, writer's cramp, and blepharospasm.

b. Signs and symptoms. There is a cracking, straining, and harshness to the voice with episodic laryngeal spasm. When extreme, this spasm can lead to stridor. Spastic dysphonia appears to be a variant of laryngeal spasm. Sound production is difficult and staccato in nature. Associated movements, including facial grimacing, frequently accompany attempted phonation.

c. Diagnosis. Indirect laryngoscopy is normal. However, accompanying straining and grimacing are noticeably present and should make the diagnosis suspect. Videolaryngeal stroboscopy is helpful.

d. Therapy

(1) A **neurologic examination** is a necessity to ensure that neurogenic causes (e.g., brainstem) are not present.

(2) **Speech therapy** is of value. However, patients with true spastic dysphonia respond poorly to either speech therapy or psychotherapy.

(3) **Unilateral sectioning of the recurrent laryngeal nerve** has been advocated for spastic dysphonia. Initial benefit has been observed in many cases, yet it does not persist in many instances.

(4) Reports of successful use of botulinum toxin have emerged from a number of centers, although the technique, dosage, and frequency are not uniformly accepted. This can be performed in an outpatient setting with very gratifying results. Side effects of vocal breathiness and aspiration do occur, but are rare.

V. Respiratory obstruction

A. Airway obstruction. See Chap. 1, I–VII.

B. Vocal cord paralysis

1. **Pathophysiology**

   a. **The recurrent laryngeal nerve** is the primary motor innervation to the intrinsic laryngeal musculature. The cricothyroid is the only motor muscle supplied by the superior laryngeal nerve. Recurrent laryngeal nerve damage results in paralysis of the ipsilateral vocal cord with fixation in the median or paramedian position. The voice is usually breathy until the unaffected vocal cord compensates and approaches the paralyzed cord during phonation. If the vocal cord is in the median position, the vocal quality approaches normalcy. If both recurrent laryngeal nerves are affected, the cords may be midline in position, causing airway obstruction with dyspnea and respiratory distress. With bilateral involvement and subsequent lateralization, protection of the tracheobronchial tree may become problematic. The final position that the vocal cord assumes has very little relationship to the etiology of the paralysis. Even with normal cord mobility on the opposite side, there may be some dyspnea on exertion if the vocal cord is fixed in the adducted position.

   b. **Superior laryngeal nerve.** Malfunction of the superior laryngeal nerve affects laryngeal sensation. This nerve also innervates the cricothyroid muscle, a vocal cord tensor. There is resultant hypesthesia with possible aspiration and decreased ipsilateral vocal cord tension, potentially resulting in a lowered pitch with associated weakness. The vocal cord may be bowed as a result of the unopposed action of the thyroarytenoid muscle. With bilateral superior laryngeal involvement, aspiration is more likely.

2. **Etiology and diagnosis.** In 90% of the cases, the cause of the vocal cord paralysis is a peripheral nerve injury, while only 10% are due to central nervous system pathology. Involvement may be bilateral or unilateral, affecting the abductor muscles, the adductors, or the tensors. The diagnosis is made by examination of vocal cord mobility, using any of the indirect techniques described (see **II.A.**). Laryngeal electromyography (EMG) may also be helpful in establishing the diagnosis. If the etiology is not apparent in the older age groups, direct laryngoscopy is necessary to palpate the cricoarytenoid joint for fixation and to definitively rule out malignancy.

   a. **Congenital** vocal cord paralysis can be either unilateral or bilateral. Although present at birth, it may not be recognized until stridor or respiratory distress develops, usually after an upper respiratory tract infection.

      (1) **Bilateral** vocal cord paralysis, a less frequent occurrence than unilateral disease, is often associated with respiratory distress, since the vocal cords are close to the

midline. The cry may be normal, occasionally leading to a delay in the appropriate diagnosis. Stridor is obvious. Bilateral cord paralysis is most often associated with central nervous system disease involving the motor nucleus of the tenth cranial nerve (nucleus ambiguous). Brain damage, hydrocephalus, meningomyelocele, trauma to the brainstem, and peripheral neuropathies have been implicated.

(2) Unilateral vocal cord paralysis may occur on either side. Left cord paralysis is most often due to a congenital vascular malformation impinging on the left recurrent nerve as it enters the mediastinum. Other mediastinal lesions, as well as surgery to repair cardiovascular abnormalities, have also been implicated. Right-sided lesions are more often associated with peripheral neuropathies. Symptoms associated with a unilateral vocal cord paralysis may go unnoticed. Hoarseness or a weak cry may be present, with stridor occurring less often. Respiratory obstruction is rarely a problem.

(3) Diagnosis. Congenital paralysis in the neonate or young infant can be difficult to diagnose. Routine radiographs are of little value, but fluoroscopy is occasionally helpful. Direct visualization is mandatory and often may be achieved with a small flexible fiberoptic laryngoscope. Direct laryngoscopy may on occasion be necessary. Although sedation may be used, general anesthesia is not required. It is imperative to place the tip of the laryngoscope within the vallecula so that the supraglottic and glottic structures can be visualized during movement with respiration and phonation. A skilled endoscopist is essential to establish the correct diagnosis. Videolaryngeal stroboscopy is invaluable in evaluating the degree of vocal movement impairment; it is also used for comparison to the results of treatment.

b. Iatrogenic

(1) Vocal cord paralysis may occur as a consequence of surgical procedures in the neck, chest, or following endoscopy. Thyroidectomy still rates as the most frequent iatrogenic cause of both unilateral and bilateral vocal cord paralysis. Paralysis can occur after cardiac surgery, or carotid surgery. Either or both nerves can be injured after anterior approaches to the cervical spine. Prolonged or traumatic intubation can cause injury to the arytenoids or the cricoarytenoid joint with secondary nerve injury, fixing the vocal cords.

(2) Obtaining a history of external or internal trauma is mandatory if the appropriate diagnosis is to be made. Palpation of the vocal cords and arytenoid cartilages may be necessary after intubation to assess the mobility of the cricoarytenoid joint.

c. Neurogenic

(1) Central nervous system disorders affecting vocal cord function can arise at the cerebral cortex or the brainstem. Laryngeal manifestations rarely occur in isolation. Space-occupying lesions, trauma, cerebrovascular accidents, or thrombosis as well as a myriad of diffuse neurologic disturbances; poliomyelitis, multiple sclerosis, syringomyelia, Friedreich's ataxia, recurrent icterus, or encephalitis are but a few of the possible etiologies.

(2) Involvement of the tenth cranial nerve (vagus) may occur anywhere along its course. At the base of the skull, this involvement can be due to tumors of the nasopharynx, metastatic lesions, trauma, or congenital deformities such as the Arnold-Chiari syndrome (with herniation of the cerebellum into the foramen magnum) or impingement on the jugular foramen. As the nerve crosses through the parapharyngeal space, it can be disrupted by tumors of the parotid gland, by neurogenic tumors such as neurilemmoma or neruofibroma, or by carotid body tumors. Direct invasion in the neck can result from spread of carcinoma of the esophagus or hypopharynx, and from extranodal extension of metastatic tumor in the cervical chain.

Within the mediastinum, the recurrent laryngeal nerve may be affected as it crosses the aortic arch on the left or the subclavian artery on the right. Most often, carcinoma of the lung or breast, metastatic to the mediastinal nodes, will interrupt laryngeal nerve function. This disruption can also occur with lymphoma or other neoplastic processes. As both right and left nerves return to the larynx, via the tracheoesophageal groove, they may once again be involved by tumors arising from the upper aerodigestive tract. In this area, involvement of the nerve can occur from a thyroid lesion, be it goiter or malignancy.

(3) A peripheral vagal neuropathy may be due to diabetes mellitus, chronic alcoholism, toxicity from lead or mercury, or inflammatory processes (syphilis or tuberculosis). Inflammatory neuritis may be viral in origin (herpes simplex, herpes zoster, influenza, or Coxsackie) and may occur in isolation or with other neuropathies.

Guillain-Barré syndrome sometimes causes laryngeal paralysis. Carcinoma of the larynx itself may limit vocal cord motion by infiltration of the thyroarytenoid muscle, by fixation of the cricoarytenoid joint, or by infiltration of the recurrent laryngeal nerve. Any of the latter would stage a carcinoma of the larynx as T_3.

d. Idiopathic.

When all of the possible causes of vocal cord paralysis have been ruled out, there remains a group for whom the diagnosis is not established. Idiopathic paralysis occurs in approximately 30% of patients.

3. Evaluation. Not every patient requires every test, since the etiology of vocal cord paralysis may be apparent. Certain diagnostic procedures appear to be of particular value. These procedures include a complete blood count, urinalysis, chest and skull base x rays, and a barium swallow. More specific procedures, as well as endoscopy, must be individualized.

4. Complications of vocal cord paralysis. The adverse effects of cord paralysis depend largely on their final position.

   a. If one vocal cord is affected, the most frequent symptom is hoarseness without serious sequelae. Difficulty arises when the vocal cord that is mobile does not compensate and reach the paralyzed cord. A breathy voice may ensue, should the vocal cord lateralize, causing further air escape. A lateral cord may be associated with aspiration if glottic incompetence exists. It is compounded by an associated superior laryngeal nerve paralysis.

   b. In patients with bilateral cord paralysis and lateralization of both, marked breathiness may occur, with aspiration being a significant problem. If the vocal cords are both fixed near the midline, however, the glottic aperture may be less than 3 mm, not affording the adult an adequate glottic aperture. Dyspnea and hypoxia may ensue. Intervention is usually necessary.

5. Therapy

   a. Unilateral vocal cord paralysis usually requires no therapy. Most cases tend to compensate within 6 months to 1 year after onset. With speech therapy, the vocal quality achieved is quite acceptable. If the larynx has not regained adequate function, however, and hoarseness, breathiness, an ineffective cough, or aspiration persist, further therapy should be considered.

   (1) Vocal cord injection. The paralyzed vocal cord can be medialized by an injection of glycerine into the paraglottic space. A permanent result can be obtained with an injection of Teflon paste. Synthetic collagen preparations are currently being evaluated. These substances may produce less vocal cord stiffness, fibrosis, and allow for increased precision in amount and location of injected material. The laryngoscopic procedure is performed under local anesthesia with adjunct sedation. The injections are most effective when there is atrophy of the thyroarytenoid muscle or when aspiration due to mild glottic incompetence is a problem. Shortcomings of this procedure are possible granuloma formation, displacement of the injected material, local infection, and overcorrection. Any significant degree of laryngeal incompetence is difficult to correct by this technique.

   (2) Surgical medialization. If the defect is too large to be corrected by Teflon alone, muscle, cartilage, or bone can be introduced via an external approach.

(3) **Nerve-muscle pedicle reinnervation.** This surgical procedure has been described by Tucker. It attempts to restore adduction of the paralyzed cord by reinnervating it with the ansa-hypoglossi nerve in conjunction with the omohyoid muscle. This nerve muscle pedicle is transferred into the lateral thyroarytenoid muscle, the major laryngeal adductor. If cricoarytenoid joint fixation has occurred, the procedure is of no value. Moreover, even in the best situation, 4–6 months must elapse before vocal cord motion returns. The efficacy of the procedure remains controversial.

(4) **Hypoglossal to recurrent nerve transposition,** alone or in conjunction with other techniques, may induce reinnervation and improve voice and cord function.

(5) **Laryngeal framework surgery** (laryngoplasty), as initially described by Ishiki, has gained increasing attention and popularity. It is an external surgical procedure, done under local anesthesia, in which the thyroid cartilage is visualized and a window created in the lamina on the affected side. A block of cartilage or Silastic is inserted through the window that medializes the vocal cord. Positioning is assisted by simultaneous fiberoptic visualization. The benefits of this procedure are potential improved vocal quality, less fibrosis, and potential reversibility (with removal of the tissue or silastic block). Shortcomings include the need for an external incision and greater technical difficulty than with endoscopic vocal cord injection. Thyroplasty finds its greatest utility in those patients who can anticipate longevity and not in those in whom the vocal cord paralysis is due to metastatic pulmonary cancer.

b. **Bilateral abductor vocal cord paralysis** usually requires intervention, since limitation of the airway frequently restricts physical activity. Initially, if there is not an acute airway problem, a waiting period of 6 months may be in order to see if cordal motion returns. If not, the following procedures are applicable.

(1) **Tracheotomy** will bypass the obstructing glottis, but adds the additional need for care of the tracheotomy tube. New, fenestrated tracheotomy tubes with a one-way breathing valve, as well as tracheotomy buttons designed to fit the trachea fenestra, have allowed adequate voice with an improved airway.

(2) **Surgical lateralization.** Displacing the vocal cord laterally with removal of the arytenoid cartilage improves the airway at the expense of vocal quality. The procedure can be performed either from an external approach or endoscopically, removing the arytenoid by microdissection or with the laser. Also a cricoarytenoid arthrodesis with lateralization and pinning of the arytenoid cartilage has been shown to be of value.

(3) Nerve-muscle pedicle reinnervation. This technique, much as the one described in **a.(3)**, was originated by Tucker. Again, using a small portion of the omohyoid muscle with the attached ansa-hypoglossal nerve, an attempt is made to reinnervate the posterior cricoarytenoid muscle, the only abductor of the vocal cord. If successful, this procedure produces a return of some muscle function. As stated, few surgeons have had such success; therefore, its value remains in doubt.

c. Surgery for aspiration

(1) Occasionally, **chronic aspiration** may become an intractable problem. Although vocal cord paralysis plays a significant role, other etiologies exist. These causes include intracranial catastrophes, e.g., hemorrhage, trauma, tumor, inflammation, and degenerative diseases. Also extracranial-neurologic disorders can be implicated.

(2) Frequently, a tracheotomy and gastronomy will prevent inanition, aspiration, and pneumonia. When these techniques fail, laryngeal closure is warranted. Suturing the epiglottis over the laryngeal introitus is the procedure of choice and is reversible.

VI. Hemoptysis

A. Etiology. Although hemoptysis is usually secondary to pathology below the level of the vocal cords, a head and neck source must be ruled out. Many sites in the aerodigestive tract can give rise to hemoptysis.

1. History

a. A patient may be able to differentiate the sensation of blood draining from the posterior pharynx that causes coughing from blood arising from within the chest. Associated epistaxis raises the suspicion of pathology within the nose, nasopharynx, or paranasal sinuses.

b. Lesions within the oral cavity rarely cause hemoptysis.

c. Varices at the base of the tongue may give rise to painless hemoptysis.

d. Hemoptysis with dysphagia or voice change should raise the suspicion of hypopharyngeal malignancy. Patients with laryngeal neoplasia have hoarseness or respiratory distress more often than hemoptysis as a presenting complaint.

2. Diagnosis

a. The examination should include visualization of the nasal chambers, nasopharynx, hypopharynx, and larynx. Blood identified in the subglottis on indirect laryngoscopy usually indicates that the origin is pulmonary or bronchial.

b. Chest radiographs or CT scanning of the lung help localize pulmonary pathology.

c. Bronchoscopy, using a flexible fiberoptic endoscope, affords peripheral pulmonary washings and microbiopsies of suspicious mucosal lesions.

Selected Readings

American Joint Committee on Cancer: *Staging of Cancer of the Head and Neck Sites and of Melanoma,* 1980 (revised 1987).

Batsakis, J. G. *Tumors of the Head and Neck* (2nd ed.). Baltimore: Williams & Wilkins, 1979.

Bless, D., Hirano, M., and Feder, R. J. Videostroboscopic evaluation of the larynx. *Ear Nose Throat J.* 66:289, 1987.

Blitzer, A. B., Brin, M. F., Fahn, S., and Lovelace, R. E. Localized injections of botulinum toxin for the treatment of focal laryngeal dystonia (spastic dysphonia). *Laryngoscope* 98:193, 1988.

Brin, M. F., Blitzer, A., Fahn, S., Gould, W., and Lovelace, R. E. Adductor laryngeal dystonia (spastic dysphonia): Treatment with local injection of botulinum toxin (Botox). *Mov. Disorders* 4:287, 1989.

Cohen, S. R., et al. Papilloma of the larynx and tracheobronchial tree in children: A retrospective study. *Ann. Otol. Rhinol. Laryngol.* 89:497, 1980.

Cotton, R. Management of subglottic stenosis in infancy and childhood: Review of a consecutive series of cases managed by surgical reconstruction. *Ann. Otol. Rhinol. Laryngol.* 87:649, 1978.

Cotton, R. T. The management and prevention of subglottic stenosis in infants and children. *Adv. Otolaryngol. Head Neck Surg.* 1:241, 1987.

Crelin, E. S. Development of the upper respiratory system. *Clin. Symp.* 28:1, 1976.

Crumley, R. L. Teflon injections versus nerve transfer: A comparison. *Ann. Otol. Rhinol. Laryngol.* 99:759, 1990.

DeSanto, L. W., Devine, K. D., and Lillie, J. C. Cancers of the larynx: Glottic cancer. *Surg. Clin. North Am.* 57:611, 1977.

DeSanto, L. W., Lillie, J. C., and Devine, K. D. Cancers of the larynx: Supraglottic cancer. *Surg. Clin. North Am.* 57:505, 1977.

Elman, A. J., et al. *In situ* carcinoma of the vocal cords. *Cancer* 43:2422, 1979.

Fink, B. R., and Demarest, R. J. *Laryngeal Biomechanics.* Cambridge, Mass.: Harvard University Press, 1978.

Fried, M. P. (ed.). *The Larynx: Otolaryngolic Clinics of North America.* Philadelphia: Saunders, 1984.

Fried, M. P. A survey of the complications of laser laryngoscopy. *Arch. Otolaryngol.* 110:31, 1984.

Fried, M. P. *The Larynx: A Multidisciplinary Approach.* Boston: Little, Brown, 1988.

Fried, M. P., and Shapiro, J. Acute and Chronic Laryngeal Infections. In M. M. Paparella, D. A. Shumrick, J. L. Gluckman, and W. L. Meyerhoff (eds.), *Otolaryngology: Head and Neck* (vol. III, 3rd ed.). Philadelphia: Saunders, 1991. Pp. 2245–2256.

Gall, A. M., Sessions, D. G., and Ogura, J. H. Complications following surgery for cancer of the larynx and hypopharynx. *Cancer* 39:624, 1977.

Grillo, H. C. Tracheal tumors: Surgical management. *Ann. Thorac. Surg.* 26:112, 1978.

Hart, C. W. Functional and neurological problems of the larynx. *Otolaryngol. Clin. North Am.* 3:609, 1970.

Holinger, L. D. Etiology of stridor in the neonate, infant, and child. *Ann. Otol. Rhinol. Laryngol.* 89:397, 1980.

Holinger, L. D., Holinger, P. C., and Holinger, P. H. Etiology of bilateral abductor vocal cord paralysis: A review of 389 cases. *Ann. Otol. Rhinol. Laryngol.* 85:428, 1976.

Holinger, L. D., and Wolter, R. K. Neurologic Disorders of the Larynx. In G. M. English (ed.), *Otolaryngology* (vol. 3). Hagerstown, Md.: Harper & Row, 1990. Chap. 42.

Hybels, R. L. Selected new techniques of laryngeal surgery. *Surg. Clin. North Am.* 60:637, 1980.

Isshiki, N., Taira, T., Kojuma, H., and Shoji, K. Recent modifications on thyroplasty type I. *Ann. Otol. Rhinol. Laryngol.* 98:777, 1989.

Kleinsasser, O. *Microlaryngoscopy and Endolaryngeal Microsurgery.* Baltimore: University Park Press, 1979.

Landing, B. H., and Dixon, L. G. Congenital malformations and genetic disorders of the respiratory tract (larynx, trachea, bronchi, and lungs). *Am. Rev. Respir. Dis.* 120:151, 1979.

Ludlow, C. L. Treatment of speech and voice disorders with botulinum toxin. *JAMA* 264:2671, 1990.

McGill, T. J., and Healy, G. B. Congenital and acquired lesions of the infant larynx: A refresher survey. *Clin. Pediatr.* (Phila.) 17:584, 1978.

Proctor, D. F. The upper airways: II. The larynx and trachea. *Am. Rev. Respir. Dis.* 115:315, 1977.

Rothman, K. J., et al. Epidemiology of laryngeal cancer. *Epidemiol. Rev.* 2:195, 1980.

Sagel, S. S., et al. High resolution computer tomography in the staging of carcinoma of the larynx. *Laryngoscope* 91:292, 1981.

Sasaki, C. T. Physiology of the Larynx. In G. M. English (ed.), *Otolaryngology* (vol. 3). Hagerstown, Md.: Harper & Row, 1980. Chap. 7.

Silver, C. E. Surgical management of neoplasms of the larynx, hypopharynx, and cervical esophagus. *Curr. Probl. Surg.* 14:2, 1977.

Thomas, R. L. Non-epithelial tumors of the larynx. *J. Laryngol. Otol.* 93:1131, 1979.

Tucker, H. M. Management of the patient with an incompetent larynx. *Am. J. Otolaryngol.* 1:47, 1979.

Vaughan, C. W. Transoral laryngeal surgery using the CO_2 laser: Laboratory experiments and clinical experience. *Laryngoscope* 88:1399, 1978.

Vrabec, D. P., and Davison, F. W. Inflammatory Disease of the Larynx. In G. M. English (ed.), *Otolaryngology* (vol. 3). Hagerstown, Md.: Harper & Row, 1990. Chap. 37.

Weber, A. L. (ed.). Symposium on the larynx and trachea. *Radiol. Clin. North Am.* 16:181, 1978.

Appendix: Voice Evaluation and Rehabilitation

Otolaryngologists examine many patients who experience chronic dysphonia or vocal fatigue. For many, changing the behaviors that led to the development and maintenance of their dysphonia allows them to eliminate their symptoms and their pathology. Speech-language pathologists can help patients decrease their vocal abuse and misuse through speech/voice therapy. Generally, the goal of voice therapy is to return the voice to the best possible level, within the patient's anatomic and physiologic capabilities, with the least amount of effort.

To increase the success of treatment, the speech pathologist and otolaryngologist help each other determine which patients are appropriate for vocal rehabilitation. All patients who receive voice treatment are required to have an examination by an otolaryngologist to ensure that their dysphonia is not a sign of more serious disease.

I. **Patients who may benefit from voice therapy.** The otolaryngologist often has initial contact with dysphonic patients. He or she determines if they should be seen for a thorough voice evaluation by the speech-language pathologist, who then determines their candidacy for voice therapy. Patients who report chronic voice abuse, overuse, or misuse (pushing or straining) need behavioral intervention. Physicians should be aware of the vocal benefits available to patients evidencing the following:

A. **Hyperfunction,** generally defined as using too much effort to phonate. It is characterized by excess musculoskeletal tension. The following may be observed when viewing hyperfunction under laryngeal videostroboscopy: excessive ventricular or false vocal cord movement (ventricular phonation in extreme cases), excessive arytenoid tilting, excessively tight or stiff vocal cords, persistently small glottis when phonating, and/or a narrowing of the laryngeal space. Hyperfunction is the most common problem exhibited by patients receiving vocal rehabilitation. Patients with hyperfunction sound hoarse, harsh, strained, and/or diplophonic. They often complain of vocal strain, vocal fatigue, or discomfort. Hyperfunction is common in dysphonic patients with **no vocal cord pathology** and in patients evidencing a variety of **vocal pathologies,** including the following:

1. **Vocal nodules, polyps, chronic edema, or erythema**

2. **Renke's space edema, contact ulcer/granulomas, papillomas, and cysts** are diagnoses that often require surgical intervention. If the patient's dysphonia remains after surgery, it is often due to maintained hyperfunction. Voice therapy helps reduce this vocal misuse and decrease the chance of recurrence of pathology.

3. Patients with **spasmodic dysphonia** may experience some improvement from voice therapy that is aimed at educating the patient regarding the disorder and at providing relaxation

techniques. Severe or advanced cases require medical treatment such as **botulinum toxin** injections.

4. Patients with **vocal fold paralysis** may develop extensive hyperfunction in an effort to compensate for vocal fold weakness.

B. **Hypofunction** is an inability to approximate the vocal cords that causes decreased loudness and an excessively breathy voice. Patients with vocal **cord paralysis or paresis, arthritis of the arytenoid cartilages, and some neurological disorders (causing dysarthria)** may benefit from voice rehabilitation.

C. **Resonance disorders.** The otolaryngologist may encounter patients who complain of hyper- or hyponasality—often as a result of injury. Through training, these patients can improve their resonance. If a prosthesis is necessary, proper referrals are facilitated.

D. **Laryngectomy, supraglottic laryngectomy, and hemilaryngectomy** all can cause unique problems with speaking and swallowing.

1. **Preoperative counseling** is valuable to help prepare the patient regarding what speech, swallowing, and breathing changes are expected.

2. **Postoperative training** for alaryngeal speech training, for learning to swallow supraglottically, or for learning to use the voice optimally with a reconstructed vocal fold is usually necessary.

II. **Laryngeal videostroboscopy or strobovideolaryngoscopy** is a clinical tool that is used for viewing and evaluating detailed laryngeal anatomy and physiology. It allows immediate imaging of the presence or absence of vocal cord pathology and allows the vibratory characteristics of the vocal cords to be analyzed in depth, significantly adding to what one can view with the naked eye (because the vocal folds vibrate too rapidly).

A. **Stroboscopy works** by attaching a camera to a light source that provides pulsed light, synchronized with the patient's fundamental frequency, illuminating segments of vocal fold vibration. This appears on a monitor as apparent slow motion. The procedure is videotaped and kept as a permanent record. A rigid scope is used for analyzing vocal fold vibration on a sustained vowel sound. A flexible fiberoptic scope is used to analyze conversational speech.

B. **Benefits of stroboscopy** include providing permanent documentation of pathology and of vibratory characteristics of the vocal cords, allowing more accurate diagnoses to be formed, allowing viewing of cord mucosa and approximate degree of any cancerous infiltration, providing excellent patient education by viewing recordings, providing documentation of any changes from therapy or surgery, allowing monitoring of a lesion or of therapy progress, providing a means for choosing treatment options, allowing repeated viewing of a single event, and allowing difficult cases to be viewed by numerous professionals.

C. **Indications for use** are to determine the cause of a disorder, to determine the degree and extent of underlying disease, to evaluate the degree of disturbance of phonatory function, to help determine prognosis, to establish a therapy program, to monitor results of treatment, and to monitor status of pathology.

D. Patients to refer include those with chronic hoarseness of unknown pathology, those with known laryngeal pathology who need further documentation of the lesion, those with suspected laryngeal paralysis or paresis, and those patients undergoing surgery or voice rehabilitation who need pre- and post-documentation and analysis of vocal fold structure and function.

E. Laryngeal videostroboscopy protocol. Laryngeal videostroboscopy is not meant to replace traditional laryngeal examinations, but rather to supplement them. All patients receiving stroboscopy should have a complete head and neck examination from a physician prior to the stroboscopic examination. Laryngeal videostroboscopy may be completed by a speech-language pathologist or by a physician (protocol varies among facilities). Analysis of **vocal fold structure and function** is completed by both an otolaryngologist and a qualified speech pathologist.

    1. Analysis of vocal fold structure and vocal pathology is completed by a physician.

    2. Analysis of vocal fold function includes features such as glottic closure, supraglottic activity, mucosal wave, amplitude, phase closure, phase symmetry, regularity of cord vibration, nonvibrating portion of the vocal folds, and vertical level of vocal fold approximation. These parameters provide information about how the voice is being used, as well as information about the extent and invasiveness of a disease process.

F. Ultra–high-speed photography and electroglottography may also be used for evaluating vocal fold vibration.

III. A voice evaluation is completed on any patient referred for voice therapy.

    A. Interview. The initial interview is an important part of the voice evaluation and gives the clinician additional insight regarding possible contributors and causes to the patient's dysphonia. It also allows the clinician to observe the patient's typical vocal and postural habits. The interview should include:

        1. Medical history, including history of sinus problems, postnasal drip, allergies, esophageal reflux, asthma, thyroid dysfunction, temporomandibular joint dysfunction, history of surgery with intubation, arthritis, neurologic dysfunction, as well as any other medical problems.

        2. Patient's description of the disorder, including the time of onset, the perceived severity, perceived cause, and variability of the voice problem.

        3. Patient's typical voice use, including use at work, at home, socially, professionally (for singing or theater), with hearing-impaired individuals, etc.

4. **Patient's vocally abusive behaviors,** including frequent throat clearing or coughing, talking over noise, lecturing without amplification, voice use during exercise, speaking in stressful situations, excessive singing, excessive talking when the larynx is irritated, etc.

5. **Exposure to or use of irritants,** including smoking (direct or environmental), alcohol use, caffeine use, and exposure to dust or other irritants in the environment.

B. **Acoustic measurements** comprise the objective part of a voice evaluation. Different facilities may use different specific measurements, but certain measures are common across facilities.

1. **Fundamental frequency** (Fo), typically measured as average pitch (measured in hertz) for a sustained (as close to 9 seconds as possible) "ah." Average male Fo ranges from 105–150Hz. Average female Fo ranges from 190–240 Hz. Female pitch tends to lower with age, averaging from 180–240 Hz, whereas the male pitch may become higher, 100–160 Hz. Fo may vary with the language used.

2. **Pitch range** is the lowest tone the patient can reach up to the highest tone. The amount of the tone that is voiced versus unvoiced is important to note. The average frequency range is 38 semitones for a male and 32 semitones for a female.

3. **Pitch perturbation or jitter** is defined as cycle-to-cycle variations in the periods of glottal cycles. It correlates to the perceptual judgement of hoarseness or roughness.

4. **Shimmer** is defined as cycle-to-cycle variations in amplitude.

5. **Habitual pitch,** usually measured during a counting task and/or during a conversational sample or reading passage.

6. **Optimal pitch,** the pitch where the voice is produced most efficiently with the least amount of effort.

7. **Average loudness,** measured in decibels (dB), usually done during a reading passage.

8. **Maximum loudness** is usually completed on a yelled word, such as "hey" or "one."

9. A **spectograph** can be used to measure **periodicity,** the regularity of opening and closing of the vocal folds, and **formants,** relating to the size and shape of resonating cavities of the vocal tract.

C. **Perceptual vocal assessment** is completed as the patient participates in a variety of speech samples, including spontaneous speech, paragraph reading, and vowel prolongation. All speech samples should be tape recorded on a high-quality tape recorder.

1. **Vocal quality** is judged and described as hoarse, harsh, breathy, diplophonic, aphonic, hypernasal, or hyponasal. Speech may contain glottal fry, hard glottal attacks, pitch breaks, and/or phonation breaks. An experienced clinician can distinguish these vocal characteristics by their sound.

2. **Pitch and loudness** are judged according to their appropriateness, considering the patient's age and sex.

3. **Speech rate, fluency, and average phrase length** are also judged.

4. **Breath support, musculoskeletal tension, and posture** are observed.

D. **Respiratory evaluation** measures may be used as part of voice evaluation, given the close relationship between breath and phonation.

1. **Sustained s/z production** task helps measure phonatory and respiratory efficiency. Normal prolongation of "s" and "z" is approximately 20 seconds. It decreases as age increases.

2. **Mean flow rate** is the rate at which air is expelled from a patient's mouth during sustained vowel production, and is measured in milliliters per second. It provides information regarding the volume of air passing through the glottis. Special equipment is needed for this measurement.

3. **Subglottic pressure, vital capacity, tidal volume, inspiratory reserve volume, expiratory reserve volume, and air-flow pressure** may also be measured.

E. **Oral motor examination** is completed and includes observation of lips, tongue, and jaw strength and range of motion. Palatal movement, observation of dentition, and strength of cough and throat clear are also included.

F. **Stimuability measurements** are taken in order to help determine the method of treatment best suited to a particular patient. The patient is educated about the disorder, about the anatomy and physiology of respiration, about the effects of vocal abuse and misuse, and about the goal of treatment.

IV. **Treatment.** Voice treatment is specialized to meet patient's needs and varies across disorders; however, some general goals remain fairly consistent. Again, the overall goal is to return the patient's voicing to its best possible level. Candidates for therapy must be chosen carefully. All patients participating in voice therapy must be motivated to improve their voice quality, because therapy is hard work and involves diligent participation outside of the clinic.

A. **Hyperfunction treatment**

1. **Education and increasing patient awareness of voice use.** The patient is educated regarding the anatomy and physiology of phonation and respiration. He or she is also educated regarding the effects of vocal abuse and misuse.

2. **Decreasing vocal abuse.** The clinician and patient work together to set goals for decreasing abusive vocal behavior such as yelling or screaming, coughing or throat clearing, talking over noise, speaking loudly when tense, singing loudly with the radio, etc.

3. **Improving vocal hygiene.** The patient is advised to drink 6 to 8 glasses of water daily, because it is important to maintain hydration in order to prevent mucous membranes from drying. A humidifier may be used in dry climates. The patient should quit smoking, decrease alcohol intake, and decrease caffeine intake.

4. **Decreasing vocal misuse.** This involves teaching the patient to use the voice appropriately and naturally.

   a. **Decreasing head and neck tension** is an important step toward decreasing hyperfunction. This is done primarily through stretching exercises, through guided imagery for relaxation and, if necessary, through direct deep-muscle massage, requiring referral to a physical therapist.

   b. **Improving breath support** is critical for reducing hyperfunction. Many patients begin "pushing" their voices out because of inadequate breath support. The patient is trained to use more efficient diaphragmatic breathing versus habitual clavicular or thoracic breathing.

   c. **Decreasing laryngeal tension during phonation** involves training the patient to become aware of using breath for phonation while completely eliminating any direct muscular effort from the larynx.

   d. **Improving vocal placement** involves training the patient to resonate the voice out the front of the mouth rather than directly from the throat (which tends to create more muscle tension and reduces vocal flexibility).

5. **Improving vocal flexibility** includes improving ability to project in a nonabusive way and improving vocal range.

6. **Providing counseling and support** for patients as they complete the often difficult task of changing their previously automatic vocal habits.

7. **Making appropriate referrals** to other professionals, i.e., psychiatrists, stress reduction programs, marriage counselors, smoking cessation programs, voice and/or singing coaches, allergists, etc., is often necessary. Some of these referrals must be agreed on by the physician in advance.

B. **Hypofunction treatment**

1. **Increasing breath support and projection** with the least amount of muscular effort possible.

2. **Vocal augmentation.** The speech pathologist, the patient, and the otolaryngologist work together to determine the best method of cord augmentation for that patient's age, general health, voice use, etc.

C. **Treatment of resonance disorders** involves palatal exercises, focus on oral resonance, and possibly work with a prosthetic device.

D. **Laryngectomy treatment** includes alaryngeal speech training.

1. **Electrolarynx.** Patients need assistance with placement, articulation, and phrasing using an electrolarynx.

2. **Esophageal speech** is alaryngeal speech in which the air supply for phonation is injected from the oral cavity to the upper portion of the esophagus, where it is then ejected to produce sound (the pharyngoesophageal segment functions as a neoglottis). Esophageal speech is typically difficult to learn and requires extensive training by a speech pathologist.

3. **Mymucosal shunt or tracheoesophageal puncture** has allowed for fairly good quality speech with less effort than it takes to learn esophageal speech. The speech pathologist assists the patient in fitting and placement of a voice prosthesis, if such is necessary, and in coordinating voicing. Patients need to cover their stoma (with their thumb or with a "no hands" valve) to divert air through the shunt or the prosthesis into the esophagus, where vibration of the pharyngoesophageal segment occurs.

4. **Supraglottic or hemilaryngectomy** patients may require voice and/or swallowing intervention.

Selected Readings

Aronson, A. E. *Clinical Voice Disorders: An Interdisciplinary Approach.* New York: Decker, 1980.

Bastian, R. Factors leading to successful evaluation and management of patients with voice disorders. *Ear Nose Throat J.* 67:6, 1988.

Bless, D. M., Hirano, M., and Feder, R. Videostroboscopic evaluation of the larynx. *Ear Nose Throat J.* 66:7, 1987.

Boone, D. Expanding perspectives in care of the speaking voice. *Journal of Voice* 5:2, 1991.

Cooper, M. *Modern Techniques of Vocal Rehabilitation.* Springfield, Ill.: Charles C Thomas, 1973.

Hirano, M. Objective evaluation of the human voice: Clinical aspects. *Folia Phoniatr.* 41:2, 1989.

Hirano, M., and Bless, D. *Stroboscopic Evaluation of the Larynx.* College Hill Press, 1986.

Hirano, M., Hibi, S., Terasawa, R., and Fujiu, M. Relationship between aerodynamic, vibratory, acoustic and psychoacoustic correlates in dysphonia. *Journal of Phonetics* 14, 1986.

Ludlow, C. Treatment of speech and voice disorders with botulinum toxin. *JAMA* 264:20, 1990.

Prater, R., and Swift, R. *Manual of Voice Therapy.* Boston: Little, Brown, 1984.

Prytz, S. Laryngeal videostroboscopy. *Ear Nose Throat J. Suppl.* 1987.

Sataloff, R. T. Professional singers: The science and art of clinical care. *Am. J. Otolaryngol.* 2:3, 1981.

Sataloff, R. T., and Spiegel, J. R. Objective evaluation of the voice. In *Medical Problems of Performing Artists.* Philadelphia: Hanley and Belfus, 1988.

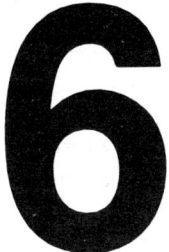

Salivary Glands

The major salivary glands are the paired parotid, submandibular, and sublingual glands, with the minor salivary glands found diffusely through the mucous membranes of the upper aerodigestive tract (Fig 6-1). They are subjected to endogenous and exogenous influences. Although the pathology of salivary gland disorders is complex, the clinical presentation for such a diverse etiologic group is remarkably similar, being either a mass or a diffuse enlargement. Therefore, the clinical evaluation must stress the history, primarily with the physical examination, laboratory data, radiography, and biopsy when indicated, serving to confirm the initial clinical considerations.

I. Anatomy

A. Parotid gland and facial nerve.
The parotid gland lies above the posterior aspect of the mandible anterior and inferior to the ear. It is divided into lobes and compartments by the deep cervical fascia. The deep portion of the gland is in proximity to the lateral pharyngeal space, which allows infections to spread from the gland into the neck. The distinction of superficial and deep lobes is based only on the relationship to the facial nerve, rather than on true anatomic divisions.

The parotid (or Stensen's) duct arises from the anterior portion of the parotid with the intraoral portion protruding at the level of the maxillary second molar. The punctum may be difficult to visualize.

The vessels of the parotid are the external carotid artery, which divides into the superficial temporal and internal maxillary arteries. The external jugular vein arises from the superficial temporal and internal maxillary veins, which join to form the posterior facial vein, as well as a branch from the postauricular vein.

The nerve supply to the gland is from the auriculotemporal nerve, a branch of the mandibular division of the trigeminal nerve. This is a parasympathetic secretomotor nerve arising from the otic ganglion. The otic ganglion receives branches from the lesser petrosal nerve and from the tympanic plexus, derived from the glossopharyngeal nerve.

The parotid gland is rich in lymph nodes, lying both superficial and deep to the glandular substance.

The facial nerve leaves the temporal bone at the stylomastoid foramen, entering into the posterior aspect of the parotid gland. It divides at the pes anserinus into the temporal, zygomatic, buccal,

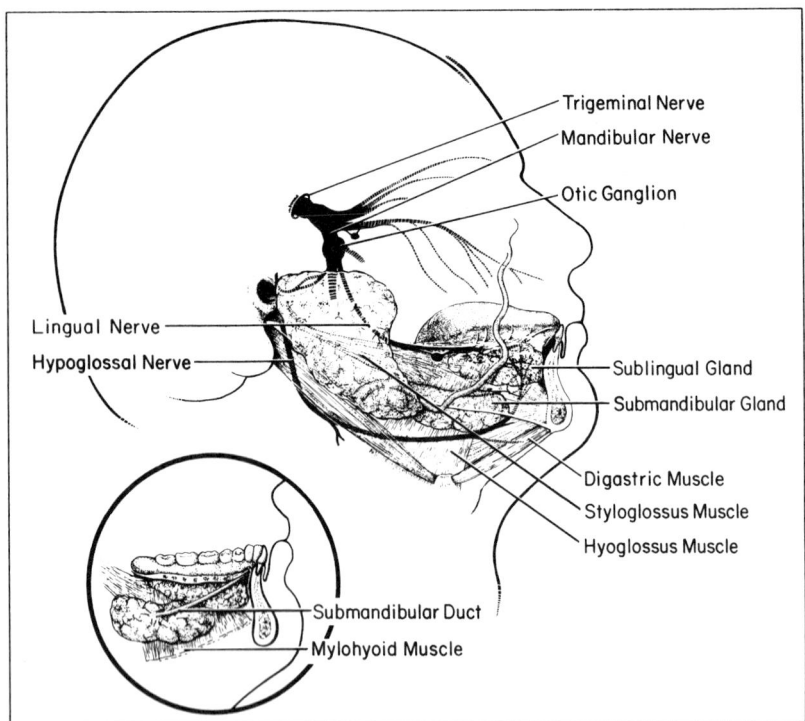

Fig. 6-1. The major salivary glands with spatial and anatomic relationships. (From D. E. Peterson, et al. [eds.], *Head and Neck Management of the Cancer Patient*. Amsterdam: Martinus Nijhoff, 1986.)

mandibular, and cervical branches. These provide motor function to the musculature of the face.

The greater auricular nerve is derived from the roots of C2 and C3 through the cervical plexus and is sensory to the auricle and the tragus.

B. **Submandibular gland.** This gland lies below the body of the mandible, between the anterior and posterior bellies of the digastric muscle. The marginal mandibular nerve lies superficial to it, as does a group of lymph nodes. The hypoglossal and lingual nerves are found deep to the submandibular gland. The duct of the submandibular gland lies above the mylohyoid muscle coursing along the anterior floor of the mouth and terminating in a punctum just posterior to the symphysis of the mandible. Parasympathetic innervation is by the chorda tympani nerve, a branch of the facial nerve, with sympathetic supply through the lingual nerve.

C. **Sublingual gland.** The sublingual glands are found in the anterior floor of the mouth, superficial to the mylohyoid muscle and deep to the oral mucosa. Multiple small ducts arise from the gland penetrating into the oral mucosa.

D. Minor salivary glands

Minor salivary glands can be found throughout the mucosa of the oral cavity and pharynx, opening individually to the mucosa.

II. Embryology

The salivary glands appear in the fetus at 6–8 weeks and by birth all are functional.

III. Physiology

One to four liters of saliva can be produced daily. The parotid is primarily a serous gland; the sublingual gland primarily mucinous, secreting mostly mucoproteins. The submandibular is a mixed mucous and serous gland. The major protein in parotid secretion is amylase, but many other enzymes are produced as well. The greater the mucin content, the more viscous the saliva. Over 90% of total saliva is produced by the parotid and submandibular glands.

A. Increased salivary flow may be due to cigarette smoking, oral inflammation, heavy metal poisoning, oral muscular activity, or ingestion of highly seasoned foods.

B. Decreased Flow

1. Diminished salivary flow that causes xerostomia can be due to emotion (depression, fear, excitement), organic disease (brain tumors), or drugs.

2. Obstruction, infection, radiation therapy, or disorders such as Sjögren's syndrome may also decrease salivary flow.

3. Metabolic disorders such as diabetes insipidus, cardiac failure, uremia, or edema may decrease saliva flow.

4. Drugs responsible for xerostomia include analgesics, anticonvulsants, antihistamines, antihypertensives, diuretics, decongestants, muscle relaxants, and a number of psychotropic medications.

Evaluation

I. **History** must include the following: time of onset, periodicity, duration and extent of enlargement, nature of secretions, associated systemic pathology, and medications. Inquiry as to facial nerve function and trismus should be made. It is important to assess whether one or multiple glands are involved, whether there is pain or tenderness, whether the swelling has occurred only once, is persistent or recurrent, or if the patient has noted an isolated mass.

II. **Physical examination.** The normal parotid occupies the preauricular space extending from the zygomatic arch to beneath the earlobe. The **normal gland is not palpable.** Therefore, any palpable enlargement is by definition abnormal. The submandibular glands may be palpated below the body of the mandible, particularly in elderly patients, who may have ptotic glands. The glands should be symmetrical in size and location. Inspection and palpation are most important diagnostically. The puncta must be assessed, and the character of the saliva denoted. Specifically, paucity, ropiness, turbidity, and purulence must be recorded.

III. **Laboratory data** is history directed for these pathologic entities. Whenever indicated, cultures and microscopic evaluation of collected secretions should be obtained. Cultures should be submitted for aerobes and anaerobes as well as for tuberculosis, atypical mycobacteria, and fungi.

IV. **Imaging** studies are useful primarily in confirming clinical impressions, more so than establishing a diagnosis. Two notable exceptions are the findings of sialectasia, denoting a major diagnostic etiologic group, and enhanced radionucleotide uptake by a suspected tumor mass, suggesting either an oncocytoma or a Warthin's tumor

A. **Plain films**

1. Used primarily for the detection of calculi.

2. Eighty percent of submandibular and 40% of parotid stones are radiopaque.

B. **Contrast sialography**

1. **Indications.** Recurrent inflammation or recurrent enlargement of the parotid gland suggests a ductal stricture, calculus, or sialectasia. The diagnosis of these abnormalities can often be confirmed by sialography. A normal gland expels most contrast material within 5 minutes; retained dye indicates a functional abnormality. Sialography is inadequate for assessing space-occupying lesions.

2. **Contraindications** include acute inflammation or a known sensitivity to iodides.

3. **Interpretation.** The normal sialogram is best described as looking like a "bare tree." The normal ductal system progressively tapers, thins, and branches.

a. **Scout films** often show calculi. Calculi rarely fill the lumen totally; therefore, contrast flows around them. Radiolucent calculi show as a filling defect, and only meticulous technique ensures that the abnormality observed is not an air bubble.

b. **Strictures** are frequently multiple and easily detected.

c. **Sialectasia** has been classified as punctate, globular, or cavitary. One stage does not necessarily progress to another, and, with fulminant infection, intermediate stages may be bypassed. Sialectasia is not a diagnostically specific finding. It can be congenital, and in such cases all the salivary glands are involved. Purulent infection, benign lymphoepithelial lesions, and Sjögren's syndrome are additional causes.

d. **Sialography** has limited merit as an isolated procedure in the evaluation of neoplasms, since little practical information is obtained. Some patients with neoplasms develop post-injection obstruction, inflammation, or both, which could delay necessary operative intervention. CT and MRI imaging have largely replaced sialography.

C. Radionucleotide scanning

1. Technetium (Tc^{99}) is the most commonly used isotope for studying salivary gland pathology. As a rule, its use does not meaningfully influence the management of nonneoplastic lesions of the salivary glands.

2. With tumors, an excision will give all the needed information, although scanning can define a mass lesion as to its approximate size and depth. If the lesion is "hot," this finding suggests that the lesion is benign. If the lesion is irregular, destruction is suggested and therefore malignancy.

D. Contrast-enhanced computed tomography (CT)

1. Contrast-enhanced CT scanning is useful in differentiating deep lobe parotid tumors from other parapharyngeal space tumors.

2. Subtle masses can be detected as to their salivary gland origin. Parameters that suggest a benign diagnosis include well-defined tumor borders, homogeneous appearance, and high density.

3. The extent of malignant salivary lesions and their relationship to adjacent structures is suggested and may in fact alter surgical considerations.

E. Ultrasonography allows assessment of the solid/cystic nature of salivary gland masses. Sensitivity is high in detecting a mass; however, the specificity is poor in the characterization of inflammatory lesions. Its use is infrequent.

F. Magnetic resonance imaging (MRI)

1. Useful in defining the location of salivary gland masses (intraparotid versus extraparotid) and also the relationship of the tumor to the facial nerve.

2. Benign neoplasms and low-grade malignancies often have clearly defined margins, whereas high-grade parotid malignancies tend to have poorly defined margins. Preoperative diagnosis of high-grade tumors allows for an accurate assessment of the degree of surgical treatment needed.

3. MRI with gadolinium-enhanced contrast allows for the greatest soft tissue detail, does not expose the patient to radiation, and is valuable in evaluating the extent of deep parotid lesions, particularly in the parapharyngeal space.

V. Biopsy

A. Excisional biopsy. For mass lesions, definitive biopsy remains excision and must include a generous margin of the surrounding gland.

B. Aspiration biopsy. Needle (22-gauge) aspiration biopsies are as good as the pathologist reading them. They are easy to perform but more difficult to interpret. Seeding along the needle tract has not been a problem. This procedure is indicated for most tumors as an aid to surgical planning (extent of resection) for the patient who is a poor surgical risk and when a diagnosis is essential prior to initiating a multimodality therapeutic plan.

C. Incisional biopsies are rarely performed for salivary gland lesions. If needle aspiration fails diagnostically for the poor-risk patient or for one with extensive neoplasia, incisional biopsy may be warranted.

Clinical Categories

Categorizing salivary gland lesions into five major groups makes differentiation easier. Inflammations are characterized as either obstructive or nonobstructive and can be further subdivided into acute and chronic. Metabolic abnormalities, endocrinopathies, neoplasms, and trauma complete the diagnostic quintet.

I. Inflammations

A. Acute nonobstructive

1. Viral

a. Etiology. Mumps serves as the prototype for this group. However, other viral agents have been documented serologically by acute and convalescent titers. These include Coxsackie, ECHO, and cytomegalic viruses.

b. Prodrome. A known contact, a winter or spring tendency, and a 2- to 3-week incubation period are frequent. Most patients are 5–15 years old.

c. Signs and symptoms. A mild temperature elevation and malaise can precede the sudden onset of acute distention with associated pain. Deep parotid involvement is associated with trismus. More than one salivary gland may be infected.

d. Physical examination. The affected gland is diffusely enlarged, tense to bimanual palpation, and tender. The puncta are acutely swollen and congested. **The saliva is clear.**

e. Diagnosis is made by the history and by the finding of an abrupt onset of an enlarged salivary gland.

Laboratory data. Confirmation is enhanced by an elevated serum amylase determination. The white blood cell count shows a relative lymphocytosis. Acute and convalescent sera show increased S & V titers.

f. Therapy. The disease is self-limited. Supportive measures are all that should be necessary. Hydration is the most important consideration, with analgesia as warranted.

g. Clinical course

(1) **Immunity.** One episode is believed to confer lifelong immunity in most instances. Sporadic documented cases of secondary infection have been reported, but serologic documentation is essential to make this diagnosis.

(2) **Sequela.** Unilateral sensorineural hearing loss is a known complication. Pancreatitis, meningitis, and gonadal involvement can occur but are infrequent.

2. Bacterial

a. Child. Acute bacterial sialadenitis of childhood may initially present a pattern similar to mumps.

(1) **Signs and symptoms.** The onset is marked by sudden painful swelling of the involved gland. Frequently, there is an associated temperature elevation. Bilateral involvement is not uncommon.

(2) **Physical examination.** The involved gland is firm, indurated, and tender. There may be associated trismus. The pertinent differentiating feature from a similar illness of viral origin is the observation of purulent salivary secretions.

(3) **Diagnosis. Laboratory data.** The secretions should be cultured. *Staphylococcus aureus* and *Streptococcus pneumoniae* are the most frequent organisms identified. A white blood cell count is elevated with the initial episode. Although recurrent episodes occur more frequently in children, a serum immunoprotein analysis is warranted. **Radiographic studies** are **normal** after the acute episode subsides.

(4) **Therapy.** Most children may be treated as outpatients. Severe trismus with poor hydration requires hospitalization, but the necessity for such is rare.

Antibiotic coverage is ultimately predicated on culture documentation. Although *S. pneumoniae* are common causative organisms, coverage must also include penicillinase-producing *S. aureus*. Amoxicillin clavulinate is a good initial drug. Hydration is essential, and fluids must be forced. Heat to the area is indicated. A heating pad or hot water bottle qid for 30 minutes is sufficient. Warmth is often soothing, and the patient may choose more frequent applications. Gentle massage 4–5 times daily is essential to help express purulent secretions.

(5) **Clinical course.** In childhood, repeated attacks are not infrequent and may span many years. These attacks often subside around puberty. Good oral hygiene, judicious dilatations in selected instances, and premeal massage frequently decrease the recurrence of attacks. Surgery is rarely indicated.

A variation of this pathology occurs in premature neonates. The organism involved in this setting is almost uniformly *Staphylococcus,* and the severity lies in the potential for abscess formation. High doses of a staphylococcus-specific antibiotic (i.e., oxacillin administered IV along with hydration) usually leads to resolution. If there is no improvement after 3–4 days, as evidenced by decreased swelling, tenderness, and temperature elevation, drainage will have to be considered. This specific variant (acute neonatal bacterial sialadenitis), once adequately treated, is not prone to recur.

b. The **adult** variant is similar in both signs and symptoms to that of the child, yet it is not as prone to recurrence. One-third of the cases in the adult are associated with the postoperative state. These patients are often septic.

(1) **Etiology.** Predisposing considerations include debilitation, confinement to bed, and dehydration, often secondary to inadequate intraoperative fluid management.

(2) **Diagnosis.** Blood cultures should be obtained for the febrile patient. Stensen's duct should be cultured. In addition, a white blood cell count should be obtained and is usually markedly elevated. MRI is valuable in assessing the degree of involvement or presence of an abscess.

(3) **Treatment.** Penicillin-resistant *S. aureus* is the most common organism in this setting. IV oxacillin is imperative. For the penicillin-sensitive patient, clindamycin or a first-generation cephalosporin may be substituted in an appropriate dosage. IV hydration is essential and must be predicated on the patient's general status.

Progressive induration and continued temperature elevation unresponsive to appropriate antibiotic management requires the consideration of surgical drainage. A fluctuant mass is a rarity in the parotid, even in the most advanced stages of suppuration because of vertical fibrous septa within the gland. Thus, the clinical course dictates the appropriate time for surgical intervention; MRI is of exceptional assistance.

3. **Secondary acute inflammatory disease**

a. **Drugs.** Two types of responses are noted—direct and idiosyncratic.

(1) Iodides and heavy metals such as mercury and bismuth are known precursors. **Signs and symptoms.** A diffuse, tender enlargement is noted; on occasion, this enlargement occurs several days after exposure. The swelling frequently takes several days to resolve. For the **clinical course** the saliva remains clear, and spontaneous resolution usually occurs. Identification of the offending agent is essential to prevent recurrence.

(2) An idiosyncratic effect is related frequently to a diminished salivary flow. Atropine, as well as phenylbutazone and the phenothiazine derivatives that exhibit an atropinelike effect, can cause recurrent salivary gland enlargement. Discontinuing the offending agent will effect resolution.

(3) Allergens. Allergic phenomena are not infrequent precursors of sudden parotid enlargement.

    (a) Etiology. Detailed considerations of food idiosyncrasies, such as berries and fish, and a positive family history are essential. Detecting "craving" for a specific food and eliminating such from the diet will often lead to resolution.

    (b) Signs and symptoms. The period between contact and symptomatology is brief. Pain and associated sudden enlargement of the salivary glands are characteristic.

    (c) Physical examination. All the salivary glands can be diffusely involved and tender. Mucous plugs may be expressed from the puncta.

    (d) Laboratory. Eosinophils can in some instances be isolated from the saliva, and a white blood cell count differential may similarly show elevated eosinophils.

    (e) Therapy. The illness resolves rapidly over several hours. Treatment is supportive, including hydration and analgesia only, because of the brief clinical course. Identification of the offending allergen is critical for management.

4. Necrotizing sialometaplasia is a benign inflammatory lesion of unknown etiology that usually affects the minor palatal salivary glands. It begins as a mucosal ulceration. It can be mistaken for malignancy both clinically and histologically. The lesion is self-healing, requiring no therapy; however, biopsy may be needed to rule out more serious disorders.

B. Chronic nonobstructive

1. Childhood benign lymphosialadenopathy. In childhood, this condition usually arises after age 5 years. The clinical picture differs somewhat from that of the adult, but the histologic findings are similar. The parotids are most often involved. The etiology is unknown, but an autoimmune mechanism is hypothesized.

    a. Signs and symptoms. The onset is usually abrupt and associated with discomfort. A slight temperature elevation is not infrequent.

    b. Physical examination. With the acute episode, tenderness and enlargement are noted. After several days, the tenderness resolves as does the degree of firmness. Enlargement frequently persists for weeks, and, after several recurrences, nodularity may be noted. Parotid massage frequently elicits turbid secretions.

c. Adjunctive studies

   (1) Culture. *Streptococcus viridans* may be cultured, but often the saliva is sterile.

   (2) Radiography. Sialography may be normal in the early stages of the disease. Classically, punctate sialectasia is observed both in the clinically involved and in the uninvolved glands. Cavitary change is rarely observed. Delayed emptying is frequently detected. CT or MRI reveals only diffuse glandular enlargement, frequently with cavitary changes.

   (3) Pathology. Although biopsy is infrequent, it must evidence ductal metaplasia and parenchymal replacement by a chronic inflammatory infiltrate to be consistent with benign lymphosialadenopathy.

d. Therapy. Management should be conservative in most cases.

   (1) Acute. Penicillin or a cephalosporin should be administered PO whenever turbid secretions are present. Massage and heat are indicated in the acute and subacute stages as well as for prophylaxis. Routine premeal massage is important, and increased hydration is mandatory.

   (2) Chronic. Intraoral sites of irritation must be eliminated. Oral appliances or bite plates should be suggested for nighttime "grinding," particularly when interdentigerous ridges are present. Good oral hygiene is essential.

e. Clinical course. The frequency of recurrence has been correlated with the age of onset, an early onset heralding an increased incidence. With recurrent episodes, the amount of residual enlargement can progress, posing a cosmetic problem. If isolated nodularity persists, excision is warranted. In the childhood variant, spontaneous resolution is the rule during the teenage years, and progression to a full Sjögren's syndrome is unusual.

2. Adult benign lymphosialadenopathy. The adult features are similar to those of childhood, with the following exceptions:

a. Contrast to childhood disease

   (1) The majority of adults suffer from chronic recurrent parotitis and do not develop more serious pathology.

   (2) The disease tends to persist.

   (3) Few develop a full Sjögren's syndrome.

   (4) A smaller number develop aggressive lesions of either the epithelial components, e.g., poorly differentiated carcinomas, or of the lymphoreticular apparatus. The development of lymphoma is not necessarily associated with evidence of a systemic autoimmune process.

(5) Having the childhood variant, a self-limited process, does not increase the probability of developing the adult form.

3. Bacterial

a. Etiology. Chronic recurrent bacterial sialadenitis most characteristically affects the parotids. Many clinical conditions, both local and systemic, are potential precursors. Three factors are common to most predisposing conditions: decreased salivary flow, stasis, and altered secretions. Thus, ductal obstruction, benign lymphosialadenopathy, recurrent acute bacterial sialadenitis, allergy, medications, fluid restriction, and psychic considerations (e.g., bulimia) can be associated with this disease entity.

b. Signs and symptoms. Recurrent swelling, frequently while eating, often associated with mild to moderate discomfort, is suggestive.

c. Physical examination. The involved glands are initially tense and occasionally tender. With chronicity, the glands remain firm between exacerbations. Bimanual palpation reveals a diminished salivary flow. During acute episodes, pus may be expressed from the puncta.

d. Laboratory

(1) Cultures. When present, purulent secretions often yield a staphylococcal or a streptococcal organism.

(2) Radiography. Sialography shows ductal changes, with dilatation and sacculation of the ducts distal to areas of obstruction, caused by fibrosis. The retention of contrast for days to weeks is not uncommon in advanced disease. MRI discloses diffuse glandular enlargement.

e. Therapy

(1) Conservative therapy is the cornerstone of management. Judicious ductal dilatations with lacrimal dilators may provide protracted periods of relief. Hydration is essential. Four 8-oz glasses of water/day is the minimum for an affected adult. Sialagogues such as sour lemon candy maintain salivary flow, reducing stasis. Massage as often as possible, but at least 6 times daily, is essential. Adult exacerbations are treated as acute suppurative sialadenitis.

(2) For refractory disease, a consideration of surgical intervention must be predicated on a thorough understanding of the frequency, severity, and morbidity of the process.

Total parotidectomy remains the surgical procedure of choice. Dense fibrosis and increased vascularity make this procedure the most difficult of parotid surgery.

Experience with the operating microscope is essential i
preservation of facial nerve function is to be accom
plished. Only total removal will ensure resolution.

Tympanic neurectomy disrupts the preganglionic para
sympathetic innervation of the parotid. Therefore, secre
tory activity should cease, with resultant atrophy. The
theory is sound, but clinically its effectiveness is limited
consequently, tympanic neurectomy is not advocated.

Radiation therapy has been suggested by some in smal
doses to minimize inflammation. The associated addi
tional fibrosis makes definitive surgery for radiotherap
failures all the more difficult. Therefore, radiation ther
apy is not recommended.

Ligation of Stensen's duct has not been successful in ad
vanced cases. This procedure has also been associated
with significant morbidity and acute distention, and
therefore is not recommended.

4. **Granulomatous disease**

   a. **Etiology.** The more common granulomatous diseases affecting the salivary glands include tuberculosis, cat-scratch
   fever, atypical mycobacteria, and actinomycosis. The presenting pattern does have some specificity, and variations
   from the reference base should be thoroughly investigated.

   b. **Signs and symptoms.** As a group, the presentation is essentially that of a localized area of swelling within the gland.
   The enlargement is frequently present for a protracted period. Enlargement is slow, marked tenderness is uncommon,
   and significant associated external inflammation is unusual. In some instances, however, there may be mild superficial erythema that denotes underlying suppuration with
   cavitation. Spontaneous drainage and fistulization may
   occur.

   c. **Physical examination.** A localized palpable mass is usually
   denoted. Tuberculosis (TB) may be present in two forms: (1
   a chronic mass lesion or (2) in the acute stage with acute inflammation and distention of the entire gland.

   d. **Special studies**

      (1) **Skin tests** are essential when this group of diseases i
      suspected. TB is readily identified, whereas atypical my
      cobacteria are more difficult to document.

      (2) **Sialography,** in most instances, reveals a normal ducta
      system unless there are specific site aberrations associ
      ated with pressure.

      (3) **Fine-needle aspiration of fluctant lesions** with staining
      and appropriate cultures can identify TB, atypical my
      cobacteria, and actinomycosis.

(4) For **chronic nodularity,** an excisional biopsy is warranted to establish the diagnosis.

e. Therapy

(1) Tuberculosis. If detected early, medical management will suffice. In chronic cases, surgical extirpation of the granuloma, in conjunction with appropriate antibiotic medication is necessary.

(2) Actinomycosis. In most instances, adequate doses of penicillin will control the disease. Limited adjunctive surgery rarely proves necessary.

(3) Atypical mycobacterial infection responds to excision. Curettage in conjunction with rifampin has been reported as being therapeutic, but known failures have led the authors to recommend excision as the treatment of choice for isolated parotid disease.

(4) Cat-scratch fever frequently resolves spontaneously. With suppuration, drainage and curettage usually suffice.

5. Sjögren's syndrome

a. Sjögren's syndrome is an autoimmune disorder that affects the major and minor salivary glands; it is usually associated with rheumatoid arthritis, although can be seen with other connective tissue disorders, such as systemic lupus erythematosus or polyarteritis nodosa.

b. Signs and symptoms involve the salivary glands, producing xerostomia, abnormal taste, dry tongue, and lingual papillary atrophy, and intermittent unilateral or bilateral salivary gland (usually parotid) enlargement. When the lacrimal apparatus is affected, xerophthalmia and keratoconjunctivitis sicca occurs.

c. Diagnosis. Laboratory studies reflect an abnormal immune response with elevated rheumatoid factor, antinuclear antibody, and salivary duct antibody often being present. Sialography demonstrates bilateral punctate sialectasia of the parotid and submandibular glands, with prolonged retention of contrast medium. A gallium scan shows increased uptake by the salivary and lacrimal glands. Because the minor salivary glands are affected in over 70% of cases, a biopsy of the labial, nasal mucosal, or palatal glands is often diagnostic.

d. Therapy is symptomatic. Artificial saliva may be helpful. Good dental hygiene is important. Xerophthalmia may require artificial tears or taping the eyelids shut at night to prevent exposure corneal ulceration.

6. Sarcordosis is a granulomatous disease of unknown etiology, and salivary gland involvement may occur in up to one-third of cases. Uveoparotid fever (Heerfordt's disease) is a manifestation of sarcordosis characterized by fever, parotid and lacrimal gland swelling, and uveitis. Associated cranial neuropathies, particularly facial nerve paralysis, are found. It begins in the third to fourth decade of life and may last months to years. Minor salivary glands may be involved, and biopsy of these may be diagnostic. Rarely, the major salivary glands are biopsied.

C. Obstructive: acute and chronic

1. Calculi

a. **Etiology.** Calculi represent both a cause and sequelae of recurrent sialadenitis. Mucous plugs or cellular debris are thought to form a nidus for the deposition of inorganic calcium and phosphate salts. Submandibular gland stones are generally believed to occur far more frequently than those in the parotid. This belief may be skewed by the fact that nearly 80% of submandibular stones are seen on radiographic studies, whereas only 35–40% of parotid stones are radiopaque. However, the submandibular gland is more predisposed to radiopaque calculus formation because of the mucoserous nature of the secretion, its concentration of organic salts, and it anatomic structure that may create salivary stasis from uphill positioning and length of Wharton's duct.

b. **Signs and symptoms.** Food ingestion is associated with a sudden painful enlargement of the affected gland. Further eating increases the distention. If the obstruction is not relieved, secondary infection soon occurs. Small fragments of stone may be passed intermittently.

c. **Physical examination.** Bimanual palpation may detect a calculus during a quiescent interval. Point tenderness may be denoted near the hilum. A diffusely enlarged tense gland is evident during acute obstruction.

d. **Special studies**

   (1) Panorex or oblique soft tissue films may detect a stone in the submandibular glands.

   (2) Sialography may show partial or complete filling defects, depending on the size and associated reaction. In longstanding cases, peripheral ductal change may also exist. Contrast retention on evacuation films is expected.

e. **Complications** include salivary fistulas, acute abscess formation, sinus formation, and stricture secondary to fibrosis.

f. **Therapy**

   (1) Removal of the stone intraorally is recommended for stones within approximately 1 cm of the puncta. This removal is readily accomplished under local anesthesia for the submandibular glands and with somewhat more difficulty for the parotid.

(2) Beyond 2 cm, internal removal is not indicated, as the lingual nerve's relationship to Wharton's duct and the buccal nerve's association with Stensen's duct render each subject to injury.

(3) Multiple stones occur in 25% of patients who present with an initial calculus. An association with renal stones should suggest hypercalcemia.

(4) With longstanding disease, appropriate removal of involved parenchyma must be considered.

2. Stricture

a. Etiology. Both external and internal strictures must be considered. Dental trauma from grinding, ill-fitting dentures, and poor hygiene are associated with external strictures, whereas anomalous development, infection, trauma, calculi, and neoplasms may be associated with internal strictures.

b. Signs and symptoms. Periodic painful swelling with eating is frequent. Prolonged distention and infection may occur.

c. Physical examination. Usually, a diffusely swollen gland is present initially. Recurrent attacks lead to chronic enlargement.

d. Special studies. Sialography should be diagnostic.

e. Therapy

(1) External. Recognizing and eliminating known precursors are essential. Dilatations, judiciously performed under local anesthesia, are often all that is necessary. In the extreme, sialodochoplasty is effective.

(2) Internal. The therapeutic considerations are similar to those of chronic refractory sialadenitis (see **B.3.e.**).

3. Cysts

The parotid is the site of most salivary gland cysts, which account for up to 5% of parotid masses. Most are unilateral in children, and most cysts are benign and can be a lymphangioma, hemangioma, dermoid, or branchial cleft cyst (which arise from the first branchial cleft).

In the adult, either benign or malignant conditions may be cystic. Recurrent infections or ductal obstruction may lead to a cyst. They have also been found in association with tumors such as pleomorphic adenoma, adenoid cystic carcinoma, mucoepidermoid carcinoma, and cystadenoma lymphomatosum (Warthin's tumor). Cystic lesions of the parotid have been associated with HIV infections.

Minor salivary glands may become obstructed, producing dilatation. A ranula is such a condition of the sublingual gland, found in the floor of the mouth.

II. Metabolic and endocrine. Asymptomatic enlargement represents the typical clinical pattern for the entire group of metabolic and endocrine disorders. Although rare, early in the clinical course, size fluctuation may be evident. Pain and inflammation are most infrequent in this subset.

A. Metabolic-malnutrition. Dietary deficiencies are felt to be etiologic in the parotid enlargement associated with starvation, bulemia, and Laennec's cirrhosis. The size of the gland frequently correlates with the clinical status of the primary disease. Improvement in the disease as a whole may be associated with a decrease in size.

   1. Physical examination. The involved glands are diffusely enlarged, soft, and nontender to palpation. The saliva is of normal consistency, and Stensen's duct is normal in appearance.

   2. Laboratory. With radiography the ductal system is normal on sialography. Amylase levels are frequently increased in alcoholic cirrhosis.

   3. Therapy. Correcting the condition leading to the deficiency state must be the hallmark of management. Adjunctive supportive measures accomplish little. Surgery, except for rare diagnostic purposes, is not usually indicated. When size becomes of cosmetic significance, parotidectomy may become necessary.

B. Endocrine. Thyroid disease, diabetes, and aberrations of the pituitary adrenal axis are the most common conditions associated with parotid enlargement.

   1. Thyroid. Parotid enlargement secondary to hypothyroidism does not relate to the magnitude of the deficiency but represents a true hypertrophy.

   2. Diabetes. Although the association is reported, the evidence for a specific relationship remains inconclusive.

   3. Cushing's disease has been associated with fatty infiltration of the gland.

III. Trauma. Lacerations represent the most significant form of injury to the salivary glands, and to the parotid in particular. The facial nerve, ductal, and parenchymal injury all warrant consideration.

A. Facial nerve

   1. Signs and symptoms. The function of all branches must be assessed as soon as possible. Deficits can be compared to the normal side.

   2. Testing. For the unconscious patient, the main trunk and peripheral branches can be assessed with a transcutaneous facial nerve stimulator.

   3. Repair

   a. Early repair is most desirable and should be performed (if possible) at the time of glandular and skin closure. If performed within 48–72 hours, the nerve stimulator will assist in localizing distal segments.

   b. Delayed. Marking the distal branches is mandatory if delayed repair is a necessity. Surgical clips are readily identified at a later time. Parotidectomy aids in delayed repair by facilitating identification. The microscope and 8–0—10–0 monofilament sutures are recommended for the repair.

B. Ductal injury should be suspected when saliva is seen in the wound.

1. **Diagnosis.** Cannulating the duct intraorally and observing saliva in the wound confirms the diagnosis.

2. **Repair**

   a. **Direct.** Suturing over a polyethylene catheter is the procedure of choice.

   b. **Secondary**

   (1) When primary closure is impossible, suturing the distal end to the buccal mucosa should be attempted.

   (2) When the duct is severely traumatized, suturing a Penrose drain from the parotid adjacent to known ductal remnants into a large stab wound through the buccal mucosa frequently creates a permanent functioning fistula into the oral cavity. The drain must be left for a minimum of 2 weeks. This procedure is preferable to ligating the ductal segments.

C. Parenchyma

1. **Isolated lacerations** require meticulous debridement, being cognizant of Stensen's duct and the facial nerve. The closure should be layered. Multiple lacerations in a contaminated field may be best managed with parotidectomy.

2. **Blunt injury.** Following blunt injury to the side of the face in association with fracture of the maxilla or mandible, dysfunction can be anticipated in 80% of the cases. A pressure dressing is warranted to decrease complications.

   Sialocele, or salivary cysts, can be treated with repeated aspiration and pressure dressings. If this fails, excision of the cyst, gland, or both may become necessary.

   Chronic external fistulas can be excised.

   Large fistulas. Intraoral diversion of saliva must be effected and pressure dressings applied. Soft tissue collections of saliva require aspiration after establishing an oral conduit. Tympanic neurectomy may provide a decrease in salivary flow to enable closure of the larger fistula. If more conservative measures fail, parotidectomy is indicated. Medications to reduce salivary flow have not been a meaningful adjunct. Radiation to decrease flow is not warranted for this condition.

IV. **Neoplasia.** The neoplasms affecting the salivary glands are sufficient in pathogenic complexity to make a complete discussion of such impractical for this text. The various types of salivary gland tumors have different biological courses, but in general tend to be slow growing.

Table 6-1. Classification of salivary gland tumors

I. Benign lesions
   A. Mixed tumor (pleomorphic adenoma)
   B. Papillary cystadenolymphoma (Warthin's tumor)
   C. Oncocytosis-oncocytoma
   D. Monomorphic adenoma
      1. Basal cell adenoma
      2. Glycogen-rich adenoma and clear cell adenoma
   E. Sebaceous adenoma
   F. Sebaceous lymphadenoma
   G. Papillary ductal adenoma
   H. Benign lymphoepithelial lesion

II. Malignant lesions
   A. Carcinoma ex pleomorphic adenoma (carcinoma arising in/from a mixed tumor)
   B. Mucoepidermoid carcinoma
      1. Low grade
      2. Intermediate grade
      3. High grade
   C. Hybrid basal cell adenoma/adenoid cystic carcinoma
   D. Adenoid cystic carcinoma
   E. Acinous cell carcinoma (acinic carcinoma)
   F. Adenocarcinoma
      1. Mucus-producing adenopapillary and nonpapillary carcinoma
      2. Salivary duct carcinoma (ductal carcinoma)
   G. Oncocytic carcinoma (malignant oncocytoma)
   H. Clear cell carcinoma
   I. Epithelial/myoepithelial carcinoma of intercalated ducts
   J. Squamous cell carcinoma
   K. Undifferentiated carcinoma
   L. Miscellaneous (including sebaceous, Stensen's duct, melanoma, and carcinoma ex lymphoepithelial lesion)
   M. Metastatic carcinoma

Source: Data from J. G. Batsakis, *Tumors of the Head and Neck: Clinical and Pathological Considerations* (2nd ed.). Baltimore: Williams & Wilkins, 1979.

A. Epidemiology

Salivary gland tumors account for 5% of all head and neck neoplasms (excluding skin). Most are benign. The predominant site is the parotid, followed by the submandibular, sublingual, and the minor salivary glands. Benign tumors comprise 80% of parotid growths but less than half of tumors in the other glands. A prior history of radiation exposure, even in the distant past, can predispose to the onset of a salivary gland tumor.

B. A classification of tumors of the salivary glands appears in Table 6-1 with staging shown in Table 6-2.

C. Diagnosis is based on history and examination, with the addition of imaging studies and biopsy by fine-needle aspiration, which often are exceptionally valuable (see **I–V**).

D. Tumors of the parotid gland

Eighty percent of parotid tumors are benign; 20% are malignant. The highest incidence of benign tumors is in the fifth decade of life, with malignancy being more predominant in the sixth decade.

Table 6-2. American Joint Committee on Cancer staging of salivary gland tumors, 1988

Tumor size
  T_1: less than 2 cm
  T_2: 2–4 cm
  T_3: 4–6 cm
  T_4: > −6 cm
    All T categories are subdivided
    (a) no local extension
    (b) local extension (clinical or macroscopic evidence of invasion of skin, soft tissues, bone, or nerve)
Nodal states
  N1: single ipsilateral lymph node less than 3 cm
  N2a: single ipsilateral lymph node 3–6 cm
  N2b: multiple ipsilateral lymph nodes less than 6 cm
  N2c: bilateral/contralateral less than 6 cm
  N3: greater than 6 cm
Stage
    I: T1a/T2a NOMO
   II: T1b/T2b/T3a NOMO
  III: T1/T2 NOMO
      T4a/T3b NOMO
   IV: T4b, any N, MO
      Any T, N2/N3, MO
      Any T, any N, M1

1. **Mixed tumor (pleomorphic adenoma).** The benign mixed tumor accounts for nearly two-thirds of all parotid tumors and occurs predominantly in females. These are slow-growing, painless, well-circumscribed masses, often found in the tail of the parotid. Examination reveals a smooth, firm, mobile lesion, usually with normal facial nerve function. There is often an absence of other symptoms, and these tumors may grow to a considerable size before patients seek medical care. Treatment is by parotidectomy with a cuff of surrounding normal tissue that encompasses the microscopic outgrowths. Recurrence rate is low if this treatment plan is adhered to.

2. **Papillary cystadenoma lymphomatosum (Warthin's tumor).** This lesion represents the second most common benign tumor of the parotid gland. It appears to originate from both ductal and lymphoid elements. Clinically, it presents as a round, smooth, mobile, firm mass in the tail of the parotid. Males are affected five times more than females. Although usually isolated, multiple tumors have been found, and surgical excision (parotidectomy) is the treatment of choice.

3. **Oncocytoma and monomorphic adenoma.** These two benign tumors are usually derived from a single cell type and represent a minority of benign lesions most often found in the parotid gland. They may appear in other salivary gland sites and are usually well circumscribed. Minimal associated symptoms occur, and total excision is usually required.

4. **Mucoepidermoid carcinoma** is the most common malignancy of the parotid gland. They may be slowly growing or quite aggressive. Low-grade tumors are usually well localized, rarely metastasizing; whereas distant spread occurs in 50% of the high-grade variety. They may occur in any age group and equally in the sexes. Survival is over 90% for low-grade tumors and only 20–30% for the more aggressive types. Surgical treatment is required, with wide resection, and at times sacrifice and grafting of the facial nerve are necessary. Postoperative radiation may also be needed for high-grade tumor types.

5. **Adenoid cystic carcinoma** is the most common malignant tumor of the submandibular, sublingual, and minor salivary glands. It accounts for less than 5% of all parotid neoplasms and over 30% of those in the minor glands. Symptoms are usually of a progressively enlarging mass with occasional associated pain and often with facial nerve weakness. The adenoid cystic carcinoma tends to invade nerve sheaths. Although slow growing, it has a high recurrence rate, with frequent local and systemic spread. Distal metastases have been found in 15% of patients, with the lungs most frequently affected. The course tends to be prolonged, and recurrences are common. Treatment is surgical, with nerve resection and grafting performed as needed. Neck dissection for palpable nodes should be considered. Radiation therapy is a valuable adjunct for positive surgical margins, local control for inaccessible tumors, and for patients not able to withstand large surgical procedures. Although a 5-year survival rate of 75% has been reported, by 20 years this diminishes to approximately 10%.

6. **Adenocarcinoma** represents various histologic patterns and occurs in up to 15% of parotid malignancies. No sex or age predilection occurs. Usually, the facial nerve function is normal.

7. **Malignant mixed tumor (carcinoma expleomorphic adenoma)** represents the malignant transformation of primarily the epithelial elements of a benign mixed tumor. A mass may be present for many years that suddenly will grow rapidly, accompanied by facial pain and weakness—both ominous signs. The recurrence rate is high and prognosis poor, even with therapy that is aggressive. Nodal metastases have been found in over 10% of patients and in distant sites (lung, bone, brain) in up to 30% of patients.

8. **Acinic cell carcinoma** is less common than other major types of salivary gland tumors. It is usually found in the parotid. It tends to be slowly progressive, painless, and rarely produces facial nerve weakness. It presents most often in women 60–70 years of age and is low grade in nature.

9. **Squamous cell carcinoma** is an uncommon cancer that presents in the parotid as a firm, hard mass fixed to the surrounding structures and skin. It is highly malignant, rapidly growing, producing facial pain and nerve paralysis with cervical lymphatic involvement in half of patients. Less than 20%

5-year survival rate occurs, despite radical therapy of resection, radiation, and chemotherapy.

10. **Lymphoma of the parotid gland** is rare, but may arise in extranodal tissue. Symptoms are nonspecific and usually mimic sialoadenitis. A complete evaluation for staging is mandatory prior to the beginning of treatment, because local disease requires radiation and a disseminated process mandates chemotherapy. Patients with Sjögren's disease exhibit a higher incidence of intraparotid lymphoma.

E. **Tumors of the submandibular gland**

Tumors of the submandibular gland comprise only 10% of all salivary gland neoplasms; however, up to 50% of submandibular gland tumors are malignant. Of the benign tumors, the overwhelming majority are pleomorphic adenomas.

Most lesions of the submandibular gland are inflammatory, with symptoms and signs of pain, erythema, intermittent swelling, and purulent secretions from Wharton's duct. Chronic inflammation may be difficult to differentiate from neoplasia. Nerve weakness is uncommon; however, paralysis of the marginal mandibular nerve with weakness of the corner of the mouth is seen in malignant tumors. Despite this, only 10% of submandibular malignancies manifest nerve involvement. Cervical lymph node metastases are not uncommon. Treatment requires wide surgical excision with contiguous resection of lymphatics, when appropriate.

F. **Tumors of the sublingual and minor salivary gland** are the rarest of the growths but are important in that malignancy is more common. Presentation is often a result of a slowly growing mass. Treatment requires resection with preservation of maximal function for low-grade malignancies. As with other tumors, high-grade and advanced lesions require adjunctive radiation therapy for improved local control.

G. **Ancillary treatment measures.** Neutron beam irradiation appears to have efficacy for advanced, unresectable, or recurrent malignant salivary gland neoplasms. With progress in surgical rehabilitative techniques and adjunctive therapies, significant local and regional control is achievable. Chemotherapy is under investigation and, in certain settings, may have beneficial effects. Clearly advanced squamous cell carcinoma and high-grade mucoepidermoid carcinomas should be considered for neoadjuvant chemotherapy.

Selected Readings

Bailey, H. The surgical anatomy of the parotid gland. *Br. Med. J.* 2:245, 1948.

Batsakis, J. G. *Tumors of the Head and Neck: Clinical and Pathological Considerations* (2nd ed.). Baltimore: Williams & Wilkins, 1979.

Byrne, M., et al. Preoperative assessment of parotid masses: A comparative evaluation of radiologic techniques to histopathologic diagnosis. *Laryngoscope* 99:284, 1989.

Casselman, J. W., and Mancuso, A. A. Major salivary gland masses: Comparison of MR imaging and CT. *Radiology* 165:183, 1987.

Casterline, P. F., and Jacques, D. A. The surgical management of recurrent parotitis. *Surg. Gynecol. Obstet.* 146:419, 1978.

Conley, J. *Salivary Glands and the Facial Nerve.* New York: Grune & Stratton, 1975.

Curtin, H. Assessment of salivary gland pathology. *Otolaryngol. Clin. North Am.* 21:547, 1988.

Fried, M. Neoplasms of the Salivary Glands. In Peterson, et al. (eds), *Head and Neck Management of the Cancer Patient.* Amsterdam: Martinus Nijhoff, 1986. Pp. 201–229.

Hecht, D. W., and Work, W. P. Surgery for nonneoplastic parotid disease. *Arom. Otolaryngol.* 92:463, 1986.

Johns, M. E., and Goldsmith, M. Current management of salivary gland tumors. *Oncology* 3:85, 1989.

Johns, M. E., and Nachlas, N. E. Salivary Gland Tumors. In M. M. Paparella, D. A. Shumrick, J. L. Gluckman, and W. L. Meyerhoff (eds.), *Otolaryngology* (vol. 3, 3rd ed.). Philadelphia: Saunders, 1991. Pp. 2099–2127.

Nichols, R. D. Surgical treatment of chronic suppurative parotitis: A critical review. *Laryngoscope* 87:2066, 1977.

Rice, D. H. Non-neoplastic Diseases of the Salivary Glands. In M. M. Paparella, D. A. Shumrick, J. L. Gluckman, and W. L. Meyerhoff (eds.), *Otolaryngology* (vol. 3, 3rd ed.). Philadelphia: Saunders, 1991. Pp. 2089–2097.

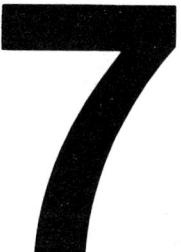

Head and Neck

I. Introduction

The neck mass mirrors a host of pathologic entities. A workable diagnostic approach necessitates a basic reference frame both for the varied clinical considerations and for the ability to correlate the neck mass with the regional anatomy (Fig. 7-1).

A. Physical examination

1. **Location.** The relationship of the neck mass to the sternocleidomastoid muscle (anterior, posterior, or deep) is essential to document. Noting the relationship to other identifiable structures is important (i.e., juxtaposed to the larynx, eleventh nerve, carotid artery, or supraclavicular fat pad). Making diagrams is essential.

2. **Character.** Defining such parameters as the size, degree of firmness, tenderness, fluctuation, encapsulation, mobility, margins, pulsation, bruits, response to swallowing, and Valsalva markedly narrows the diagnostic spectrum.

B. Diagnostic studies

1. A routine, complete clinical head and neck evaluation frequently makes the diagnosis and must precede any other studies.

2. Soft tissue films in selected instances may have merit, but their yield is low, expense considerable, and therefore they are of relatively low priority.

3. Computed tomography (CT) and magnetic resonance imaging (MRI) are of increasing importance in defining the depth of the neck mass as well as in defining relationships to the carotid sheath and other vital structures.

4. Aspiration biopsy is an increasingly important diagnostic modality for tumor identification. It is only as good as the pathologist interpreting the specimen. Aspiration biopsy should be considered after a complete head and neck evaluation, and definitely before an open biopsy. Ultrasonographic-guided needle aspiration cytology is improving the diagnostic accuracy of this sampling technique. Similarly, the limits of MRI-guided aspiration cytology for more difficult anatomic sites is being explored. If a malignancy is suspected, endoscopy and blind biopsies of the nasopharynx, tongue base, and tonsil should precede any consideration of open biopsy.

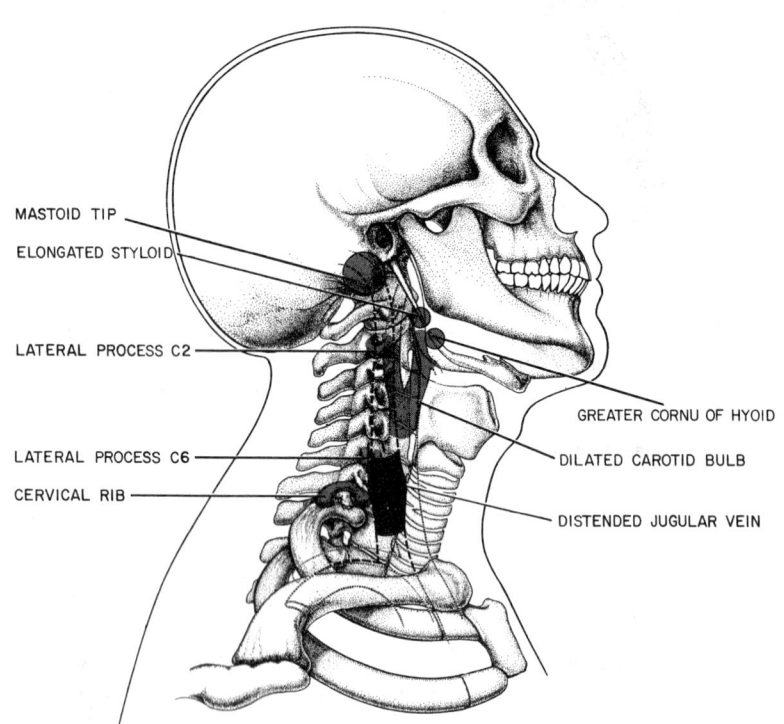

Fig. 7-1. Variations of normal anatomy in areas depicted may be misinterpreted clinically.

    5. Culture obtained by aspiration is essential when infection is a possibility and should be considered when blood and stomal cultures leave the diagnosis in doubt.

II. Branchial cleft anomalies result from an arrested development of the first four clefts, pouches, or remnants thereof. Most branchial cleft cysts presenting in the neck are devoid from clefts 2 and 3 (Fig. 7-2).

A. Branchial cysts

    1. Signs and symptoms

        a. An asymptomatic swelling, often developing after an upper respiratory tract infection, at the anterior border of the sternocleidomastoid muscle is characteristic. A family history is not infrequent. Typically, these cysts present in the late teens, but they may arise at any age. Pain is infrequent unless a secondary infection occurs. Associated abscesses are infrequent, but, when present, spontaneous or surgical drainage may create a persistent fistula. Dyspnea, with or without stridor, and dysphagia are rare associations, depending primarily on the location and size of the cyst.

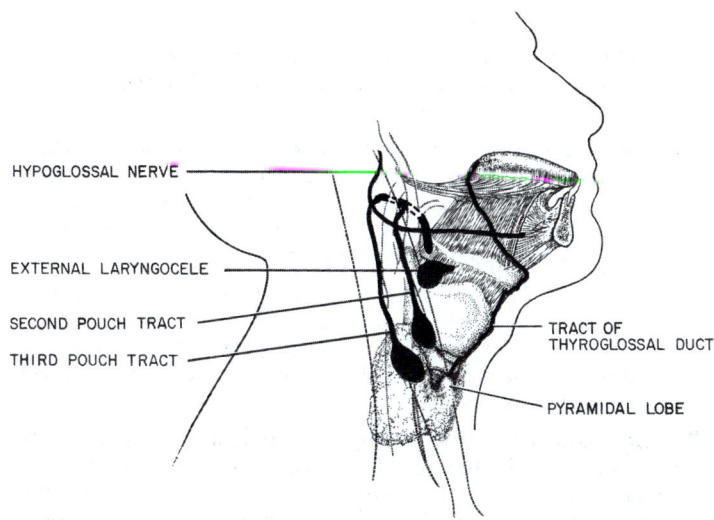

HYPOGLOSSAL NERVE

EXTERNAL LARYNGOCELE

SECOND POUCH TRACT

THIRD POUCH TRACT

TRACT OF
THYROGLOSSAL DUCT

PYRAMIDAL LOBE

Fig. 7-2. Embryological cervical vestiges found in the adult.

B. Fistulas. Signs and symptoms. Usually an asymptomatic fibrous cord is noted at the anterior edge of the sternocleidomastoid muscle. Three forms exist:

1. **External.** A fistula ending at the skin but not entering the pharynx.

2. **Internal.** Entering the pharynx but not extending to the skin.

3. **Complete.** Extending from the skin to the pharynx.

   The three types of fistulas are responsible for symptoms as diverse as chronic cough (internal), persistent or intermittent mucoid discharge (external), or food particles visualized at the neck puncta (complete). In all three, inflammation may be noted with an upper respiratory tract infection.

C. Physical examination: cysts and fistulas. The size and state of the cyst or fistula determine the palpable configuration. Noting the neck locale enables a prediction of which pouch cleft system is involved, and thus the relationship to other vital structures (i.e., first-cleft aberrations are often intimately associated with the facial nerve and external auditory canal).

D. Differential diagnosis. Differentiation must be made from hemangiomas, lymphangiomas, thymic cysts, lymphomas, metastatic thyroid carcinoma, and dermoids.

E. Special studies. A fistulagram using a radiopaque media frequently details the course of a fistula; however, CT and MRI are more commonly performed.

F. Therapy

1. **Medical.** Antibiotics are essential in the management of an infected cyst or fistula. Penicillin or a cephalosporin should be the initial drug of choice.

2. **Aspiration,** not surgical drainage, should be the first therapeutic manipulation. It affords culture material, immediately reduces the mass size, and, in contrast to surgical drainage, does not have the same potential for creating a fistula or infected tract that subsequently could prove difficult to excise.

3. **Surgery.** Total extirpation is the preferred management and is essential to prevent enlargement, recurrent infection, and the rare malignant degeneration. Surgery is best performed in a quiescent period. As a rule, children do not require surgery before age 2 years.

III. Thyroglossal duct cysts. During migration of the embryonic thyroid, a duct is formed. Failure of obliteration, which normally occurs at the tenth development week, results in a tract or cyst in immediate association with the hyoid bone. The cysts comprise 70% of congenital neck anomalies. Most are diagnosed by age 30 years.

A. Signs and symptoms. Usually midline at or just beneath the hyoid bone, the cysts are frequently first noted in conjunction with an upper respiratory infection.

B. Physical examination. A midline mass, smooth and well demarcated, is most suggestive. Motion superiorly is noted with deglutition and is considered diagnostic.

C. Special studies. When a normal thyroid is not palpable, a thyroid scan is indicated. If the entire thyroid is aberrant in position, its removal along with the cyst is not indicated unless the thyroid is otherwise abnormal.

D. Differential diagnosis. Other considerations include dermoid cysts, benign lymphadenopathy, and sebaceous cysts.

E. Therapy. Surgical excision is recommended because of the potential for infection and malignant transformation. Although malignancy is rare, papillary carcinoma has been reported. If recurrence is to be avoided, the hyoid in its midportion must be removed at the time of extirpation.

IV. Dermoids, by definition, contain skin appendages. Although potentially found in any area of the neck, they are most often midline. Detection by the second decade is usual.

A. Signs and symptoms. A painless, slowly enlarging midline mass is characteristic.

B. Physical examination. A dermoid is well demarcated, nontender, and rubbery to palpation; it is not mobile on swallowing.

C. Therapy. Complete surgical excision is the management of choice.

V. Inflammation. Adenopathy, inflammatory in origin, is the single most common neck mass. Frequently, the source of the infection can be found in adjacent regions of the head and neck.

A. Acute inflammatory adenopathy

1. **Signs and symptoms.** The adenopathy is frequently secondary to a regional inflammation (i.e., furuncles or fissures around the oral commissures lead to submental or submandibular nodes). Upper respiratory tract infections, such as pharyngotonsillitis, nasopharyngitis, or gingival inflammation are the most frequent considerations. In the pediatric population, the site of origin may go undetected.

2. **Physical examination.** A relatively rapid increase in size makes inflammatory nodes tender to palpation. In addition, in the acute stage the nodes are firm, with fluctuation occurring secondarily. Usually, multiple nodes can be detected.

3. **Studies**

   a. **Culture.** Routine examination of the nose, oropharynx, and hypopharynx usually suggests the origin of the adenopathy, which is the most appropriate site for culture.

   b. A white blood cell count and differential smear aid in identifying a viral versus a bacterial syndrome.

   c. **Aspiration.** If the site of origin cannot be identified for culture and if there is no response to the initial antibiotic regimen, aspiration for culture and sensitivity can be beneficial.

   d. Gram stain of the cultured areas can provide initial direction for the choice of antibiotics.

4. **Therapy**

   a. **Acute**

      (1) **Viral.** If the history, examination, and adjunctive studies are suggestive of viral illness, only supportive measures are warranted. These measures involve an increased amount of rest and hydration. Antipyretics can decrease the morbidity of myalgia and temperature elevation. Antihistamine-vasoconstrictor preparations also can provide symptomatic relief.

      (2) **Bacterial.** The specific antibiotics, whenever possible, should await culture direction. The very symptomatic patient should be started on an appropriate dose of penicillin prior to obtaining culture results.

      (3) **Incision and drainage.** A node increasing in dimension, with resolution at the primary site, suggests abscess formation. Aspiration confirms its presence and, on occasion, can be therapeutic. More frequently, incision and drainage are required in this setting.

B. **Chronic inflammatory adenopathy.** Adenopathy is chronic when it persists or increases in dimension beyond the latency period for an acute infection. It must be recognized, however, that it may take weeks for adenopathy to resolve following an acute process. The key is continued resolution. Adenopathy persisting without an identifiable site of origin or without a defined time of onset must be conceptualized as being chronic. In patients more than 45 years of age, all nodes must initially be considered as part of a malignant process. The most common chronic inflammatory considerations must include tuberculosis (TB), atypical mycobacteria, cat-scratch fever, actinomycosis, toxoplasmosis, sarcoidosis, and syphilis.

Using the differential diagnosis as a reference frame and adhering ing to the testing outlined earlier (see **I.B.**) will establish the correct diagnosis. Only atypical mycobacterial infections are best managed with complete removal of the involved nodes; the other inflammatory conditions respond to a medical or combined approach.

VI. **Neoplasms.** As with other anatomic regions, neoplasms of the neck fall into the categories of benign and malignant. Age is a significant determinant; neck masses developing in patients over 40 years of age have a vastly increased probability of malignancy.

A. **Benign neck masses.** Congenital cysts have been discussed (see sec. **III**), and cellular neoplasms will be considered. Although many of their physical characteristics are similar, differentiation is often possible clinically when all the pertinent considerations of the history and physical examination are collected.

1. **Cystic hygromas** are benign congenital lesions of lymphatic derivation. Ninety percent are detected by age 2 years.

   a. **History.** Usually, an asymptomatic enlarging mass is noted by the parents. Size fluctuation is not infrequent with upper respiratory tract infections. If sufficiently large, the airway can be narrowed with associated stridor.

   b. **Physical examination.** Cystic hygromas are soft, multilobular, and usually ill-defined. They can occur in any anatomic region of the head and neck.

   c. **Diagnostic studies**

      (1) Aspiration produces a straw-colored fluid.

      (2) Transillumination: these lesions do transilluminate.

      (3) CT or MRI scanning helps define areas of involvement.

   d. **Therapy.** Ill-defined borders and a disregard for facial planes make this lesion very difficult to excise. Total removal is rarely effected. There is risk to adjacent vessels and nerves. Recurrent infection, severe disfigurement, and increased growth may necessitate surgery.

2. **Hemangiomas** usually present soon after birth. They involve the skin alone in two-thirds of patients, the remainder being subcutaneous alone or mixed. Hemangiomas are the most common childhood parotid neoplasms.

   a. **History.** There is usually no history of consequence, the lesion being readily perceptible.

   b. **Physical.** Many of the cutaneous lesions are extremely red leading to the term *strawberry hemangioma*. The deeper lesions frequently blanche with pressure. A thrill or bruit may be detected.

c. **Therapy.** Ninety percent of hemangiomas resolve spontaneously in the first 2 years or are in the process of doing so. With continued involution, surgery is not indicated. When resolution does not occur, recurrent bleeding and cosmesis are reasons for considering judicious extirpation.

3. **Carotid body tumors.** These tumors are nonchromaffin paragangliomas derived from chemoreceptors at the carotid bifurcation. Some carotid body tumors are functionally active and secrete catecholamines.

a. **History.** The symptoms are most often that of a slowly enlarging mass in the area of the carotid bifurcation. Carotid body tumors usually present between the third and sixth decades. There may be a familial predisposition. Multiple associated lesions have been reported. Pain is infrequent, usually occurring with large tumors.

b. **Physical examination.** Classically, these tumors are firm rubbery masses at the carotid bifurcation. There can be lateral movement, but superior and inferior motion is limited at best. A bruit may be audible. Neural invasion or associated adenopathy is suggestive of malignancy.

c. **Diagnostic studies.** Angio-MRI will sufficiently delineate the lesion and confirm its presence.

d. **Therapy.** Surgery is the only certain means of eradication. If the perceived morbidity and mortality is excessive for a given patient, radiation therapy may be warranted as the initial therapeutic consideration. Signs of malignancy, rapid growth, patients less than 50 years of age, and disturbances in swallowing, breathing, or both are the principal factors mandating surgical consideration. Only the most expert surgeon should attempt this technically demanding procedure.

B. **Malignant.** Although primary malignancies do arise in the thyroid, malignant lesions in lateral neck sites most often represent metastatic disease. By far the most common cell type metastasizing to the cervical lymph nodes is squamous cell carcinoma. The primary site is usually in the head and neck, with tongue, tonsil, and larynx being most frequent (Fig. 7-3). Distant primaries are the origin in approximately 10% of neck metastases, and occult primaries represent less than 5%.

Failure to initiate an immediate investigation of a suspicious mass in the older patient almost always adversely influences the morbidity and mortality, should the lesion prove to be squamous cell carcinoma. Similarly, the premature open biopsy of a node containing squamous cell carcinoma can reduce survival statistics by as much as 50%. Therefore, a carefully conceived protocol must be followed for all suspicious lesions.

1. The **history** is frequently not accurate as to the onset of symptoms. Also, the magnitude of alcohol consumption is usually

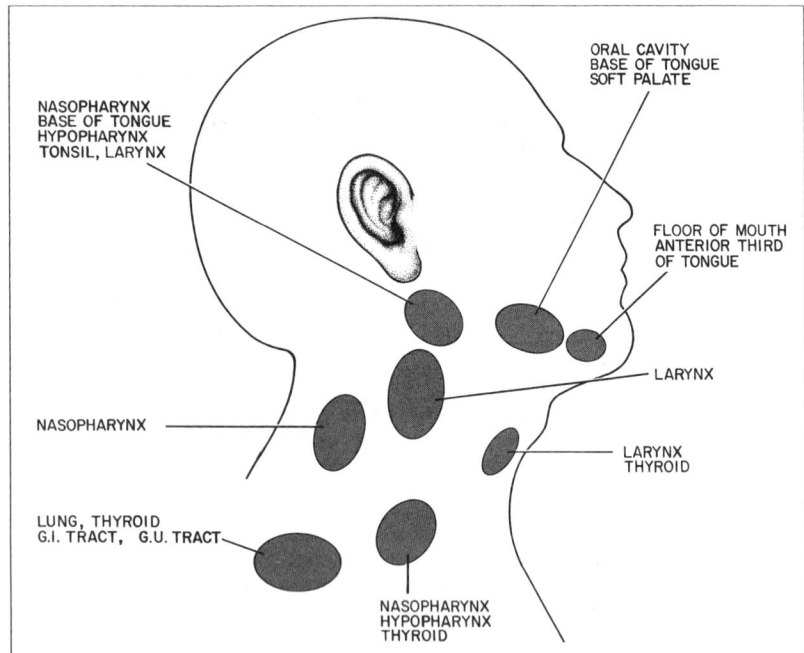

Fig. 7-3. Sites of origin of cervical nodal metastases.

minimized. A responsible family member will often be candid. Smoking is a known precursor. The magnitude and duration of smoking should be recorded, as they impact decidedly on therapeutic considerations via the effect on pulmonary function. Eliciting a history of pharyngalgia, referred otalgia, hoarseness, aspiration, and symptoms of airway obstruction frequently helps define the primary site. Having had a prior head and neck malignancy is of obvious significance. Childhood irradiation can predispose to thyroid and salivary gland neoplasms.

2. **Physical examination.** Although the site of involved nodes, their number, and size all impact on therapeutic considerations, in general a clinically positive node decreases the survival for a site-specific lesion by 50%. Also, no matter how experienced the examiner, mobile nodes less than 2 cm in size, with an identified head and neck primary, will be reactive or inflammatory 20% of the time. It is understood that a complete examination of the head and neck is essential in the presence of an identified neck mass.

3. **Diagnostic approach**

   a. If a head and neck primary is identified on physical examination, the patient is admitted for mapping biopsies.

      (1) Preoperative studies include liver function tests and coagulation determinations to rule out alcohol-induced

disease and to screen for metastases. An albumin-globulin ratio and total protein analysis serve as nutritional guides. A TB skin test, both for breakdown of a primary complex and for the potential for anergy, is evaluated. Other blood studies should be performed as warranted by the history.

(2) X-ray studies

(a) A barium swallow is ordered to rule out the presence of a second head and neck primary, which can occur in as many as 20% of patients.

(b) A chest film is done to rule out another primary or metastases.

(c) A CT or MRI scan preoperatively adds to the dimensional conceptualization of a lesion.

(3) Needle aspiration biopsy (see **I.B.4.**) will often disclose whether the neck mass is malignant. This is of particular importance for further evaluation, but often will not, unto itself, preclude other studies. The latter are needed to seek the primary (location, size) and to discern the presence of second primary lesions.

(4) The lesion is palpated under general anesthesia. The lack of secondary muscle splinting often affords a more accurate clinical assessment. Invariably, the dimensions of the lesion increase when the evaluation is performed in this manner. Bronchoscopy and esophagoscopy are performed; the examiner looks for small second primaries. If the primary is found, appropriate biopsies are taken. Based on the resultant data, a therapeutic plan is formulated.

(5) If a head and neck examination does not uncover the primary, the preoperative evaluation remains the same, but intraoperative random biopsies are taken from the nasopharynx and tongue base. The tonsil, if present on the side of the lesion, is removed. If the primary still remains undetected and a fine-needle aspiration of the node is nondiagnostic, an open biopsy follows, proceeding immediately to a radical neck if the biopsy proves to be squamous cell carcinoma. Further management is based on the data obtained. Thyroid carcinoma, lymphomas, and sarcomas can also be identified using this approach. Their management is beyond the scope of this text.

4. Therapy

a. Social factors. Often overlooked is the patient's mental health relative to his or her family, job, and potential for rehabilitation following massive ablative surgery. The functional and psychic cripple alive and well at 5 years cannot be considered a therapeutic triumph. In-depth discussions with the patient and family are frequently necessary to choose the appropriate therapeutic plan—be it surgery, radiation therapy, chemotherapy, or combinations thereof. A 10% difference in survival, although clinically significant, may have little meaning for a given patient. It is the mature physician's responsibility to lucidly present all the available data and to assist a fellow human being in reaching a decision that is most appropriate for a given psychologic and social set.

The actual management of cervical metastases depends to a great extent on the primary site, be it in the head and neck, distant or unknown. Radiation therapy, surgery, and chemotherapy have all made significant advances in the past decade. An in-depth discussion of each is beyond the scope of this text. However, combinations of two or more of these modalities are commonplace in the management of stage 3 and 4 squamous cell carcinoma of the head and neck.

b. Radiation. Radiation therapy is very effective in controlling microscopic neck disease. The N_0 neck with the high likelihood of microscopic disease is most often treated with radiation therapy. Similarly, recognizing that postoperative radiation therapy is as effective as preoperative treatment for most head and neck carcinoma (when a combination of surgery and radiation therapy is indicated), the trend is toward postoperative radiation therapy. With this approach, the morbidity and mortality of the complications associated with extensive obliterative surgery are decreased. In addition, if microscopic positive margins are identified on permanent section, the radiation therapeutic plan can be so directed.

Implants, when feasible, are getting more emphasis to increase local dosage, and twice-a-day radiation therapy is gaining proponents.

c. Surgery. Surgery has made major advances in reconstruction. Myocutaneous flaps—skin islands transposed on an underlying muscle bed with an intact blood supply—now are the standard for reconstruction. Flap loss is diminished, primary healing improved, and cosmesis enhanced using these flaps. Incorporating bone in these flaps has furthered the concept of immediate reconstruction, with the emphasis on function and cosmesis. Microvascular surgery has improved reconstructive efforts. Large islands of tissue can be transposed as free grafts, the blood supply being reestablished rapidly with microtechniques. The required level of technical expertise for free flap transfer makes the use of regional tissue the primary consideration, yet free tissue transferred techniques are clearly the future.

When replacing the entire pharynx, jejunum transposed using microvascular techniques has many theoretic advantages, making it a reasonable therapeutic consideration.

The laser (CO_2, KTP, Nd-YAG) is receiving increased attention in the management of head and neck malignancies. It is an excellent choice in the primary management of many early lesions. In intraoral ablative procedures, the laser can decrease blood loss and increase the precision with which the resection is performed. Its further application in neck surgery is being explored.

   d. Chemotherapy. Advances in chemotherapy may ultimately have a great impact on the management of head and neck cancer. Multiple trials are currently being performed. Currently, the drugs most effective for squamous cell carcinoma are being evaluated in different doses, sequencing, and combinations. They include cisplatin, 5-fluorouracil, and methotrexate. If used, they appear to be most effective when instituted as the first form of therapy. Ongoing trials are investigating the benefit of induction chemotherapy for extensive neoplasms. Currently, if there is no response in the larger lesion to induction chemotherapy, the outlook for survival is extremely poor. The long-term risk-benefit ratio awaits definition.

Selected Readings

Batsakis, J. G. The pathology of head and neck tumors: The occult primary and metastases to the head and neck. *Head Neck Surg.* 3:409, 1981.

Coates, H. L., et al. An immunologic basis for detection of occult primary malignancies of the head and neck. *Cancer* 41:912, 1978.

Fried, M. P., et al. Cervical metastases from an unknown primary. *Ann. Otol. Rhinol. Laryngol.* 84:152, 1975.

Fried, M. P. Evaluation of the adult neck mass. *Med. Times* 110:96s, 1982.

Martin, H., and Morfit, H. M. Cervical lymph node metastasis as the first symptom of cancer. *Surg. Gynecol. Obstet.* 78:133, 1944.

Martin, H., and Romieu, C. The diagnostic significance of a "lump on the neck." *Postgrad. Med.* 11:491, 1952.

McGuirt, W. F., and McCabe, B. F. Significance of node biopsy before definitive treatment of cervical metastatic carcinoma. *Laryngoscope* 88:594, 1978.

Miller, D., et al. The differential diagnosis of the mass on the neck: A fresh look. *Laryngoscope* 11:140, 1981.

Paparella, M. M., Shumrick, D. A., Gluckman, J. L., and Meyerhoff, W. L., eds. *Otolaryngology—Head and Neck* (vol. III, 3rd ed.) Philadelphia: Saunders, 1991.

Shapshay, S. M., et al. Simultaneous carcinomas of the esophagus and upper digestive tract. *Otolaryngol. Head Neck Surg.* 88:372, 1980.

Sismanis, A., Strong, M. S., and Nerriam, J. Fine-needle aspiration biopsy diagnosis of head masses. *Otolaryngol. Clin. North Am.* 13:421, 1980.

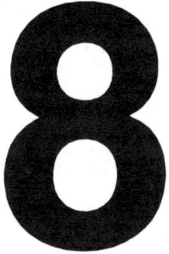

Otolaryngological Manifestations of AIDS

Acquired immunodeficiency syndrome (AIDS) first came to medical attention in the early 1980s, when an isolated number of deaths from rare lung infections (*Pneumocystis carinii* pneumonia [PCP]) and unusual skin tumors (Kaposi's sarcoma) were noted in previously healthy homosexual men in California and New York. In the 1990s, AIDS has become an epidemic. As of January 1990, the Centers for Disease Control (CDC) has reported more than 121,500 cases of AIDS and approximately 72,500 AIDS-related deaths in the United States. Fifty-nine percent of all reported cases of AIDS as of October 1989 have died, with current estimates of a 100% mortality rate between 3 and 5 years after diagnosis.

I. HIV

The causative agent of AIDS is the human immunodeficiency virus (HIV). HIV infection manifests itself in a wide range of disease processes: constitutional abnormalities (Table 8-1), opportunistic infections (Table 8-2), and secondary cancers (Table 8-3).

A. Pathophysiology

HIV is a retrovirus that attacks CD4 receptors found on T-helper cells, macrophages, central nervous system (CNS) cells of monocytic origins, and other antigen-presenting cells. As a result, a T cell immunodeficiency occurs and the host becomes susceptible to many opportunistic infections and neoplastic conditions.

Because of the multiple systemic manifestations of AIDS, the CDC divided the spectrum of HIV infections into four stages (Table 8-4).

Other classification systems for HIV infection do exist, such as the Walter Reed staging system, which uses both clinical and laboratory indicators (number of peripheral CD4+ lymphocytes and levels of HIV antigen) to monitor disease progression. To date, CD4+ cell count is the most clinically useful measure of immune function in the HIV-infected individual. When the count falls below 200 cells/mm^3, the host becomes most susceptible to opportunistic infections.

B. Transmission

HIV has been isolated from a number of body fluids, including blood, semen, saliva, tears, urine, cerebrospinal fluid, breast milk, and cervical and vaginal secretions. Transmission of the virus has been reported from sexual intercourse (anal and vaginal),

Table 8-1. Constitutional abnormalities associated with HIV

Diarrhea
Fever
Generalized lymphadenopathy
Hepatosplenomegaly
Night sweats
Weight loss/wasting syndrome

Table 8-2. Opportunistic infections associated with AIDS and HIV infection

Pneumocystis carinii pneumonia
Candida albicans (bronchial, esophageal, or pulmonary)
Cryptococcus neoformans (extrapulmonary)
Coccidioides immitis (extrapulmonary)
Disseminated histoplasmosis
Disseminated toxoplasmosis (after 1 month of age)
Disseminated *Mycobacterium tuberculosis*
Disseminated *Mycobacterium* species (*M. avium intracellulare* or *M. kansasii*)
Chronic isosporiasis
Extraintestinal strongyloidiasis
Nocardiosis
Cytomegalovirus infection outside of liver, spleen, and lymph node (after 1 month of age)
Progressive multifocal leukoencephalopathy

Table 8-3. Secondary cancers associated with AIDS and HIV infection

Kaposi's sarcoma
Primary lymphoma of the brain
B-cell non-Hodgkin's lymphoma

parenteral innoculation (e.g., IV drug abuse, blood transfusion, organ transplantation), and from HIV-infected mother to child. Latency between HIV infection (seropositivity) and full-blown AIDS has a reported mean of 10 years.

C. Epidemiology

As of January 1990, the CDC reported more than 121,645 cases of AIDS in the United States; 97.9% of these cases occurred in adults, 0.4% in adolescents (aged 13 to 19 years), and 1.7% in children (aged <13 years). Approximately 72,500 of reported cases have ended in death as of January 1990. The current estimates predict that 31% of persons with AIDS have died within 1 year of initial diagnosis, 56% at 2 years, 76% at 3 years, and nearly 100% at 5 years.

Major risk groups for HIV infection include male homosexuals, IV drug abusers, persons receiving unscreened blood transfusions or

Table 8-4. CDC stages of HIV infection, 1986

Group 1	Acute infection (often an EBV-like syndrome with or without aseptic meningitis)
Group 2	Asymptomatic
Group 3	Persistent generalized lymphadenopathy
Group 4[*]	
Subgroup A	Constitutional disease (e.g., with weight loss, fever, diarrhea)
Subgroup B	Neurological disease
Subgroup C1	Secondary infectious diseases (12 specific diseases), including PCP pneumonia, toxoplasmosis, and esophageal or pulmonary candidiasis
Subgroup C2	Secondary infectious disease (another 6 specified diseases), including hairy leukoplakia and oral candidiasis
Subgroup D	Secondary cancers, including Kaposi's sarcoma, Hodgkin's lymphoma, and non-Hodgkin's lymphoma
Subgroup E	Other conditions, e.g., chronic lymphoid interstitial pneumonitis

[*]Only patients in group 4, subgroups C1 and D fulfill the criteria for AIDS.

blood products, and sexual partners of the above groups. As of 1990, the breakdown of AIDS cases reported in the United States was 68% homosexual men (7% with history of IV drug abuse), 21% heterosexuals with a history of IV drug abuse, 5% heterosexuals without a history of IV drug abuse, 2% associated with blood transfusions or blood products, and 1% were hemophiliacs.

African-Americans and Hispanics represent greater than 40% of AIDS cases. Women and children of minority populations are markedly over-represented among persons with AIDS.

Cumulative data based on three large cohort studies including more than 1200 health care workers with HIV exposure due to accidental needlestick injury estimate the rate of infection as 0.4%. Additionally, case reports of transmission from HIV-infected doctors to patients have also been reported. More data are needed on this aspect of transmission and epidemiology.

II. Manifestations of AIDS in otolaryngology

Patients with AIDS often present with diseases of the head and neck. Different studies have indicated that greater than 40% of patients with HIV present initially with otolaryngological manifestations.

A University of California at San Francisco study conducted from 1980 to 1984 revealed that out of 399 AIDS presentations, 165 (41%) initially presented with head and neck manifestations. Of the presenting symptoms, 35% had cutaneous, oral, and pharyngeal lesions of Kaposi's sarcoma; 22% had chronic cough and shortness of breath; 8% had rapidly enlarging neck masses; and 4% had herpes simplex virus. Two additional European studies revealed that 68% and 88% of AIDS patients manifested head and neck symptoms.

Manifestations of AIDS can be classified into three groups: (1) opportunistic infections caused by immunosuppression, (2) tumors resulting from immunosuppression, and (3) direct effects of HIV infection. This section examines the otologic, rhinologic, and oral manifestations of HIV, as well as lymphadenopathy in AIDS patients. Many patients with the listed conditions may follow a similar clinical course as the immunocompetent individual.

A. Otologic manifestations

HIV infection may predispose to a variety of otologic infections by immunosuppression, hastening preexisting disease or development of opportunistic infections. However, most otologic diseases associated with AIDS parallel disease in the immunocompetent host.

1. Infections

a. **External otitis.** *Pseudomonas aeruginosa* is a common pathogen. Cases of fungal external otitis have been reported.

b. **Acute otitis media.** As in the immunocompetent host, *Pneumococcus* and *Haemophilus influenzae* are the organisms most frequently cultured in HIV-infected patients.

c. **Serous otitis media.** Increased eustachian tube dysfunction in HIV-infected patients may occur secondary to nasopharyngeal masses, recurring viral infections, and allergy.

d. **Chronic otitis media.** Cases of extrapulmonary PCP-infected aural polyps have been reported.

e. **Herpes zoster oticus (Ramsay Hunt syndrome).** Bullous myringitis-type lesions have been reported.

f. **Otosyphilis.** Accelerated development of otosyphilis from its latent state may occur in HIV-infected patients.

2. Neoplasms

a. **Kaposi's sarcoma.** Prior to HIV, Kaposi's sarcoma was a rare malignant disease found mainly in elderly-Caucasian men. It is a mesenchymal tumor, and clinically appears as red-purple plaques and nodules. The sarcomatous lesions may involve the external auricle, nasopharynx, or both.

3. HIV-induced hearing loss

The hearing deficit in HIV-infected individuals can be divided into sensorineural and conductive hearing losses.

a. **Sensorineural hearing loss.** This is the most frequent cause of hearing loss in HIV-infected patients, usually in the high-frequency range. Possible causes include:

(1) CNS and end-organ involvement, with tumors, infections (CNS toxoplasmosis, neurosyphilis, tuberculosis, and bacterial, viral or cryptococcal meningitis), or HIV drug regimen side effects.

(2) HIV virus neurotropism could conceivably involve the eighth cranial nerve.

(3) Central demyelination from HIV infection. Auditory brainstem-evoked responses with conduction delays greater than two standard deviations and a degraded waveform have been noted in patients with AIDS and in healthy seropositive patients.

b. Conductive hearing loss. This is less common. Causes include PCP granulomas and Kaposi's sarcoma of the external auditory canal, external otitis, and otitis media.

B. Rhinologic manifestations

1. Infections

a. Sinusitis. The incidence of sinusitis has ranged from 10–68% in AIDS patients. Because the frequency of sinusitis is so high in this population, patients presenting with fever, headache, or URI symptoms should be evaluated for sinusitis. The most common pathogens are *Staphylococcus aureus, Pneumococcus,* and *Pseudomonas aeruginosa.*

Immunologic factors. B-cell dysfunction also occurs in AIDS patients, and patients are therefore at higher risk for recurrent bacterial infections than the general population. IgG subclass deficiencies found in some AIDS patients have been associated with increased frequency of infections, including otitis media, sinusitis, and bronchopneumonia. Deficiencies in the subclasses IgG2 and IgG4 exist in a subgroup of AIDS patients, predisposing this population to recurrent bacterial sinopulmonary infections. In addition, progressive elevation of IgE levels in association with an increase in histamine release has been reported in certain AIDS patients. This may be relevant when considering the frequent drug reactions seen in this population; this may also predispose patients to recurrent rhinosinusitis.

b. Herpes reactivation. Seventy-three percent of patients at high risk for AIDS who presented with herpes zoster were found to be HIV seropositive upon testing, and an additional 15% became HIV positive during follow-up. Latent activation of varicella zoster virus in the dorsal root ganglion, thought to be secondary to deficient cell-mediated immunity, may occur more often than in the immunocompetent host. Here, patients may present with giant herpetic nasal ulcers that begin in the vestibule and extend onto the septum or face.

c. Candidiasis. Nasopharyngeal candidiasis is often part of a spectrum of diffuse pharyngeal candidiasis (see **II.C.**).

2. Neoplasms

a. Nasopharyngeal lymphoid masses. Nasopharyngeal masses, which on biopsy reveal benign lymphoid hypertrophy, have been reported. Patients may present with nasal obstruction and otitis media with serous effusions.

b. **Lymphoma.** Cases of high-grade, undifferentiated, large-cell lymphomas and high-grade, small, noncleaved, B-cell lymphomas in the nasal cavity and antrum have been reported. Patients present with nasal obstruction, foul-smelling nasal discharge, and alar flaring.

c. **Kaposi's sarcoma.** This malignancy has been reported on the nasal skin, vestibule, cavity, septum, and nasopharynx.

3. **HIV-associated diseases with rhinologic manifestations**

   Idiopathic thrombocytopenia. Patients with this complication can present with epistaxis.

C. **Oral manifestations**

   Oral lesions appear to represent an early indication of immunosuppression. Because HIV-infected people are immunocompromised, these lesions may represent the first presentation of AIDS.

1. **Infections**

   a. **Candida.** Candida is the most common intraoral fungal infection in HIV-positive patients and may represent the earliest sign of HIV infection. Prevalence is 30–90% among HIV-positive patients. Forms of this infection include:

      (1) **Pseudomembranous infection (thrush).** Clinically, it appears on the oral mucosa as a creamy plaque resembling mild curd; it wipes off easily, but often leaves a bleeding surface.

      (2) **Hyperplastic candidiasis (leukoplakia candidiasis).** Clinically, this appears as a white firm plaque that cannot be wiped off.

      (3) **Erythematous candidiasis (atrophic candidiasis).** Patients present with red patches on the buccal mucosa, hard and soft palate, or dorsum of tongue.

      (4) **Angular cheilitis.** This is a perioral manifestation of the disease and presents as a fissuring, cracking erythema, or ulceration, at the corner of the mouth.

   b. **Cryptococcus neoformans**

   c. **Histophasmonia.** Cases have been reported.

   d. **Bacterial infections.** Streptococcal species, *Staphylococcus aureus*, and less commonly *Klebsiella pneumoniae, Enterobacter cloacae, Mycobacterium avium intracellulare, Actinomyces*, and *Escherichia coli* have been reported. These bacterial infections cause severe periodontal and gingival disease in the oral cavities of AIDS patients. Clinically, these infected, colonized patients experience severe pain, hyperemic gingiva, and spontaneous bleeding that results in gross destruction of soft tissue and bone.

   e. **Hairy leukoplakia (associated with Epstein-Barr virus).** Oral hairy leukoplakia is an asymptomatic hyperkeratotic lesion often found in the oral cavity and oropharynx of the immunocompromised, including HIV-infected patients. Clinically, it appears as a white patch, sometimes corrugated, usually on the lateral margins of the tongue. Cases have been reported on the floor of the mouth, buccal mucosa, oropharyngeal mucosa, and soft palate. Candida overgrowth occurs frequently on the surface of these lesions.

f. **Herpes simplex virus.** Symptoms differ in HIV-infected patients and healthy patients. In the immunocompetent host, lesions are usually restricted to attached tissues and appear as small vesicles that coalesce in a few days to shallow ulcers, most lasting 7 to 14 days. However, lesions in HIV-infected patients may occur throughout the mouth, especially on the palate, lips, and perioral areas. Ulcers are deep and painful and may persist for several weeks.

g. **Other herpes viruses.** Few cases of herpes zoster and cytomegalovirus (CMV) have been reported.

h. **Human papilloma virus.** This virus is common in the HIV-infected patient and produces oral manifestations of focal epithelial hyperplasia, warts, and condyloma acuminatum.

2. **Neoplasms**

a. **Kaposi's sarcoma.** Kaposi's sarcoma is the most common intraoral neoplasm associated with AIDS. The hard palate is most commonly involved; however, cases involving the gingiva, buccal mucosa, and soft palate have been reported. Candida-infected sarcomatous lesions have been reported.

b. **Non-Hodgkin's lymphoma.** The location and symptoms can mimic Kaposi's sarcoma.

c. **Squamous cell carcinoma.** Although this is the most common intraoral malignancy in non–HIV-infected patients, it is less common than both Kaposi's sarcoma and non-Hodgkin's lymphoma in AIDS patients. The tongue is the most frequently involved site in HIV-positive patients.

3. **HIV-associated diseases with oral manifestations**

a. **Parotid disease.** Parotid enlargement is very common in HIV-infected patients, and evidence of xerostomia has been reported in 6–10% of this population. Clinically, a cystic enlargement of the parotid gland, which often accompanies a syndrome of persistent generalized lymphadenopathy, is observed. Parotid masses caused by HIV infection usually occur as unilateral or bilateral multicystic, nontender parotid enlargements.

b. **Sjögren's-like syndrome.**

c. **Recurrent apthous stomatitis.** These ulcers are larger and more painful in the HIV-infected individual. They can interfere with speech and swallowing.

Table 8-5. Head and neck sites of adenopathies in HIV-infected patients

Site	Percentage	Site	Percentage
Posterior cervical	86	Submandibular	37
Preauricular	51	Submental	26
Postauricular	47	Supraclavicular	26
		Jugular	17

d. **Idiopathic thromboctyopenia.** Like the rhinologic manifestations of epistaxis, patients may present with oral ecchymosis, petechiae, and spontaneous gingival bleeding.

e. **Oral mucosal hyperpigmentation.** These lesions are spots or striations in buccal mucosa, hard palate, gingiva, and tongue often seen in HIV-infected patients.

f. **Tonsillar abnormalities.** Tonsillar abnormalities, secondary to tumor (Kaposi's sarcoma and lymphoma) and infections have been reported.

g. **Vocal cord edema.** Hoarseness, secondary to true vocal cord edema usually from chronic cough, previous radiation therapy, or lymphatic obstruction from Kaposi's sarcoma has been reported.

h. **Recurrent laryngeal nerve paralysis.** CMV infection of the recurrent laryngeal nerve can occur.

D. **Lymphadenopathy in AIDS**

Most HIV-infected patients have marked lymphadenopathy, seen mainly in the head and neck (Table 8-5).

Lymph node enlargement, a hallmark of HIV infection, occurs in all stages of the disease. Causes for lymphadenopathy range from benign lymphadenopathy to neoplastic and opportunistic infections. Causes include:

1. **Persistent generalized lymphadenopathy (PGL).** PGL is found in early HIV infection and is an unexplained lymphadenopathy of 3 or more months' duration involving two or more extrainguinal sites in an individual at risk for developing AIDS.

2. **Non-Hodgkin's lymphoma.** The majority of HIV-positive patients with lymphoma have high-grade B-cell tumors, including immunoblastic lymphoma, diffuse large-cell lymphoma, and small noncleaved Burkitt's and non-Burkitt's lymphoma.

3. **Hodgkin's lymphoma.** Cases have been reported in HIV positive patients, but do not appear to occur in increased frequency compared to non–HIV-positive patients.

4. **Kaposi's sarcoma**

5. *Mycobacterium avium intracellulare*

6. *Mycobacterium tuberculosis*

7. *Histoplasma capsulatum*

III. Pediatric AIDS: Specific ENT problems

HIV infection has been well documented in children. Like adults, children suffer the ravages of this disease, including:

A. Cervical adenopathy. Nodes are soft, regular, and nonadherent (see **II.D.**).

B. Parotid gland enlargement. This enlargement is common, usually bilateral and painful. Course waxes and wanes. See **II.C.**

C. Oroesophageal candidiasis. Most HIV-infected children develop mucocutaneous candidiasis (thrush). As in adults, the most common form is pseudomembranous candidiasis. See **II.C.**

D. Oral hairy leukoplakia. This has also been noted in the pediatric setting. See **II.C.**

E. Bacterial infections. There is an increased incidence of bacterial infections in children with AIDS. Otitis and sinusitis occur frequently. See **II.A.** and **II.B.**

F. Viral infections. Upper respiratory tract infections caused by viruses are common in HIV-infected children and usually run a self-limited course. Herpes simplex and varicella zoster have been reported in HIV-infected children. See **II.C.**

G. Thrombocytopenia. As in adults, some children with HIV have associated thrombocytopenia and may present with petechiae of the palate and head and neck, as well as epistaxis. See **II.B.** and **II.C.**

Selected Readings

Brahim, J. S., and Roberts, M. W. Oral manifestations of human immunodeficiency virus infection. *Ear Nose Throat J.* 69:464, 1990.

Buchbinder, A. Virology of the human immunodeficiency virus type 1. *Ear Nose Throat J.* 69:376, 1990.

Chanock, S. J., and McIntosh, K. Pediatric infection with the human immunodeficiency virus: Issues for the otorhinolaryngologist. *Otolaryngol. Clin. North Am.* 22:637, 1989.

Chow, J. H., Stern, J. C., Kaul, A., Pincus, R. L., and Gromish, D. S. Head and neck manifestations of the acquired immunodeficiency syndrome in children. *Ear Nose Throat J.* 69:416, 1990.

Corey, J. P., and Seligman, I. Otolaryngololgy problems in the immune compromised patient—An evolving natural history. *Otolaryngol. Head Neck Surg.* 104:196, 1991.

Davidson, B. J., Morris, M. S., Kornblut, A. D., and Macher, A. M. Lymphadenopathy in the HIV-seropositive patient. *Ear Nose Throat J.* 69:478, 1990.

Falloon, J. Current treatment for human immunodeficiency virus infection. *Ear Nose Throat J.* 69:487, 1990.

Hadderingh, R. J., Tange, R. A., Danner, S. A., et al. Otorhinolaryngological findings in AIDS patients: A study of 63 cases. *Arch. Otorhinolaryngol.* 244:11, 1987.

Hamburg, M. A. The epidemiology of human immunodeficiency virus infection and acquired immunodeficiency syndrome in the United States. *Ear Nose Throat J.* 69:394, 1990.

Herdman, R. C., Foster, S., Stafford, N. D., and Pinching, A. J. The recognition and management of the otolaryngological manifestations of AIDS. *Clin. Otolaryngol.* 14:323, 1989.

Marcusen, D. C., and Sooy, C. D. Otolaryngologic and head and neck manifestations of acquired immunodeficiency syndrome (AIDS). *Laryngoscope* 95:401, 1985.

Meiteles, L. Z., and Lucente, F. E. Sinus and nasal manifestations of the acquired immunodeficiency syndrome. *Ear Nose Throat J.* 69:454, 1990.

Morris, M. S., and Prasad, S. Otologic disease in the acquired immunodeficiency syndrome. *Ear Nose Throat J.* 69:451, 1990.

Paparella, M. M. *Otolaryngology* (vol. 1, 3rd ed.). Philadelphia: Saunders, 1991.

Polis, M. A. Occupational transmission of human immunodeficiency virus. *Ear Nose Throat J.* 69:401, 1990.

Rarey, K. E. Otologic pathophysiology in patients with human immunodeficiency virus. *Am. J. Otolaryngol.* 11:366, 1990.

Rubin, J. S., and Honigberg, R. Sinusitis in patients with the acquired immunodeficiency syndrome. *Ear Nose Throat J.* 69:460, 1990.

Sperling, N. M., and Lin, P. Parotid disease associated with human immunodeficiency virus infection. *Ear Nose Throat J.* 69:474, 1990.

Wenig, B. M., Kuruvilla, A., Goldrich, M. S., Heffner, D. K., and Tuur, S. Pathologic manifestations of acquired immunodeficiency syndrome in the head and neck. *Ear Nose Throat J.* 69:406, 1990.

Index

The Little, Brown **Spiral**®Manual Series
The Little, Brown Handbook Series
AVAILABLE AT YOUR BOOKSTORE

☐ **MANUAL OF ACUTE BACTERIAL INFECTIONS,** 2nd Edition – Gardner & Provine (#303895)

☐ **MANUAL OF ACUTE ORTHOPAEDIC THERAPEUTICS,** 3rd Edition – Iversen & Clawson (#434329)

☐ **MANUAL OF ACUTE RESPIRATORY CARE –** Zagelbaum & Pare (#984671)

☐ **MANUAL OF ALLERGY AND IMMUNOLOGY,** 2nd Edition – Lawlor & Fischer (#516686)

☐ **MANUAL OF ANESTHESIA,** 2nd Edition – Snow (#802220)

☐ **MANUAL OF CLINICAL EVALUATION –** Aronson & Delbanco (#052108)

☐ **MANUAL OF CLINICAL ONCOLOGY,** 2nd Edition – Casciato & Lowitz (#130672)

☐ **MANUAL OF CARDIAC ARRHYTHMIAS –** Vlay (#904767)

☐ **MANUAL OF CARDIOVASCULAR DIAGNOSIS AND THERAPY,** 3rd Edition – Alpert & Rippe (#035203)

☐ **MANUAL OF CLINICAL HEMATOLOGY –** Mazza (#552178)

☐ **MANUAL OF CORONARY CARE,** 4th Edition – Alpert & Francis (#035130)

☐ **MANUAL OF DERMATOLOGIC THERAPEUTICS,** 4th Edition – Arndt (#051829)

☐ **MANUAL OF ELECTROCARDIOGRAPHY,** 2nd Edition – Mudge (#589187)

☐ **MANUAL OF EMERGENCY AND OUTPATIENT TECHNIQUES –** Washington University Department of Surgery: Klippel & Anderson (#498688)

☐ **MANUAL OF EMERGENCY MEDICINE,** 2nd Edition – Jenkins & Loscalzo (#460559)

☐ **MANUAL OF ENDOCRINOLOGY AND METABOLISM –** Lavin (#516503)

☐ **MANUAL OF GASTROENTEROLOGY –** Eastwood & Avunduk (#203971)

☐ **MANUAL OF GYNECOLOGIC ONCOLOGY AND GYNECOLOGY –** Piver (#709360)

☐ **MANUAL OF INTENSIVE CARE MEDICINE,** 2nd Edition – Rippe (#747122)

☐ **MANUAL OF INTRODUCTORY CLINICAL MEDICINE,** 2nd Edition – Macklis, Mendelsohn, & Mudge (#542474)

☐ **MANUAL OF MEDICAL CARE OF THE SURGICAL PATIENT,** 4th Edition – Coussons, McKee, & Williams (#774936)

☐ **MANUAL OF MEDICAL THERAPEUTICS,** 27th Edition – Washington University Department of Medicine: Woodley & Whelan (#924202)

☐ **MANUAL OF NEONATAL CARE,** 3rd Edition – Cloherty & Stark (#147621)

☐ **MANUAL OF NEPHROLOGY,** 3rd Edition – Schrier (#774863)

☐ **MANUAL OF NEUROLOGY,** 4th Edition – Samuels (#769940)

☐ **MANUAL OF NUTRITIONAL THERAPEUTICS,** 2nd Edition – Alpers, Clouse, & Stenson (#035122)

☐ **MANUAL OF OBSTETRICS,** 4th Edition – Niswander (#611735)

☐ **MANUAL OF OCULAR DIAGNOSIS AND THERAPY,** 3rd Edition – Pavan-Langston (#695475)

☐ **MANUAL OF OTOLARYNGOLOGY,** 2nd Edition – Strome, Fried, & Kelley (#819689)

☐ **MANUAL OF OUTPATIENT GYNECOLOGY,** 2nd Edition – Havens, Sullivan, & Tilton (#350982)

☐ **MANUAL OF PEDIATRIC THERAPEUTICS,** 4th Edition – The Children's Hospital Department of Medicine, Boston: Graef (#138886)

☐ **MANUAL OF PSYCHIATRIC EMERGENCIES,** 2nd Edition – Hyman (#387193)

☐ **MANUAL OF PSYCHIATRIC THERAPEUTICS –** Shader (#782203)

☐ **MANUAL OF RHEUMATOLOGY AND OUTPATIENT ORTHOPEDIC DISORDERS,** 3rd Edition – Paget, Beary, Christian, & Pellicci (#688460)

☐ **MANUAL OF SURGICAL INFECTIONS –** Gorbach, Bartlett, & Nichols (#320706)

☐ **MANUAL OF SURGICAL THERAPEUTICS,** 8th Edition – Nyhus & Condon (#153672)

☐ **MANUAL OF UROLOGY –** Siroky & Krane (#792969)

☐ **PROBLEM-ORIENTED MEDICAL DIAGNOSIS,** 5th Edition – Friedman (#293873)

☐ **PROBLEM-ORIENTED PEDIATRIC DIAGNOSIS –** Barkin (#081027)

☐ **MANUAL OF CLINICAL PROBLEMS IN ADULT AMBULATORY CARE,** 2nd Edition – Dornbrand, Hoole & Pickard (#190195)

☐ **MANUAL OF CLINICAL PROBLEMS IN CARDIOLOGY,** 4th Edition – Hillis, Lange, Wells, & Winniford (#364053)

☐ **MANUAL OF CLINICAL PROBLEMS IN DERMATOLOGY, –** Olbricht, Bigby, & Arndt (#094250)

☐ **MANUAL OF DIAGNOSTIC IMAGING,** 2nd Edition – Straub (#818593)

☐ **MANUAL OF CLINICAL PROBLEMS IN GASTROENTEROLOGY –** Chobanian & Van Ness (#138975)

☐ **MANUAL OF CLINICAL PROBLEMS IN INFECTIOUS DISEASE,** 2nd Edition – Gantz, Gleckman, Brown, & Esposito (#303526)

☐ **MANUAL OF CLINICAL PROBLEMS IN INTERNAL MEDICINE,** 4th Edition – Spivak & Barnes (#807389)

☐ **MANUAL OF CLINICAL PROBLEMS IN NEPHROLOGY –** Rose & Black (#756377)

☐ **MANUAL OF CLINICAL PROBLEMS IN NEUROLOGY,** 2nd Edition – Mohr (#577480)

☐ **MANUAL OF CLINICAL PROBLEMS IN OBSTETRICS AND GYNECOLOGY,** 3rd Edition – Rivlin, Morrison, & Bates (#747742)

☐ **MANUAL OF CLINICAL PROBLEMS IN ONCOLOGY,** 2nd Edition – Portlock & Goffinet (#714259)

☐ **MANUAL OF CLINICAL PROBLEMS IN OPHTHALMOLOGY –** Gittinger & Asdourian (#314714)

☐ **MANUAL OF CLINICAL PROBLEMS IN PEDIATRICS,** 3rd Edition – Roberts (#750026)

☐ **MANUAL OF CLINICAL PROBLEMS IN PSYCHIATRY –** Hyman (#387223)

☐ **MANUAL OF CLINICAL PROBLEMS IN PULMONARY MEDICINE,** 3rd Edition – Bordow & Moser (#102725)

☐ **MANUAL OF CLINICAL PROBLEMS IN SURGERY –** Cutler, Dodson, Silva, & Vander Salm (#165751)

☐ **MANUAL OF CLINICAL PROBLEMS IN UROLOGY –** Resnick (#740543)

THE LITTLE, BROWN HANDBOOK SERIES

Visit your local bookstore or call **1 (800) 343-9204** for these and other Little, Brown Medical Publications. In Canada, check with your local bookstore or contact Copp Clark Pitman, Ltd., 2775 Matheson Blvd., East, Mississauga, Ontario, Canada L4W 4P7

For further information write to Little, Brown and Company, Medical Division, 200 West Street, Waltham, MA 02254-9931

And don't forget . . .

M858

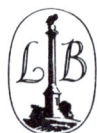